Disaster Health  nt

The second edition of this leading textbook provides the definitive guide to disaster health management. From the key concepts, principles and terminology, to systems for mitigation, planning, response and recovery, it gives readers a comprehensive overview of every aspect of this emerging field.

Split into eight parts, the book begins by drawing the parameters of disaster health management before outlining key elements such as communication, community engagement and legal issues. It then moves on to discuss preparing for potential disasters, managing and mitigating their impact, and then recovering in the aftermath. Offering key insights into evaluation, leadership and the psychosocial aspects of disaster health management, the new edition also features a range of international case studies, including those outlining the management of COVID-19.

It is essential reading for both students and practitioners engaging in this important work.

Gerry FitzGerald retired in July 2019 as Professor of Public Health at QUT and discipline Leader of Health Management and Disaster Management.

Stacey Pizzino is a humanitarian epidemiologist and global health expert focused on strengthening the evidence base for vulnerable populations impacted by disasters, armed conflict and complex humanitarian emergencies.

Penelope Burns is a General Practitioner, and a local Disaster Manager with appointments at the Australian National University and Western Sydney University.

Colin Myers has recently retired from a career in Emergency, Retrieval and Disaster Medicine and holds current appointments as adjunct Associate Professor in the Public Health Faculty at Queensland University of Technology and as Adjunct Professor, School of Public Health, Faculty of Medicine, James Cook University.

Mike Tarrant holds an adjunct appointment Associate Professor in the Public Health Faculty at Queensland University of Technology.

Ben Ryan is a Professor in the Thomas F. Frist, Jr. College of Medicine at Belmont University in Nashville, Tennessee, United States of America.

Marie Fredriksen is a senior Paramedic with the Queensland Ambulance Service and a guest lecturer in Disaster Management at QUT.

Peter Aitken is Executive Director, Disaster Management Branch, Queensland Health.

Disaster Health Management

A *Primer for Students and Practitioners*

Second Edition

Edited by
Gerry FitzGerald, Stacey Pizzino, Penelope Burns,
Colin Myers, Mike Tarrant, Ben Ryan,
Marie Fredriksen and Peter Aitken

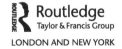

Routledge
Taylor & Francis Group

LONDON AND NEW YORK

Designed cover image: Getty Images

Second edition published 2024
by Routledge
4 Park Square, Milton Park, Abingdon, Oxon, OX14 4RN

and by Routledge
605 Third Avenue, New York, NY 10158

Routledge is an imprint of the Taylor & Francis Group, an informa business

© 2024 selection and editorial matter, Gerry FitzGerald, Stacey Pizzino, Penelope Burns, Colin Myers, Mike Tarrant, Ben Ryan, Marie Fredriksen and Peter Aitken; individual chapters, the contributors

The right of Gerry FitzGerald, Stacey Pizzino, Penelope Burns, Colin Myers, Mike Tarrant, Ben Ryan, Marie Fredriksen and Peter Aitken to be identified as the authors of the editorial material, and of the authors for their individual chapters, has been asserted in accordance with sections 77 and 78 of the Copyright, Designs and Patents Act 1988.

All rights reserved. No part of this book may be reprinted or reproduced or utilised in any form or by any electronic, mechanical, or other means, now known or hereafter invented, including photocopying and recording, or in any information storage or retrieval system, without permission in writing from the publishers.

Trademark notice: Product or corporate names may be trademarks or registered trademarks, and are used only for identification and explanation without intent to infringe.

First edition published by Routledge 2017

British Library Cataloguing-in-Publication Data
A catalogue record for this book is available from the British Library

Names: FitzGerald, Gerard Joseph, editor.
Title: Disaster health management: a primer for students and practitioners / edited by Gerry FitzGerald, Stacey Pizzino, Penny Burns, Colin Myers, Mike Tarrant, Ben Ryan, Maria Fredriksen, and Peter Aitken.
Description: Second edition. | Abingdon, Oxon; New York, NY: Routledge, 2024. | Includes bibliographical references and index.
Identifiers: LCCN 2023037816 | ISBN 9781032626611 (hbk) | ISBN 9781032139401 (pbk) | ISBN 9781032626604 (ebk)
Subjects: MESH: Disaster Planning—methods | Community Health Planning—methods | Australia
Classification: LCC RA645.5 .D56 2024 | DDC 363.34—dc23/eng/20231026
LC record available at https://lccn.loc.gov/2023037816

ISBN: 978-1-032-62661-1 (hbk)
ISBN: 978-1-032-13940-1 (pbk)
ISBN: 978-1-032-62660-4 (ebk)

DOI: 10.4324/9781032626604

Typeset in Minion
by codeMantra

Contents

Figures

Tables

Case studies

Notes on contributors

Jonathan Abrahams leads MUDRI's transdisciplinary program of research, education and collaborative projects aimed at strengthening resilience of communities in Australia and internationally. In the WHO Health Emergencies Program, he has played leading roles in advancing risk-based approaches to global policy, good practice guidance and capacity development across health systems and the whole-of-society, e.g., the WHO Health Emergency and Disaster Risk Management (EDRM) Framework and negotiations of the Sendai Framework for Disaster Risk Reduction 2015–2030. He has facilitated partnerships in health, e.g., WHO Health EDRM Research Network, and with countries, UNDRR, WMO and partners to promote the integration of public health, disaster risk management and climate change adaptation. His experience includes delivering regional training programs for country health emergency managers at the Asian Disaster Preparedness Centre, establishing emergency response teams at AusAID, managing development programs and performance standard reporting at Emergency Management Australia, and helping establish the National Centre for War-Related Post-traumatic Stress Disorder, the forerunner to Phoenix Australia.

Peter Aitken is an Emergency Physician with postgraduate qualifications in Disaster Medicine and Clinical Education. He is currently the Executive Director of the Disaster Management Branch, Queensland Health. Peter has been involved in all aspects of disaster health from leading response teams, Emergency Operations Centre, administrative and academic and research roles. He has also worked in disaster-related roles for a number of NGOs and professional organisations including St John Australia National Office; the International Federation of Emergency Medicine Disaster Medicine; the World Association for Disaster and Emergency Medicine, the Emergency Medicine Foundation and the World Health Organisation. Peter has received more than $3million in research funding with more than 100 publications, 100 presentations and as a peer reviewer for more than 14 journals. His special interests in Disaster Health include deployable teams, pre-hospital care and Emergency Medical Systems.

Nahuel Arenas-García has over 20 years of experience leading humanitarian, disaster risk reduction and development cooperation programs around the world. He is the Deputy Chief of Regional Office, Americas & the Caribbean, at the United Nations Office for

Disaster Risk Reduction (UNDRR). Before joining UNDRR in 2017, he was the Director for Humanitarian Programs and Policy at OXFAM USA. Nahuel worked for organisations like OXFAM, Action Against Hunger, and the Japan International Cooperation Agency (JICA) in the Americas, Africa and Asia-Pacific. He has a background in international politics (SOAS, University of London), crisis management (Universidad Complutense de Madrid, Spain) and public policy (FLACSO, Argentina) and is currently a PhD candidate at the Centre for Global Ethics, University of Birmingham (UK). He has been a frequent guest lecturer at many universities in the USA and contributed to different academic programs including the Harvard Humanitarian Initiative/Harvard X Course 'Humanitarian Response to Conflict and Disasters'.

Vicenzo Bollettino is the Director of Resilient Communities Program at the Harvard Humanitarian Initiative. Prior to his current appointment, Dr. Bollettino served for five years as Executive Director of the Harvard Humanitarian Initiative. His research and professional experience include disaster resilience, humanitarian action, civil-military engagement in emergencies and humanitarian leadership. He has spent the past 20 years of his career at Harvard University in administration, teaching and research. Current research focuses on disaster preparedness and resilience, humanitarian leadership, climate change and civil military engagement during humanitarian emergencies. Dr Bollettino has taught courses on research design, peace building, and international politics at the Harvard Extension School and is the author of publications related to disaster preparedness, climate change, and humanitarian action. Dr Bollettino completed his PhD at the Graduate School of International Studies at the University of Denver. Dr Bollettino currently serves as an Advisory Committee Member of the MSF Speaking Out Case Studies and is a former board member of ELRHA (Enhancing Learning and Research for Humanitarian Assistance), and former President of the ACF International Scientific Council (Action Against Hunger).

Diane Bretherton has 16 years' experience in emergency and disaster management in senior roles across state government, non-government, and corporate entities, leading key planning, capability and operational activities within Australia and internationally. A specialist in leading disaster management programs in large complex organisations and a highly regarded relationship manager, Di has a strong passion for increasing maturity emergency and disaster management capability within the health sector. Di is currently the Director of Emergency Management at Metro North Hospital and Health Services, where she has led this portfolio since 2015.

Penny Burns is a general practitioner who has worked in remote rural and urban general practice in Australia and Papua New Guinea. Dr Burns has worked in Far North Queensland with the Royal Flying Doctor Service and in Aboriginal Controlled Community Health Services. She is an academic and researcher at the Australian National University and Western Sydney University. Her research has investigated the management of animals in disasters, human safety in tunnel emergencies and GP contributions to COVID-19. She has completed a PhD on the role of General Practitioners in disasters. Dr Burns is Co-Chair of the World Association of Disaster & Emergency Medicine Primary Care Special Interest Group. Dr Burns has contributed to education, policy, and guidelines on GP disaster management. She has been involved in disaster management from frontline to GP EOC liaison through various Australian bushfire, flood, heat, and terror incidents. She is a MIMMS and an EMERGO TS instructor. Dr Burns is a member of ATAGI (Australian Technical Advisory Group on Immunisation) and the NCET-19 (National COVID-19 Evidence Taskforce). During COVID Dr Burns was a member of the ATAGI COVID Working Group and worked in a GP Respiratory Clinic, mass vaccination clinics, and in a family medicine clinic.

Graham Dodd is the associate medical director for Health Emergency Management of British Columbia (HEMBC) and the physician lead for emergency preparedness for BC's Divisions of Family Practice. He is a clinical instructor in the departments of family medicine and emergency medicine at the University of British Columbia and sits on the board of the Centre for Excellence in Emergency Preparedness (ceep.ca). Previously he served on the board of the World Association of Disaster and Emergency Medicine. He has a master's degree in emergency management from Royal Roads University. He is an avid photographer specialising in sports photography.

Weiwei Du (also known as Donald Du) is the Chief of the Division for Exchange in the Office of International Cooperation, Peking University Health Science Center. He got his PhD degree in disaster health management from Queensland University of Technology, Brisbane, Australia in 2010, and Bachelor of Arts and Bachelor of Economics from Peking University, Beijing, China in 2007. Weiwei Du currently works in the area of international collaboration projects (medical research and public health programs), medical student exchange programs, MD-PhD co-training programs etc. His research interests include public health programs, disaster health management, policy analysis, medical education, science of team science, virtual internationalisation etc.

Michel Dückers is a professor of Crises, Safety and Health at the University of Groningen and ARQ National Psychotrauma Centre. He leads the Research Programme Disasters and Environmental Hazards at the Netherlands Institute for Health Services Research (Nivel). Michel is an advisor for national and local governments in the event of calamities. He holds a Master's degree in Public Administration (Twente University), a PhD in Social and Behavioural Sciences (Utrecht University), and completed his habilitation (post-doctoral dissertation and training) dealing with the relativity of the mental health consequences of disasters (University of Innsbruck). His main areas of research are crisis management, disaster health research, mental health and psychosocial support (MHPSS) and monitoring and evaluation.

Michael Eburn is a leading commentator on the law of emergency management. His PhD was on Australia's legal arrangements for sending and receiving international disaster assistance and he consulted with the International Federation of the Red Cross on developing a model law to facilitate international disaster relief. He was the lead researcher on projects funded by the Bushfire CRC and then the Bushfire and Natural Hazards CRC looking into the policies, institutions and governance of natural hazards. Now an independent researcher, Dr Eburn continues to consult with the emergency management sector and operates a popular blog reporting on legal developments.

Gerry FitzGerald is an Adjunct Professor of Health Management in the School of Public Health and Social Work at the Queensland University of Technology. Prior to his retirement he was a discipline Leader of Health Management and Disaster Management. He was previously the Director of the Emergency Department at Ipswich Hospital, Medical Director and then Commissioner of the Qld Ambulance Service and Chief Health Officer for Qld. Since moving to QUT in 2007, he led the development of the Master of Health Management program including disaster health management courses. His research interests focus on the way in which emergency health services function under the routine challenges from a growing and ageing population and the non-routine challenges associated with disasters including those related to global warming. He has published over 170 peer-reviewed articles, a text in Disaster Health Management, eight book chapters and more than 100 conference representations. He has supervised more than 25 PhD students to completion and obtained over $5m in research grants.

Helen Foster has vast experience in risk, resilience and assurance activities in a number of public and private sector organisations, including health. She has a master's in emergency management and other post-graduate qualifications in risk and quality management. Helen has been involved in large campaign disasters and emergencies over a number of years, representing both government and industry. She is currently teaching risk and emergency management courses and is an active participant in the development of Australian Institute of Disaster Resilience (AIDR) handbooks. Helen also serves as a risk expert on the International Standards Organisation (ISO) Technical Committee for Risk Management as convenor for ISO 31000: 2018 Risk Management – Guidelines Handbook and as a member of a number of other working groups.

Richard Franklin is a pracademic who uses an evidence-based approach to developing real-world solutions to improving health, safety and wellbeing with a focus on health services, rural populations, those working in agriculture, disasters and drowning. He is a Professor of Public Health and the Director for the World Safety Organization Collaborating Centre – Injury Prevention and Safety Promotion and Co-Director of the WSO Collaborating Centre – Disaster Health, Resilience and Emergency Response at James Cook University, within the College of Public Health, Medical and Veterinary Sciences where he teaches, undertakes research and outreach work. His research interests are wide-ranging and have included epidemiological, qualitative, translational, program evaluation, product evaluation, surveillance and pure research. Current projects include: heatwaves and health services impact; farm safety; rural road safety; drowning prevention; mitigating the impact of flooding and cyclones; benchmarking WHS; quad bike safety; disaster preparedness and resilience; ageing; and horse safety.

Marie Fredriksen is a Paramedic with the Queensland Ambulance Service (QAS) with more than 25 years of experience in front-line service delivery during numerous natural and technological disasters, planning and preparedness for mass gathering events and in a number of education and training roles. While working with Emergency Management Queensland, Marie wrote and delivered training exercises and helped Disaster Management Groups at District and Local level and NGOs prepare for, respond to and recover from natural disasters. While seconded to the Queensland University of Technology, Marie was an Associate Lecturer with the Centre for Emergency and Disaster Management (CEDM). During this time, she coordinated the development of the first edition of this text. Marie's particular research interests are in emergency management systems; pre-hospital patient care and community resilience including strategies to better prepare individuals and communities for disaster events. Marie is passionate about disaster management issues, particularly improving the resilience of vulnerable populations.

Carl A. Gibson is a Director of Executive Impact Pty Ltd and undertakes research into the neuroscience of decision making under crisis situations. He is the author of publications in the areas of disease epidemiology and pathology, risk, safety, and emergency management, including a number of national and international Standards.

Angela Hamilton is the Medical Lead for the COVID-19 Vaccination Program for the Western Sydney Local Health District. She commenced working with WSLHD during the initial phase of the COVID-19 pandemic and subsequently developed, led, and managed the clinical component of the district vaccination program which included the mass vaccina4on clinic at Qudos Bank Arena, vaccination centres at Westmead & Blacktown Hospitals as well as hospital InReach and community outreach programs. Prior to this she worked as a General Practitioner across urban, rural and remote settings, primarily in Indigenous Health. Her qualifications include an MBBS, FRACGP and Bachelor of Business Management (Marketing) and she has recently commenced a Master of Health Technology Innovation. Her current interests include public health, digital health, the integra4on of technology and healthcare, governance and healthcare policy implementation.

Rosemary Hegner has worked in the field of emergency management for the past 13 years across a variety of portfolios including health, education & statewide recovery services. A key component of Rosemary's role is to build the capability and understanding across the sector and broader community of the impacts of disaster and the advantages of prior planning. Rosemary has worked across the full spectrum of emergency management in the prevention, preparedness, response and recovery areas and has coordinated agency responses to a number of incidents including the Lindt Cafe siege, NSW bushfires and recovery from the Northern NSW floods. Her current focus within the NSW Department of Education is to build generational resilience and capability.

Rose Henderson is a Director of Allied Health in New Zealand working at Te Whatu Ora Waitaha (Canterbury). She is a Life Member of the Aotearoa New Zealand Association of Social Workers and the Immediate past Global Vice President of the International Federation of Social Workers (IFSW) and Immediate Past President of IFSW Asia Pacific. Her career in Christchurch New Zealand, has seen her providing psychosocial response and recovery leadership and oversight in communities impacted by many of the various disasters the region has experienced over the last decade, ranging from the Earthquakes of 2010–2011 through to the current pandemic.

David Heslop is an Associate Professor at the School of Population Health at UNSW Sydney. He retains military responsibilities as Senior Medical Adviser for CBRNE to the Australian Army and to Australian Defence Force (ADF) leadership. He is a clinically active vocationally registered General Practitioner and Occupational and Environmental Medicine Physician. During a military career of over 15 years he has deployed into a variety of complex and austere combat environments and has advanced international training in Chemical, Biological, Radiological, Nuclear and Explosive (CBRNE) Medicine. He has experience in planning for and management of major disasters, mass casualty and multiple casualty situations. He is regularly consulted and participates in the development and review of national and international clinical and operational general military and CBRNE policy and doctrine. His research interests lie in health and medical systems innovation and research using computational modelling and simulation to address otherwise intractable problems.

Sarah Hockaday is a United States emergency medicine physician and former US Naval Special Warfare Physician specialising in dive medicine, submarine medicine, radiation health injuries. Wilderness medicine fellow with experience in austere medical treatment and evacuation. Emergency disaster medicine and global health fellow UTSW 2021–2022.

With more than 40 years of experience, **Bob Jensen** led the U.S. government's on the ground crisis communications efforts after the massive earthquake in Haiti, for the Deepwater Horizon oil spill response and for more than 30 major U.S. disasters including Hurricane Sandy. He was a spokesman for the White House's National Security Council and the U.S. Embassy in Baghdad, he also led communication efforts in Saudi Arabia, Iraq and Afghanistan during four combat zone deployments. He also provided oversight and input to risk assessments and strategy development for U.S. national security issues including cybersecurity, disasters caused by natural hazards, pandemics, counterproliferation and counterterrorism. Currently, he consults with national and state governments as well as law enforcement agencies, major corporations and international aid and development organisations globally.

Andrew Johnson has had a long career in senior roles in public and private healthcare, and in the Australian Defence Force. He has extensive experience in leadership and management of medical services, including Emergency Preparedness and Continuity Management (Disaster Management), safety and quality of services and healthcare workforce. Over recent years he has led in the application of the construct of healthcare resilience, the capacity to adapt to challenges and changes at different system levels, to maintain high-quality care. This has involved collaborative research and engagement with academic partners across a global network and has resulted in the development of frameworks for leadership in complexity, adopted in health services and education both nationally and internationally. Andrew is a Professor at James Cook University, an Honorary Professor at Macquarie University, a Distinguished Fellow of RACMA, a Pre-Eminent Staff Specialist in Queensland Health and a Group Captain in the Air Force Health Reserves.

Michael Kidd AM is Deputy Chief Medical Officer and Principal Medical Advisor with the Australian Government Department of Health and Aged Care, where he was involved in leading Australia's national primary care response to the COVID-19 pandemic. He also has an appointment as a foundation Professor of Primary Care Reform at The Australian National University. He is a general practitioner, a past president of the Royal Australian College of General Practitioners, a past president of the World Organization of Family Doctors (WONCA) and a past Dean of the Faculty of Medicine, Nursing and Health Sciences at Flinders University. Prior to returning to Australia to support the national pandemic response, he was Director of the World Health Organization Collaborating Centre on Family Medicine and Primary Care, Senior Innovation Fellow with the Institute for Health System Solutions and Innovative Care, and Professor and Chair of the Department of Family and Community Medicine at the University of Toronto in Canada.

Ingrid Larkin is an educator and researcher in business, with a special interest in work-integrated learning. In 2017, Ingrid commenced her current role as Associate Director – Work Integrated Learning, leading work-integrated learning across QUT Faculty of Business and Law. Since joining QUT, Ingrid has designed and delivered learning experiences for undergraduate, postgraduate and executive education students. Ingrid has been a coach and mentor for students participating in international business case competitions, and industry-led competitions and challenges since 2012. Prior to joining QUT Business School in 2004, Ingrid was a senior public relations and communication professional in both corporate and consulting roles for clients across Australia and internationally.

Peter Logan is an emergency physician and Senior Staff Specialist in prehospital & retrieval medicine at Retrieval Services Queensland, as well as Clinical Director at Disaster Management Branch of Queensland Health. He has a special interest in mass casualty management education and training and is a member of the Queensland AusMAT team, with whom he has deployed overseas.

Bob Lonne is a Professor II at the Department of Social Work at the Norwegian University of Science and Technology (NTNU) at Trondheim Norway and an Adjunct Professor at Queensland University of Technology (QUT). Professor Lonne has had a distinguished career with a track record that includes over $1,370,000 in research grants and an additional $3,700,000 as part of the 2022 Norwegian NORWEL research project's International Advisory Panel. He has authored/co-authored 4 books, 3 monographs, 17 book chapters, 53 refereed journal articles, and 6 major/government reports, as well as holding high-level national leadership roles. Professor Lonne has been engaged as an expert legal witness for child abuse and neglect matters involving civil litigation, as well as Coronial inquiries in several jurisdictions. Professor Lonne was the National President of the Australian Association of Social Workers during 2005–2011 and was also the Elections Officer for the International Federation of Social Workers 2008–2012.

Lidia Mayner has full academic status as an Associate Professor at Flinders University in the College of Nursing and Health Sciences and Torrens Resilience Initiative. Dr Mayner's research at Flinders University focussed on disaster-related themes, emergency department presentations during heatwaves, disaster-related terminology and climate change. The outcomes from this work included many conference and meeting presentations and peer-reviewed publications. Dr Mayner was part of the UNISDR Expert Working Group on Indicators and Terminology relating to disaster risk reduction in 2014 and the report was adopted in 2017 by the UN General Assembly. Recently, Dr Mayner contributed towards the work on hazard terminology and hazard profiles, both reports were published by the International Science Council (ISC) and the UN Office for Disaster Risk Reduction (UNDRR). Dr Mayner has recently published several book chapters on climate change and health challenges; international agreements and policies from an environmental hazards perspective and public health and disaster risk management.

Stefan M. Mazur works as a PreHospital and Retrieval physician and Medical Retrieval Consultant with the South Australian state based retrieval service, SAAS MedSTAR and as an Emergency Physician in the Royal Adelaide Hospital Emergency Department. Is a USAR Doctor with South Australian USAR team. Previously worked undertaking retrievals for NETS in Sydney, New South Wales, for CareFlight Queensland as Director of

Training and Education and spent a period in London working for London HEMS in Pre-Hospital trauma care. Has an academic position at School of Public Health at James Cook University and is an examiner in Retrieval Medicine for the Royal College of Surgeons in Edinburgh and in PreHospital and Retrieval Medicine for the Australasian College for Emergency Medicine.

Graeme McColl has over 18 years' experience in health emergency management, including roles such as Response Manager and Operations Manager in the New Zealand National Health Coordination Centre during the H1N1 pandemic response and offshore health responses, liaison officer between the Ministry of Health and Christchurch health services during earthquake responses, and Secretary for the World Association for Disaster and Emergency Medicine, Oceania Chapter. Most recently he was a member of the Canterbury Primary Response Group, a primary healthcare team working closely with other emergency responders in Christchurch and setting the standard for systematic primary healthcare involvement in disasters.

Fiona McDonald is an Associate Professor in the School of Law and the Australian Centre for Health Law Research at Queensland University of Technology, an Adjunct Associate Professor at the Department of Bioethics, Dalhousie University, Canada and a Senior Research Fellow at the New Zealand Centre for Public Law at Victoria University of Wellington, New Zealand. She undertakes research into the legal and ethical regulation of health systems, including slow disasters.

Amisha Mehta specialises in risk and crisis communication and trust at the QUT Business School. She applies this expertise in emerging industries like hydrogen energy and commercial drones and in the context of corporate, health, and natural hazard emergencies. Amisha's research has been translated into new national policy via the Australian Warnings System and new organisational practice. She leads the World Meteorological Organization's High Impact Weather trust project. Amisha's teaching and research have been recognised by national and industry associations.

Colin Myers started his career as a rural general practitioner in New Zealand supporting local volunteer Emergency Services. He moved to Brisbane and qualified as an Emergency Physician (FACEM) in 1991. He spent many years developing trauma and critical care retrieval services in both Queensland and the Northern Territory. In this role he has been the site medical commander at many major incidents and has travelled overseas as part of the Australian Government's response to a disaster on several occasions. He has been a Squadron Leader in the RAAF Reserve, instructed on MIMMS commander courses and an AUSMAT Team leader. Dr Myers was the Director of Emergency and Children's Services at the Prince Charles Hospital in Brisbane for 12 years and spent 5 years as Executive Director of Critical Care Services for Metro North HHS. During this time, he gained his FRACMA and a Masters In Public Health (Biosecurity and Disaster Response).

Carissa Oh is an emergency physician at St George Hospital, New South Wales and a pre-hospital and retrieval physician with New South Wales Ambulance. She has been involved in major incidents and disaster response through teaching Major Incident Medical Management and Support (MIMMS) and Hospital MIMMS, as well as deployments with AusMAT and Urban Search And Rescue (USAR).

David Parsons is a Director of Crisis Management Australia, Director of Response and Recovery Aotearoa New Zealand, Director of the Australian Institute of Emergency Services and Honorary Fellow of the Business Continuity Institute, David is an adjunct lecturer at Charles Sturt University and the author of the Australian Institute for Disaster Resilience Emergency Planning and Incident Management Handbooks.

Stacey Pizzino is a global health and development expert who is passionate about improving the lives of those impacted by disasters and complex humanitarian emergencies. Stacey's research draws on her background as a paramedic and focuses on strengthening the evidence base to improve outcomes for vulnerable communities affected by crises and disasters. Her PhD examining the health impacts of explosive ordnances resulted in the world's largest epidemiological analysis of casualties of landmine and explosive remnants of war.

Elizabeth Rushbrook is a Specialist Medical Administrator who graduated in Medicine from the University of Queensland in 1994. She has extensive medical and military experience and is a fellow of the Royal Australasian College of Medical Administrators. Liz initially worked in Queensland before serving in the Navy. She rose steadily through the Navy ranks as a Medical Officer to Commodore, serving ashore and afloat before returning to Queensland in 2016. Her interests include Disaster Management, Business Continuity, Medical Workforce Management and Clinical Governance. Liz is currently the Chief Medical Officer for Metro North Hospital and Health Service in Brisbane. She continues to serve in the Navy as an active reservist as a specialist health advisor. Liz is married to Andrew. They have three sons who they enjoy supporting making their way in the world.

Benjamin Ryan has experience working, researching and teaching in disaster risk reduction, environmental public health, communicable and non-communicable diseases, and community resilience. Dr Ryan has led activities in these fields across the Americas, Europe, and Indo-Pacific. He has been funded by the World Health Organization, United States Department of Agriculture, National Science Foundation, and the International Organization for Migration. Dr Ryan regularly participates in activities and initiatives led by the United Nations Office for Disaster Risk Reduction, which has included supporting the development of the public health and food system resilience scorecards. Operationally, Dr Ryan has conducted environmental public health assessments in community settings, responded to natural disasters and disease outbreaks, activated emergency operations centres and managed projects in Indigenous communities. His leadership skills were used to guide health preparations for the G20 Finance Ministers meetings in Australia, facilitate health services for asylum seekers and as part of United States delegations in engagement with the Association of Southeast Asian Nations (ASEAN) on humanitarian assistance and disaster relief. Dr Ryan has worked at all levels of government in Australia, federally in the United States, and as a consultant. He is well-published and has experience in disaster resilience processes, leading teams, and conducting local and international research.

Paul Scully is a Clinical Psychotherapist and has been a Visiting Fellow and Adjunct Associate Professor at the Centre for Emergency and Disaster Management, Queensland University of Technology, Australia. He is the founder and inaugural manager of the Staff Support 'Priority One' Mental Health and Peer Support program within the Queensland Ambulance Service (QAS), Australia. Prior to this, Paul spent many years as a Paramedic and then as a Paramedic Educator within the QAS. Paul has co-facilitated mental health research projects within the QAS and has published and co-authored articles and book chapters relating to mental health and coping within the ambulance service work setting. He has played a key role in the development of workplace Mental Health and Peer Support programs for a range of organisations including St John Ambulance Northern Territory, Ambulance Service Tasmania, as well as having been a Workplace Mental Health Consultant to international ambulance organizations such as the Scottish, London and Northumbria Ambulance Services in the UK.

Jane Shakespeare-Finch, PhD, is a Professor in the School of Psychology and Counselling at QUT. Jane's primary area of teaching and research is trauma. She has worked with emergency services in the promotion of positive post-trauma outcomes for more than 25 years and also investigated post-trauma adaptation and posttraumatic growth in other populations including survivors of sexual assault, natural disasters, bereavement, and people from a refugee background. Recent research is in transdisciplinary teams looking at a range of post-trauma outcomes using epigenetics and EEG. Jane is on the editorial board of two international trauma journals and is on the Scientific Advisory Board for the Bouldercrest Institute for Posttraumatic Growth in the USA. Jane has enjoyed supervising approximately 80 post-graduate student research projects and has published approximately 140 peer-reviewed works.

Erin Smith is the CEO of the Dart Centre for Journalism and Trauma Asia Pacific and an Honorary Enterprise Professor in the Department of Critical Care at the University of Melbourne. Erin is a Board Director of the World Association for Disaster and Emergency Medicine (WADEM) where she was formerly the convenor of the Psychosocial Special Interest Group and Deputy Convenor of the Oceania Chapter. Erin is a member of the Emergency Services Foundation (ESF) Mental Health Advisory Group, an Advisory Board member of the Australian Federal Police Shield program, and an Ambassador for the Victoria Police Health and Wellbeing Committee.

Mike Tarrant is an adjunct Associate Professor in the Public Health Faculty at Queensland University of Technology. He was an Assistant Director Education and Research at the Australian Emergency Management Institute and has worked in disaster management education and research for the past 25 years.

Vivienne Tippett OAM is an Adjunct Professor in the Faculty of Health at Queensland University of Technology (QUT). She was previously Acting Head, School of Clinical Sciences at QUT and has a long-standing research and education interest in emergency pre-hospital services and their role in emergency and disaster management.

Ghasem-Sam Toloo is a lecturer in the School of Public Health and Social Work at Queensland University of Technology (QUT). With a social science background, his research and teaching interests have been focused on social determinants of health, health behaviour and societal influences. Over the past two decades, he has pursued his passion and extended his research to understanding social-psychological determinants of inequality in decision-making, accessing and utilising emergency health services including ambulance and hospital emergency departments, as well as community vulnerability to health effects of heatwaves. He is currently teaching and coordinating Emergency and Disaster Management courses.

Robina Xavier, PhD, GAICD, is Deputy Vice-Chancellor and Vice-President (Academic) with overall responsibility for the quality and integrity of learning and teaching across the university. She has more than 25 years' experience in the tertiary sector including serving as Executive Dean, QUT Business School. Her doctoral studies were in crisis management. Prior to joining QUT, Robina worked as a consultant to both the private and public sectors, specialising in corporate and financial relations. She has served on international committees for the Association of Advanced Collegiate Schools of Business in the US and the European Foundation for Management Development including the EFMD Executive Academy. Robina is a director of Financial Services Institute of Australia, is Vice President of the Queensland Academy of Arts and Sciences and serves on Universities Australia Deputy Vice Chancellor (Academic) Executive.

C. Joris Yzermans is a sociologist. For more than 25 years his work concentrates on the (long-term) health effects of disasters and environmental incidents. He investigated health consequences of four major disasters in the Netherlands. In those studies he used data from registries of general practices, both retrospectively and prospectively. He is a senior researcher at the research program 'Disasters and Environmental Hazards' at Nivel. His main interest is the recurrence of physical symptoms and psychological problems after disasters and environmental incidences. He has also developed a questionnaire to measure symptoms and perceptions (SaP scale; Yzermans, 2016). Since 2009 he has been involved in several projects on the association between livestock farming and the health of local residents. Other projects concern potential associations between health and electromagnetic fields as well as wind turbines, the use of pesticides in the proximity of the houses of local residents, and the emissions of industrial plants.

Foreword

Disasters are important.

The unchallenged public perception is that disasters are becoming more common. Whether this perception is due to increased frequency particularly those associated with climate change, or greater awareness and reporting is subject to debate. What is not debated however is that disasters are having an increasing impact on the health and well-being of the community. In 2021 alone, there were 432 reported disasters, which caused 10,492 deaths, affected 101.8 million people and caused US$2523 billion in economic damage.[1] At the same time, the worldwide pandemic of COVID-19 led to an additional 18 million[2] deaths across the globe in the first two years. This was due to a combination of the illness, overwhelmed health systems, and reduced care for vulnerable population, leading to unmeasurable adverse health, social and economic damages.

Public awareness of, and interest in disasters has been built through the combined effects of intense media and political scrutiny of every event, and public entertainment's best efforts to dramatise (or fictionalise) the countless personal stories that epitomise the personal impact of such events. Partly, this derives from the community's lesser tolerance of adversity and their expectations about the maintenance of standards of living and quality of life even in the context of the most extreme circumstances. It may also be due to the effect that disasters have on highly complex social structures and more sophisticated and expensive infrastructure. A tsunami in South Asia, a massive earthquake in Türkiye and Syria, a mass shooting in Christchurch New Zealand or the outbreak of a novel Coronavirus in China creates millions of personal stories each speaking to the devastating impact such events have on real people and real communities. Those personal impacts can be life-changing leaving a legacy amongst those who survive which may last their entire lives.

What is clear is that there is an increasing public, media and political focus on disasters. Modern disasters are played out in real-time and on mass media with every decision and action scrutinised and disassembled by legions of armchair critics. This imposes on those tasked with managing disasters, the challenge of doing their best while under intense scrutiny, both contemporaneously and in retrospect. Disasters have significant political consequences to add to the substantial health, economic, social and environmental impacts.

There is a widespread community expectation that the 'authorities' (however so defined), should be prepared and ready to respond to the most extreme event and failure to do so has political and economic consequences. This expectation exists despite the reluctance of some members of the community to participate in any way in providing for themselves or in mitigating the risks they face. This irony is difficult to rationalise, but it does impede governments and public authorities' ability to realistically meet community expectations.

Disaster management can help reduce their impact

In the past, natural disasters were called an 'Act of God', but increasingly societies around the world have sought to demand more organised efforts to reduce risk and improve disaster management. This is predicated on the justifiable belief that effective disaster management can limit the impact of disasters on people and their communities. These efforts are not limited to responding to disasters but rather imply a range of strategies that seek to prevent and/or mitigate disasters, to prepare for and respond to disasters when they occur and to help individuals and the community to recover from or adapt to their consequences.

Traditionally communities relied solely on their own resources, but increasingly wider cooperation has characterised disaster management with resources and support being provided by neighbouring communities and often remote nations facilitated by the UN and large international aid agencies.

Nation-states retain prime responsibility for disaster management in their communities and responsibility for the establishment of local community-based arrangements and policy settings. The overwhelming number of disasters are handled by local communities with or without the assistance or involvement of national and jurisdictional resources.

The international community has also recognised the importance of effective disaster management on development. The UN General Assembly adopted the International Strategy for Disaster Reduction in December 1999 and designated the 1990s as the International Decade for Natural Disaster Reduction (IDNDR). It established the UN Office for Disaster Risk Reduction to coordinate risk reduction strategies and has facilitated the development of international frameworks, the most recent being the Sendai Framework for Disaster Risk Reduction 2015–2030 (Sendai Framework).[3] This framework focuses on less well-developed countries, complements other international co-operative approaches and identifies the importance of the core priorities of understanding disaster risk, strengthening disaster risk governance, investing in risk reduction for resilience and enhancing disaster preparedness.

The net impact has been a much greater degree of centralised control and international cooperation in both the preparation for and response to disasters. This was particularly evident during the COVID-19 pandemic.

The increasing sophistication of centralised systems of preparation, response and relief has the potential to disempower or discourage the community's own efforts. At one extreme this can lead to passive dependence. Thus, the focus of management efforts has shifted towards building community resilience as a partnership between the local community and those who may have the resources to encourage and support. This complements the other core approach which is to focus on improving disaster management throughout the continuum of prevention, preparedness, response, and recovery.

However, the political and media focus tends to concentrate on issues experienced in the response and recovery phases of a disaster rather than the prevention and preparedness. This tends to focus on the effectiveness of decision making. Following a disaster, decisions such as providing compensation payments, purchasing temporary housing and restoring community centres may be made out of concern for those affected but the implementation of these decisions needs careful evaluation. This allows improvement of future responses and leads to improved and timelier decisions in the future.

Making improvements to the system of disaster management requires leadership and effective management at all levels and this in turn is reliant on effective education and training and a common language and conceptual understanding. Disaster management involves the establishment of a temporary organisation for a specific purpose, but one which builds upon the organisations and structures that already exist. It is not about supplanting existing organisations and their roles and responsibilities, but about enhancing those roles with enhanced coordination and management.

To better understand how such structures are organised and managed, it is critical to first understand the policy, legal and organisational environment. It is also critical to have a sound understanding of the system and its guiding principles and strategies. Individuals responsible require skills to develop policies and plans, capabilities within the health system, and to strategically manage responses and system recovery. They also require common understanding and agreement of the principles of disaster management and their application to practice. This may be described as a 'common language' which forms the basis of a common understanding which aims to enable greater cooperation within and between communities.

The aim of this text

The principal aim of this text is to propose a foundational understanding that may underpin coordinated approaches to disaster management.

The contents are drawn from experience, practice and the literature. We define disasters within the context of other community events and explain the complexity of the 'management' tasks required. We distinguish the concepts of disaster management from leadership but seek to explain how these concepts complement each other.

The text is aimed at practitioners, both existing and future. It is intended to guide practice and to provide the core principles and concepts that form the basis of educational programs that seek to develop the skills of new practitioners in this field. The text is not intended to foster debate amongst experts. That is achieved by the published literature. Rather it seeks to lay the groundwork of basic principles and practice that should enable consistency of practice. Where there is significant debate, we will refer to that debate without exploring its detail and certainly without attempting to 'decide' the issue.

The text focuses on the impact that disasters have on people and the communities in which they live and therefore on management from the community and people perspective. As such it has a strong focus on the health and wellbeing of people and the communities in which they live and therefore considers how health and wellbeing may be protected and preserved. It does not seek to address risks or hazards and their prediction and management. It does aim to identify the way in which communities seek to manage the impact those hazards have on their community and on the health and wellbeing of people.

The text covers the scope of disaster management; from the core underpinning principles through to the principles of leadership that are required to ensure that the objects of disaster management are achieved within communities and organisations.

The particular aim of this second edition is to refine the material using feedback and the experience of those who have used the text and to ensure that the text is of more universal appeal by focusing on the principles of disaster management. It also seeks to include more contemporary examples.

This text is divided into eight parts in three broad sections. The first section identifies the underpinning concepts including the conceptual basis (Part 1) the key elements of disaster management (Part 2) and the healthcare considerations (Part 3). The second section addresses the continuum of disaster management through getting ready (Part 4), incident management and response (Part 5) and recovering (Part 6). The third section explores the particular challenges of selected events that complement the generic principles (Part 7) and the way in which the future may be developed strategically through leadership, education, research and future challenges (Part 8).

Each chapter outlines the objectives that we consider the reader should achieve from that chapter. We will offer examples and case studies drawn from the literature and from history to demonstrate or illuminate particular points. We summarise at the end of each chapter key points to allow the reader to consolidate and test their understanding. We also offer activities in each Chapter to help readers test their understanding or to help them consolidate their thinking. Further we seek to provide not only a basic level of understanding but also to encourage and challenge readers to go beyond accepted norms. We provide extension readings that may explore particular issues in greater depth.

This text is not intended to be prescriptive of how disaster management should occur. That would be in breach not only of our mandate but of the principles that have proven effective. The most effective disaster management for any particular community is a product of that community's history, culture, politics, economy, resources, geography, demography and people and therefore not only may arrangements vary but by necessity they should be tailored to the particular need.

We welcome you to share this journey with us!

Gerry FitzGerald, Stacey Pizzino, Penelope Burns, Colin Myers, Mike Tarrant, Ben Ryan, Marie Fredriksen and Peter Aitken

Notes

1. Centre for Research into the Epidemiology of Disasters. 2021 Disasters in Numbers accessed on 18th January 2023 at https://cred.be/disasters-numbers-2021
2. H. Wang, K.R. Paulson, S.A. Pease, S. Watson, H. Comfort, P. Zheng, A.Y. Aravkin, C. Bisignano, R.M. Barber, T. Alam, J.E. Fuller, E.A. May, D.P. Jones, M.E. Frisch, C. Abbafati, C. Adolph, A. Allorant, J.O. Amlag, B. Bang-Jensen, G.J. Bertolacci, S.S. Bloom, A. Carter, E. Castro, S. Chakrabarti, J. Chattopadhyay, R.M. Cogen, J.K. Collins, K. Cooperrider, X. Dai, … C.J.L. Murray, Estimating excess mortality due to the COVID-19 pandemic: a systematic analysis of COVID-19-related mortality, 2020–2021. *The Lancet.* 2022, **399**(10334): 1513–1536. https://doi.org/10.1016/s0140-6736(21)02796-3
3. United Nations Office of Disaster Risk Reduction. *Sendai Framework for Disaster Risk Reduction 2015–2030 (Sendai Framework)* accessed at https://www.undrr.org/implementing-sendai-framework/what-sf on 19th February 2020Disaster Health Management

Acronyms

4 R's	Reduction, readiness, response, and recovery
AADMER	ASEAN Agreement on Disaster Management and Emergency Response
ADRRN	Asian Disaster Reduction and Response Network
AEMI	Australian Emergency Management Institute
AHMPPI	Australian Health Management Plan for Influenza Pandemic
AHPPC	Australian Health Protection Principal Committee
AIDR	Australian Institute for Disaster Resilience
AIDs	Acquired Immunodeficiency Syndrome
AIHW	Australian Institute of Health and Welfare
AIIMS	Australasian Inter-Service Incident Management System
AS/NZS	Australian/New Zealand standard
ASEAN	Association of Southeast Asian Nations
AUSAID	Australian Agency for International Development
BAU	Business as usual
BCDR	Business continuity and disaster recovery
BCMS	Business Continuity Management Systems
BCP	Business Continuity Plan
BIA	Business Impact Analysis
CAS	Complex Adaptive System
CBRNE	Chemical, biological, radiological, nuclear, and explosive
CDC	Centers for Disease Control and Prevention
CHE	Complex humanitarian emergency
CHS	Core humanitarian standards
CIMS	Coordinated Incident Management System
COAG	Council of Australian Governments
COMDISPLAN	Commonwealth Disaster Plan (Australia)
COVID-19	Coronavirus disease 2019
CRED	Centre for Research into the Epidemiology of Disasters
DALA	Damage and loss assessment
DEL	Direct economic loss
DHM	Disaster health management
DMAT	Disaster medical assistance team

DRR	Disaster risk reduction
EB	Executive board
ECHO	European Community Humanitarian Office
EPCIP	European Programme for Critical Infrastructure Protection
ED	Emergency department
EHS	Emergency healthcare system
EID	Emerging Infectious Diseases
EM-DAT	Emergency Events Database
EMS	Emergency Medical Systems
EMT	Emergency Medical Team
EMSA	California Emergency Medical Services Authority
EOC	Emergency operations centre
EU	European Union
FEMA	United States of America's Federal Emergency Management Agency
FMT	Foreign medical team
FFH	Foreign field hospital
GEJET	Great East Japan Earthquake Tsunami
GFDRR	Global Facility for Disaster Reduction and Recovery
GP	General Practitioners
GPID	Guiding Principles on Internal Displacement
GPRCs	General Practitioner-led Respiratory Clinics
HAZMAT	Hazardous material
HIV	Human Immunodeficiency Virus
HICS	Hospital Incident Command System
HNO	Humanitarian needs overviews
HRP	Humanitarian response plans
I-EMT	International emergency medical team
IAEA	The International Atomic Energy Agency
IAEM	International Association of Emergency Managers
IASC	Inter-Agency Standing Committee
ICCPR	International Covenant on Civil and Political Rights
ICESCR	International Covenant on Economic, Social and Cultural Rights
ICU	Intensive care unit
IHR	International health regulations
IMS	Incident management system
IMT	Incident Management Team
IOM	International Organisation for Migration
INES	International Nuclear and Radiological Event Scale
IPC	Infection prevention and control
ISO	International Organisation for Standardisation
LGBTIQA	Lesbians, gays, bisexuals, transgenders, intersexes, queers and allies
LRS	Lower respiratory symptoms
MAO	Maximum acceptable outage
MCI	Mass casualty incident
MG	Mass gathering
MoU	Memorandum of understanding
N-EMT	National emergency medical team
NDRF	National Disaster Recovery Framework (US)

NDRRA	Natural Disaster Relief and Recovery Arrangements
NGO	Non-government organisation
OECD	Organisation for Economic Cooperation and Development
OFDA-USAID	Office of Foreign Disaster Assistance
OH&S	Occupational health and safety
PAC	Post acute COVID-19
PAHO	Pan American Health Organization
PDCA	Plan-do-check-act
PDNA	Post-Disaster Needs Assessment
PFA	Psychological First Aid
PHEOC	Public Health Emergency Operations Centres
PHSMs	Public health and social measures
PMR	Private, Mobile and Radio
PPE	Personal protective equipment
PPRR	Prevention, preparedness, response, and recovery
PTG	Posttraumatic growth
PTSD	Posttraumatic stress disorder
RAIR	Rail, air or industrial rescue
RDD	Radiological dispersion devices
RHC	Resilient health care
RTO	Recovery time objective
SARS-CoV-2	Severe Acute Respiratory Syndrome-associated Coronavirus 2
SDG	Sustainable development goal
SITREP	Situation report
SOD	Sudden onset disaster
SUMA	Supply Management
TB	Tuberculosis
TEC	Tsunami evaluation coalition
TFQCDM	Task Force on Quality Control of Disaster Management
TIEMS	The International Emergency Management Society
TQM	Total quality management
UN	United Nations
UNDAC	United Nations Disaster Assessment and Coordination
UN-DHA	United Nations Department of Humanitarian Affairs
UNDRR	United Nations Office for Disaster Risk Reduction
UNESCO	United Nations Educational, Scientific and Cultural Organisation
UNGA	United Nations General Assembly
UNHCR	United Nations High Commission for Refugees
UNISDR	United Nations International Strategy for Disaster Reduction
US	United States
USAID	United States Agency for International Development
USAR	Urban search and rescue
VOCs	Variants of Concern
WADEM	World Association of Disaster and Emergency Medicine
WASH	Water supply, sanitation and hygiene
WHO	World Health Organisation
WTC	World Trade Center

Part 1

The conceptual basis of disaster management

1
Definitions and terminology

Lidia Mayner and Erin Smith

INTRODUCTION AND OBJECTIVES

Disasters are a recurring feature of human life and the extent to which they can be identified and managed is contingent upon our collective understanding of the meaning and dimensions of the concept. So, what is a disaster? What is disaster health? How do disasters differ from other emergencies?

The aim of this chapter is to summarise the development and evolution of the definition of disasters along with other terms relevant to disaster management. On completion of this chapter, you should have:

1. Developed a detailed understanding of disasters and related terms.
2. Be able to conduct an informed discussion on the elements of these definitions and the relationships between concepts.
3. Identify ways in which disasters may be categorised and the relative benefits of these measures.

UNDERSTANDING DISASTERS

Descriptions of disasters are common throughout history as evidenced by Pliny the Younger's graphic descriptions of the eruption of Pompeii. However Canadian, Samuel Henry Prince is considered to be the pioneer of disaster research. In 1917, Prince began the formal study of disasters with his dissertation on Canada's worst catastrophe, the 1917 ship explosion in the harbour of Halifax, Nova Scotia [1]. His pioneering study and sociological exploration of the effects of disaster, stimulated further empirical and theoretical research throughout the 1930s, 1940s, and 1950s, with a resulting shift in the way that disasters were defined. Instead of referring primarily to a physical agent, definitions and descriptions of disasters began to emphasise the social impact of the event.

In 1957, Fritz and Mathewson published a study exploring convergence behaviour of victims, responders, volunteers, onlookers, and concerned members of the community during disasters [2]. The study highlighted how this type of convergence may obstruct and complicate rescue operations. Fritz [3] further proposed a sociologically based definition for disasters, claiming they were events:

DOI: 10.4324/9781032626604-2

In which a society or a relatively self-sufficient sub-division of society, undergoes severe danger and incurs such losses to its members and physical appurtenances that the social structure is disrupted and the fulfilment of all or some of the essential functions of the society is prevented.

[3]

This sociological framework focused on disruptions to the vital functioning of a society. Disasters were examined by how they affected health, social, cultural, and economic infrastructure. This emerging conceptualisation was reinforced by the work of Barker and Chapman [4], and books examining communities and behaviour during disasters [5, 6]. However, despite continued interest in disasters throughout the 1960s, a discipline encompassing disaster research was lacking.

This changed in the 1970s, when Henry Quarantelli pushed for the international recognition of disaster research as an academic speciality, and the need for a specialist journal. Quarantelli's efforts led to the creation of the Research Committee on Disasters of the International Sociological Association, and publication of the *International Journal of Mass Emergencies and Disasters* [7]. Quarantelli and his colleagues triggered the emergence of new models of approaching disasters based on the analysis of communities [8]. The next 30 years of disaster research continued to engage academics from a wide variety of disciplines to examine their nature, definition, and concepts.

These developments in the field of disaster research further highlighted an issue that had dominated the early works of pioneer disaster researchers, how to define and conceptualise the term disaster. While this greater multi-disciplinary interest in disasters led to more reflection and interpretation, a single definition defining the phenomena of disaster was still elusive with most disciplines proposing definitions that reflected their individual interests.

Al-Madhari et al. [9] examined whether a universal definition for disaster was feasible. After reviewing 27 existing definitions they concluded that one over-arching definition was not possible. Nevertheless Al-Madhari et al. [9] suggested a definition incorporating both health and economic aspects as follows:

An event localised in time and space if one or more of the following consequences occur:
1. 10 or more fatalities;
2. damage exceeds $1 million (US); and or
3. 50 or more people evacuated.

The Centre for Research into the Epidemiology of Disasters (CRED) [10] defines disasters for the purposes of standardising data collection as events in which:

Ten (10) or more people reported killed.
Hundred (100) or more people reported affected.
Declaration of a state of emergency.
Call for international assistance.

Thus, there is no single accepted definition of disasters. Disasters are defined within the context of the need for the definition. The plethora of disaster definitions tends to be specific to the circumstances of the community and the needs of the organisation crafting the definition.

Definitions of disaster vary at international, national, and local levels where organisations develop their own working definitions of disaster to meet their particular requirements. These reflect not only the professional background of the definer, but also the context of work, studies, or research.

Disaster definitions may relate to the purpose of the definer. Definitions for data collections purposes must necessarily be relatively prescriptive, but often distinctly different to those described in impact terms. A government may define disasters for the purposes of declaring a disaster and enabling response and recovery arrangements to be enacted. A response agency may define disasters built around their surge requirements.

Notwithstanding this considerable disparity, most definitions convey the essential components that constitute a disaster. It is these components that make a particular event a disaster:

- Causes serious disruption.
- Beyond the day-to-day capacity.
- Requires *special* mobilisation of resources and organisations.

The United Nations Office for Disaster Risk Reduction (UNDRR) [11] defines disaster as:

A serious disruption of the functioning of a community or a society at any scale due to hazardous events interacting with conditions of exposure, vulnerability and capacity, leading to one or more of the following: human, material, economic and environmental losses and impacts.

The International Committee of the Red Cross [12] adopted a similar definition:

Disasters are serious disruptions to the functioning of a community that exceed its capacity to cope using its own resources. Disasters can be caused by natural, man-made and technological hazards, as well as various factors that influence the exposure and vulnerability of a community.

Using these definitions, events such as earthquakes, floods, and hurricanes/cyclones are not disasters in their own right, rather, they become disasters when they adversely and seriously impact on human life, livelihoods, and property.

CASE STUDY 1.1 – SEVERE TROPICAL CYCLONE INGRID, 14–16 MARCH 2005

Severe TC Ingrid caused significant impact on the Australian coast. The only cyclone ever recorded to impact as a severe tropical cyclone on the coastline of three different states or territories. First crossing the QLD East Coast, south of Lockhart River as a Category 4, she then moved across the Gulf into the Northern Territory and impacted on the small islands north of the Arnhem Land Coast as a Category 5 cyclone. TC Ingrid then weakened slightly to Category 4 as it crossed Croker Island and the Cobourg Peninsula. As a category 3 cyclone, she traversed the Tiwi Islands

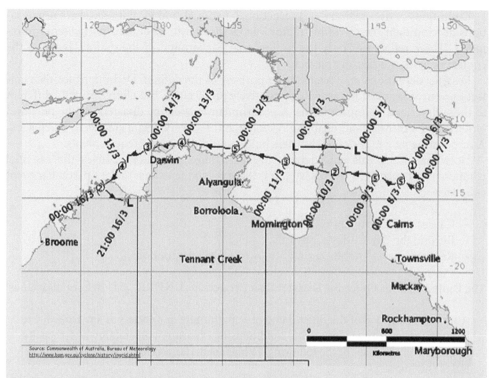

Figure 1.1 The track and intensity of Severe Tropical Cyclone Ingrid (Commonwealth of Australia, Bureau of Meteorology, 2016)

north of Darwin and finally re-intensified to category 4 before making final landfall on the West Australian Kimberley coast (Figure 1.1).

Was this a disaster?

While small in size, TC Ingrid was very intense, the remote location, sparsely populated areas, the preparedness of the communities impacted by TC Ingrid, and the accuracy and timeliness of the cyclone watches and warnings meant there was no loss of life and evacuations were not necessary. Property damage was minimal although there was significant environmental damage.

Source: Commonwealth of Australia, Bureau of Meteorology http://www.bom.gov.au/cyclone/history/ingrid.shtml

It is these elements that capture what is different about disasters, and therefore distinguishes them from other events or challenges. It is a situation or an event in which individuals, organisations, and systems have to behave or operate in a non-routine way, sometimes forging new modes of operation or creating organisational structures (e.g., disaster coordination centres) which complement routine activities.

Figure 1.2 seeks to demonstrate the relative nature of the definition of a disaster. There is no 'start or end point' but rather all events lie along a continuum with the daily

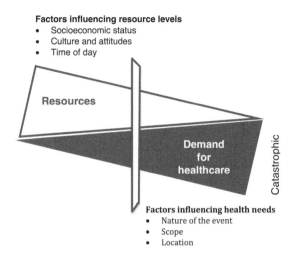

Factors influencing resource levels
- Socioeconomic status
- Culture and attitudes
- Time of day

Factors influencing health needs
- Nature of the event
- Scope
- Location

Figure 1.2 The mismatch between resources and health needs that determine a disaster

(routine) events at one end and the extreme (catastrophic) disasters, such as earthquakes, at the other. Where events place along this continuum is dependent on the context and the nature of the event. When that event becomes a disaster is dependent on the relative mismatch between the demands and the resources available to deal with the event. Thus, the extent of the challenge to the health and wellbeing of the community is determined by the nature of the event, its location, spread and impact along with the characteristics, culture, and size of the community. Even the timing of the event can determine the mismatch as it determines the available resources.

DEFINING DISASTER-RELATED TERMS

There is an extensive array of other terms that disaster management practitioners need to familiarise themselves with. The following documents identify not only the array of terms but also the variability of understandings.

A particular subclass of disaster is the Complex Humanitarian Emergency (CHE). The United Nations High Commission for Refugees (UNHCR) [13] defines a CHE as "a humanitarian crisis in a country, region or society where there is a total or considerable breakdown of authority resulting from internal or external conflict, and which requires an international response that goes beyond the mandate or capacity of any single agency and/ or the ongoing UN country programme". CHEs thus result from the interplay of macro community challenges such as population displacement, political instability, food insecurity, or military conflict. These events create massive complex challenges to health and wellbeing.

It is not easy to make sense of the huge array of terms. Differentiating emergencies from disasters is challenging. It could be argued emergencies are sudden events that may or may not be disasters depending on their scale and impact. Emergencies are often the 'business as usual' focus of emergency services including emergency health services.

Various terms are often used without careful attention to their precise meaning, or as stated above, the terms may reflect their particular focus or interest. This only adds to the confusion. For example, some people equate risk management with disaster management.

United Nations General Assembly (UNGA). *Report of the open-ended intergovernmental expert working group on indicators and terminology relating to disaster risk reduction.* 2016, United Nations Digital Library; Available from: https://digitallibrary.un.org/record/852089?ln=en

United Nations Office for Disaster Risk Reduction (UNDRR). *Hazard definition & classification review technical report.* 2020, Geneva, Switzerland; Available from: https://council.science/wp-content/uploads/2020/06/UNDRR_Hazard-report_DIGITAL.pdf

Proposed updated terminology on disaster risk reduction: A technical review. 2015; Available from: http://www.preventionweb.net/files/45462_backgoundpaperonterminologyaugust20.pdf

Prehospital and disaster medicine: Disaster terminology; Available from: http://www.preventionweb.net/files/3913_VL206323.pdf

Task Force on Quality Control of Disaster Management (TFQCDM)/World Association for Disaster and Emergency Medicine (WADEM). *Health disaster management: Guidelines for evaluation.* 2002; Available from: https://wadem.org/publications/guidelines-evaluation-research/

United Nations Educational, Scientific and Cultural Organisation (UNESCO) Office Bangkok and Regional Bureau for Education in Asia and the Pacific Glossary of basic terminology on disaster risk reduction. Document code: TH/2010/ED/009; Available from: https://unesdoc.unesco.org/ark:/48223/pf0000225784

United Nations International Strategy for Disaster Reduction (UNISDR) Geneva, Switzerland. *2009 UNISDR terminology on disaster risk reduction.* May 2009; Available from: https://www.unisdr.org/files/7817_UNISDRTerminologyEnglish.pdf

The former implies simply the management of 'potential' not the consequences. It is important in the interest of clarity of understanding and communication to develop a dictionary of terms which demonstrates their relationships to each other and to the underlying concepts. The best advice is to rely on plain English interpretations of terms rather than using technical definitions that may differ and thus confuse.

While it is not possible to deal with this diversity in a comprehensive fashion, there are important words worthy of emphasis. These concepts will be explored progressively throughout subsequent chapters.

- **Hazard** is a process, phenomenon, or human activity that may cause loss of life, injury or other health impacts, property damage, social and economic disruption, or environmental degradation [14]. Recent published reports on hazard classification describe 302 UN-accepted hazards and descriptions of each of the individual hazards [11, 15].
- **Disaster risk** refers to the potential loss of life, injury, or destroyed or damaged assets which could occur to a system, society, or a community. Disaster risk is determined probabilistically as a function of hazard, exposure, vulnerability, and capacity [14].
- **Disaster risk management** is the application of disaster risk reduction policies and strategies to prevent new disaster risk, reduce existing disaster risk, and manage residual risk, contributing to the strengthening of resilience and reduction of disaster losses [14]. Disaster risk management plans set out the goals and specific

objectives for reducing disaster risks together with related actions to accomplish these objectives. They should be guided by the Sendai Framework for Disaster Risk Reduction 2015–2030 and considered and coordinated within relevant development plans, resource allocations, and programme activities. National-level plans need to be specific to each level of administrative responsibility and adapted to the different social and geographical circumstances that are present. The time frame and responsibilities for implementation and the sources of funding should be specified in the plan. Linkages to sustainable development and climate change adaptation plans should be made where possible [14].

- **Disaster risk reduction** is aimed at preventing new risk, reducing existing disaster risk, and managing residual risk, all of which contribute to strengthening resilience and therefore to the achievement of sustainable development [14].
- The **Disaster Management Continuum** describes the fact that disaster management continues throughout the continuum of getting ready, responding, and recovering. These stages are often described in terms such as *Prevention, Preparedness, Response, and Recovery* although this description is not intended to imply that these stages are discrete and sequential but rather, they are the elements of comprehensive management that are themselves continuous and overlap.
- **Early warning system** is an integrated system of hazard monitoring, forecasting and prediction, disaster risk assessment, communication and preparedness activities, systems and processes that enables individuals, communities, governments, businesses, and others to take timely action to reduce disaster risks in advance of hazardous events [14].
- **Vulnerability** is the conditions determined by physical, social, economic, and environmental factors or processes which increase the susceptibility of an individual, a community, assets, or systems to the impacts of hazards [14].
- **Resilience** describes the inherent ability of an individual, community, or organisation to continue to function despite a challenge. This broad definition of the term incorporates four key elements:

  - The strength (the ability to take the hit) which is influenced by the design of both hard (structure) and soft (systems) infrastructure.
  - The flexibility (agility or elasticity) which implies the ability of the individual, organisation, or infrastructure to avoid the damage or bounce back
  - The responsiveness which implies the ability to react and manage the impact and restore functionality.
  - The adaptability describes the ability to alter, adjust, and build a new reality. The effectiveness of any community response to major incidents will depend on their adaptability to the new reality. Haiti or Christchurch will never be the same; too much of what was there will never be useable again. The people must adapt to a new reality.

- **Adaptive capacity** enriches resilience by describing the ability of the individual organisation or community to adapt to changing circumstances.
- **Emergency management** is a term first used in the US and effectively considered to be synonymous with disaster management. The phrase is also used to emphasise comprehensive approaches that are integrated with risk management and the management of simple emergencies.

- **Protection** is often used to imply defence against terrorism but equally, against infectious diseases.
- **Mass crowd** events capture the unique challenges of large populations, often in an environment which may be un-sustaining.
- **Mass casualty** (or **multi-casualty**) events describe those with ill-defined levels of many casualties.
- One of the critical challenges of disaster management is to understand how these various terms fit together in a rational manner which reflects clarity of understanding.

DISASTER HEALTH

Health and the ability to contribute to societal productivity and sustainability is a fundamental part of an individual's quality of life. Health is defined by the World Health Organisation (WHO) as:

a state of complete physical, mental and social wellbeing and not merely the absence of disease or infirmity.

[16]

The health system is fundamental to human life and needs to be able to support people by ensuring it can function effectively regardless of the circumstance. A critical focus of disaster management is on the preservation of **health and wellbeing**. An understanding of the challenges that face the health system is a critical component of disaster management systems.

Terms are used to convey strong messages of principle. In this context, the phrase 'disaster health' is preferred to disaster medicine. Disaster health emphasises that disaster responses are multidisciplinary by nature and not the sole domain of any single profession or expert group. Equally, the term 'health' reinforces the understanding that disaster management is not restricted to the treatment of those who may be ill or injured. The term 'health' also focuses on the preservation of health and wellbeing. Perhaps the term 'disaster medicine' is best considered a subset of disaster health, restricted to the particular aspects of clinical care that characterise the management of patients in a disaster.

Bradt [17] and Sundnes et al. [18] described the context of disaster health as involving three essential domains. These are public health, emergency and risk management, and clinical and psychological care. This speaks further to the complexity of disasters and the interrelationships between professional areas of responsibilities.

Again, strict wording is less important than understanding the common themes and ideas. For example, a hospital in a disaster may find itself in any one or combination of scenarios. It may have a surge of patients, with no damage to or loss of facilities and/or staff. The hospital may have sustained significant damage, and staff and their families are affected. It may also have sustained little internal damage but is isolated because of external infrastructure damage (power, water, gas, communications, food supplies, drugs, and all manner of consumables). In a disaster any combination of the above scenarios is possible. Stakeholders will also have different expectations of what a hospital should or should not be able to provide.

Within the health context, the distinction between a disaster and an everyday event is often difficult to make.

For example, the Australian Institute of Health and Welfare (AIHW) [19] reports that in 2020–2021, there were 8.8 million presentations to emergency departments (EDs) in public hospitals. This represents a relative utilisation of 34 per 100 population which continues to increase 3.2% per year. In 2020–2021:

- Patients aged four years and under (who make up 7% of the population) accounted for 10% of presentations.
- Patients aged 65 and over (who make up 16% of the population) accounted for 21% of presentations.
- Overall, males accounted for 49% of presentations and females 51% [19].

> *Each day hospital emergency departments in Australia treat more than 20,000 people. Australia has never had a single event with 20,000 casualties – except every day!*

This very nicely demonstrates the difference between disasters and normal days. Currently, the system (however painfully) copes with this demand. EDs are very skilled at coping with surges in demand on daily, weekly, and yearly cycles. However, a disaster for them would be when they have a situation where it is impossible to deliver the standard of care they are used to providing.

The challenge for health services is to surge its response at the same time as it deals with threats to its physical and human infrastructure.

Consider the Shizugawa hospital in Minamisanriku, Northern Japan, affected by the 2011 Tōhoku Earthquake and Tsunami. The tsunami arrived with little warning and water inundated the fourth floor of a five-story building. Imagine the array of considerations that would come into play in such a circumstance. How does a hospital prepare, respond, or recover from such an assault on health infrastructure? We have explored these issues further in Chapter 10 Health Systems (see Figure 1.3).

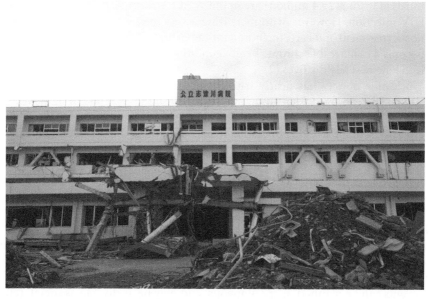

Figure 1.3 The Shizugawa Public Hospital one month after the 2011 Tōhoku Earthquake (Photo by Christopher Johnson)

The systems and structures required for everyday health responses form the cornerstone of our disaster response. Thus, disaster health responses may be integrated into business as usual and not considered another layer of planning and management. What is required are scalable arrangements, beginning with the everyday response, then scaling up to the level required for the challenge. Disaster health management is not intended to describe the management of everyday events, but rather to explore the issues that occur when these everyday events are exceeded.

> Disaster management often does not address the silent and slow-moving health disasters. It is very important to be aware of these when considering disaster management arrangements. On a global scale, some of the silent disasters have a level of impact which far exceeds any of the most dramatic catastrophic events.

- Consider Tuberculosis (TB). In 2020 an estimated 1.5 million people died from TB, including 214,000 people with HIV. Worldwide, TB is the 13th leading cause of death and the second leading infectious killer after COVID-19 (above HIV/AIDS). An estimated 10 million people fell ill with TB worldwide – 5.6 million men, 3.3 million women, and 1.1 million children. TB is present in all countries and age groups. But TB is curable and preventable but is often overlooked by health providers and can be difficult to diagnose and treat [20]. The 30 high TB burden countries accounted for 86% of new TB cases. Eight countries account for two thirds of the total, with India leading the count, followed by China, Indonesia, the Philippines, Pakistan, Nigeria, Bangladesh, and South Africa [20].
- Also consider HIV which continues to be a major global public health issue, having claimed 36.3 million [27.2–47.8 million] lives so far. There were an estimated 37.7 million [30.2–45.1 million] people living with HIV at the end of 2020, over two thirds of whom (25.4 million) are in the WHO African Region. There is no cure for HIV infection. However, with increasing access to effective HIV prevention, diagnosis, treatment and care, including for opportunistic infections, HIV infection has become a manageable chronic health condition, enabling people living with HIV to lead long and healthy lives [21].
- Worldwide obesity has nearly tripled since 1975. In 2016, more than 1.9 billion adults, 18 years and older, were overweight. Of these over 650 million were obese. Over 340 million children and adolescents aged 5–19 were overweight or obese in 2016. Most of the world's population lives in countries where overweight and obesity kills more people than underweight [22].

Within the context of disaster health there are several terms that are important to incorporate or distinguish from disaster health.

Mass gatherings

A *Mass Gathering* (MG) has been defined by the WHO as *"the concentration of people at a specific location for a specific purpose over a set period of time and which has the potential to strain the planning and response resources of the country or community"* [23]. These events can be planned or spontaneous, and may be as diverse as social, religious, cultural or sporting events or include the gathering of people as the result of natural disasters or conflict. MGs present their own unique challenges to public health and other risks.

The field of MG health is under constant development and in early 2012 the Executive Board (EB) of the WHO requested that the Director-General further develop and disseminate multi-sectoral guidance on planning, management, evaluation, and monitoring of all types of MG. This is to be developed with specific emphasis on sustainable preventive measures including health education and preparedness. The EB decision has reinforced the existing WHO strategy of working closely with Member States that are planning MGs and helping Member States to strengthen functional capacities to better utilise the International Health Regulations (2005) for MGs. This work is to be carried out by the WHO, its collaborating network, and the broader international public health community [24].

Mass casualty incident (MCI)

An MCI has been defined functionally as:

an overwhelming event, which generates more patients at a time than locally available resources can manage using routine procedures.

[25]

MCIs may result from man-made disasters such as transport, industrial, or terrorism; natural disasters such as earthquakes and bushfires; epidemics/pandemics; and the displacement of populations from their usual sources of safety and protection.

Triage

Medical triage is the process by which patients are sorted on the basis of their urgency, severity, and complexity into categories which determine their ongoing care needs and priorities. Triage was first used during the Napoleonic Wars whereby the wounded were treated according to their level of gravity of their injuries.

Triage is routinely used to sort when and where patients will be seen in an ED. Rather than operating on a 'first come, first served' system like you would expect at a restaurant, EDs use the triage system to sort patients into categories, so that they can attend to patients who need urgent help first. To support this process, EDs use standardised triage systems such as the Australasian Triage Scale.

There have been many efforts to design disaster-specific triage scales. Mostly to accommodate the different circumstances that apply in disasters. However, there is an argument to be made that those involved in disaster response should use triage systems with which they are familiar in everyday practice.

Further readings are available from the following sites:

WHO. Emergency Triage Assessment and Treatment (ETAT) Manual for participants, 2005. Available from: https://apps.who.int/iris/bitstream/handle/10665/43386/9241546875_eng.pdf?sequence=1&isAllowed=y

WHO. Emergency Triage Assessment and Treatment (ETAT) Facilitator guide, 2005. Available from: https://apps.who.int/iris/bitstream/handle/10665/43386/9241546883_eng.pdf?sequence=2&isAllowed=y

---

CATEGORISING DISASTERS

There have been many attempts to categorise disasters from the perspective of describing the nature and extent of events. Disasters are often **categorised according to the specific hazard** that led to the event. The CRED developed a classification standard for both natural and technological disasters. Natural disasters have been divided into six main disaster types, with each having a number of sub-types. The six main disaster types within this standard include meteorological, hydrological, climatological, geophysical, biological, and extra-terrestrial [26]. More recently, the UNDRR Hazard Definition and Classification Review Technical Report [15] broadly categorises hazards into meteorological and hydrological, extraterrestrial, geohazards, environmental, chemical, biological, technological, and societal. Tables 1.1–1.8 outline subtypes and examples.

Table 1.1 Hazard information profiles: **meteorological and hydrological**

Hazard cluster	Description
Convective-related	These relate to the effect of deep convection clouds that may result in sudden downburst, thunderstorms, and associated lightning strikes.
Flood	Floods may be caused by excess precipitation, displacement of stored water, rising ground water, or melting of snow or ice. • Precipitation can lead to riverine (fluvial) or estuarine flooding, or to surface water (flash) flooding. • Rising ground water may result from remote precipitation or alterations in natural drainage by debris or ice. • Displacement of stored water may occur from structural failure of water retention mechanisms or by displacement of water by an avalanche or similar incursion. Structural failure includes natural occurrences such as outbursts from glacial lakes. • Melting snow or ice may cause riverine or surface water flooding
Lithometeors	Lithometeor refers to the conglomeration of small solid particles (e.g., dust or sand) suspended in the atmosphere causing haze and the associated risks to health and to human systems. Suspended particles may include pollutants, carbon, water (fog or haze), dust, or sand.
Marine	Marine hazards relate to the composition (e.g., acidification) of sea water or to the impact of climatic or geophysical events. • Climate-induced events include rogue waves, icebergs or ice flows, storm surges and storm waves. They also include seiche which is the changes in the volume of stored water due to pressure changes in the atmosphere. • Geophysical effects include tsunami.
Pressure-related	Hazards may be caused by the changes in atmosphere pressure resulting in atmospheric depressions, tropical and extratropical cyclones (hurricanes or typhoons).
Precipitation-related	Precipitation-related hazards may relate to the absence of precipitation (drought) or to the nature of the precipitation and include acid rain, blizzards, hail, ice storms, or snow storms.

(Continued)

Table 1.1 (Continued)

Hazard cluster	Description
Temperature-related	Hazards may relate to variations in atmospheric temperature that are outside the normal range for that location and include cold (cold snap) or hot (heatwave) weather or to the impacts of associated event including icing, freezing rain or snow, or bushfires and drought.
Terrestrial	Terrestrial hazards relate to the movement of surfaces including snow (avalanche), mud, or earth and rock.
Wind-related	The movement of the air can damage both natural and built infrastructure and thus impact on human health and safety. Strong winds may occur in isolation (gales) or associated with other climatic events such as storms, cyclones, or tornadoes.

Table 1.2 Hazard information profiles: **extra-terrestrial**

Hazard cluster	Description
Extra-terrestrial	Extra-terrestrial hazards are those that are caused by external influences and include those related to solar radiation (solar storms, geomagnetic storms) and their impact on both natural and built environment and to the impact of extra-terrestrial objects both natural (meteorites) and human-built (space junk).

Table 1.3 Hazard information profiles: **geohazard**

Hazard cluster	Description
Seismogenic (earthquake)	Seismic events occur when subterranean pressure results in a sudden fracturing and movement of rock resulting in shaking of the earth (earthquake), displacement of the earth surfaces (rock or debris slide), displacement of water (tsunami), or changes to ground water containment or flow (liquefaction).
Volcanogenic (volcanoes and geothermal)	Volcanogenic hazards are those related to the pressure-related effects (earthquakes), or to the expulsion of subterranean materials (lava flows, gases, ash clouds, debris). The impact relates to the speed and extent of the event and to the impacts that hot material can have on both the natural and built environment.
Other geohazards	Other geohazards include those caused by both natural and human activities. They may include the collapse of natural structures (sinkholes, rockfalls, erosion) or to human activities (mining, explosions).

Table 1.4 Hazard information profiles: **environmental**

Hazard cluster	Description
Environmental	Environmental hazards relate to the impacts of both natural and human forces on the natural environment. These include: • Atmospheric contamination (pollution) • Land degradation and contamination • Loss and contamination of oceans and other water storage leading to disturbances to fauna (e.g., coral bleaching) • Impact on the natural biological environment through loss of biodiversity, desertification, and deforestation. • Wildfires

Table 1.5 Hazard information profiles: **chemical**

Hazard cluster	Description
Gases	Release or accumulation of gases such as ammonia, Carbon Monoxide, Phosphine, or Chlorine.
Heavy metals	Accumulation of heavy metals such as Arsenic, Cadmium, Lead, or Mercury.
Food safety	Disruptions to the level of supply or contamination of food supplies.
Pesticides	Accumulation of pesticides, insecticides or fungicides.
Persistent organic pollutants (POPs)	The accumulation of organic pollutants such as dioxins or microplastics.
Hydrocarbons	Accumulation contamination by oil or benzene.
CBRNE (chemical, biological, radiological, nuclear, and explosive)	Deliberate or accidental exposure to chemical warfare agents.
Other chemical hazards and toxins	Other chemical contaminations including asbestos, methanol, fluoride (excess or inadequate intake), or exposure to substandard and falsified medical products.
Fisheries and aquaculture	Marine toxins

Table 1.6 Hazard information profiles: **biological**

Hazard cluster	Description
Fisheries and aquaculture	Harmful algal blooms.
Insect infestation	Invasion of excess or unusual insects such as locusts, invasive weeds, or invasive species.
Human–animal interaction	Hazards related to the contact between humans and animals including the effect on humans of dangerous animals (e.g., sharks, snakes, crocodiles etc) or to the impacts human activity has on the survival or species.

(Continued)

Table 1.6 (Continued)

Hazard cluster	Description
Infectious disease (plant)	Infectious diseases may impact on the natural fauna impacting on their survival and potentially disrupting the food chain.
Infectious disease (human and animal)	An extensive array of diseases may impact on animals and on humans. The interaction between humans and animals increases the risk of animal disease being transmitted to humans. The impact and control of such diseases depend on the nature of the disease and the mode of transmission. It is difficult to generalise but the risks may be broadly defined: • Endemic diseases that have the potential to increase incidence either through failure of public health protections (e.g., vaccination programs) or as a consequence of changes to causative organisms (e.g., vaccine or treatment-resistant organisms). • Emergence of diseases not usually expected in that location such as Plague. • Resurgence of diseases previously controlled or eliminated (e.g., cholera or polio). • Novel diseases such as MERS, COVID-19, or HIV.

Table 1.7 Hazard information profiles: **technological**

Hazard cluster	Description
Radiation	The accumulation of radioactive material or waste and contamination of the physical or human environment.
CBRNE	The release or accumulation of radiation or nuclear agents.
Construction/ structural failure	Failure or damage to the built environment including structural failure or fire.
Infrastructure failure	Failure of the critical infrastructure required to support human communities including power outages, communication infrastructure failures, and water supply failure.
Cyber hazard	Challenges to electronic management, information and communication systems including design failures resulting in non-conformity and interoperability, operational failures leading to outages and disruption, deliberate or accidental release of information, malware and spyware cyber-attacks, and social misuse and cyberbullying.
Industrial failure	Industrial failure can be socially disruptive impacting on supply chains and on employment. Industrial failure may occur as a result of commercial factors, or due to the impact of failure of physical infrastructure (fires or building collapse) including the impact of natural events on industrial infrastructure (Natech). Industrial hazards also relate to the impact of industry on the natural and social environment through pollution or contamination.

(Continued)

Table 1.7 (Continued)

Hazard cluster	Description
Waste	The by-products of human and industrial activity are waste which has the potential to adversely affect the natural and human environment. Waste requires either reuse (recycling or repurposing) or disposal which creates issues with contamination. This may be general or relate specifically to particular types of waste such as electronic or biohazards. This includes waste disposed on land and in the sea creating marine debris.
Transportation	Human transportation systems create the potential for transport incidents that may impact any form of human transport, road, rail, marine or air.

Table 1.8 Hazard information profiles: **societal**

Hazard cluster	Description
Conflict	Human conflict both armed and unarmed conflict and including both wars international disputes and civil unrest. has the potential to adversely impact on human society.
Post-conflict	The impact of human conflict does not cease with the end of active warfare but rather linger as the explosive remnants of war or the environmental degradation that results from the conflict.
Behaviour	Human behaviour outside of structured conflict can impact on human wellbeing. This may result either from intentional violence or uncontrolled crowd behaviours such as human stampedes.
Economic	Adverse economic conditions can affect human health and wellbeing. Financial shocks impact on the availability and effectiveness of safety of physical and societal support mechanisms.

There is considerable debate about disaster categorisations given events are often highly complex and resist being simplified to a single hazard. For example, a cyclone (hurricane or typhoon) will produce wind damage, flooding, storm surge and in some incidents, refugees while complex humanitarian emergencies encompass unique interplays of multiple challenges. It must be recognised that disasters are social, economic, and political phenomena; the hazard is only a trigger. While segmentation of disasters into groups or categories provides a starting point for disaster managers, it is important to recognise it in the interplay between hazard and communities that is particularly relevant in understanding and managing the consequences of these disasters.

However, disaster classification provides a checklist of things to consider when identifying, evaluating, and managing the risks to the community. Furthermore, they help foster an understanding of the complex interplay of causation. Consider for example global warming and its impact on a range of hazards and vulnerabilities.

There have also been attempts to **categorise disasters on the basis of their extent and impact.** Scales have been developed on the basis of economic damage or human deaths, but there is little agreement as to the usefulness of such categorisations. In health terms, distinguishing an emergency from a disaster has often been based on the number of patients affected, the Bradford Disaster Scale for example [27]. However, it is important to note that the extent of the disaster is not only dependent on the number of people affected but also the severity and range of illnesses and injuries, and the resources available. As disasters are defined contextually, any absolute categorisation based on people affected is meaningless.

Hazard-specific severity scales have been slightly more useful.

- The Richter scale for earthquakes is almost universally recognised by the community, but has no direct correlation with the degree of damage. Rather, the extent of damage is related to the interplay between the natural forces unleased, and the community's vulnerability and the Earthquake Impact Scale is an attempt to capture both these considerations [28].
- The International Atomic Energy Agency uses a scale of 0–7 to qualify a nuclear accident. The classification depends on the consequences of the accident and not its causes. This can be confusing because some accidents such as Chernobyl are actually due to an internal error and not a natural disaster, as was the case with central Fukushima (see Figure 1.4).

The United States of America's Federal Emergency Management Agency (FEMA) seeks to categorise or describe events on the basis of the management implications [29]. The following is criteria used by FEMA:

1. Length of forewarning
2. Magnitude of impact
3. Geographical scope of impact
4. Duration of impact
5. Speed of onset

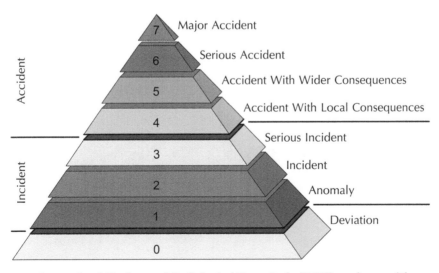

Figure 1.4 International Nuclear and Radiological Event Scale (INES) used to qualify a nuclear accident

Such criterion-based approach may help convey something of the challenge without implying a hierarchy of disasters.

APPLYING DEFINITIONS

Having explored the concept of disasters and the factors contributing to their definition, consider the following events and how they challenge your understanding of the definition of disasters.

Great East Japan Earthquake and Tsunami 2011

These events have had a lingering impact on the community. Not only because of the widespread death and devastation, but also through the damage to the nuclear power station and the ongoing concern for long-term health consequences. People in the vicinity of the power station have been evacuated, land is unavailable for agriculture, and children's education has been disrupted together with the long-term economic impacts and of a loss of confidence in Japan's agricultural products (see Figures 1.5 and 1.6).

Polluted water supply: Sydney 1998

In Sydney Australia 1998, a major capital city's water supply was contaminated with Giardia and Cytosporidium bacteria. From initial reports, it was difficult to determine if the disaster had occurred given there were no deaths associated with the crisis. However,

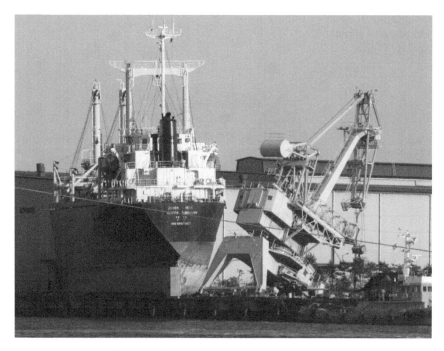

Figure 1.5–1.6 Images of the 2011 Tōhoku – Great East Japan tsunami. Top: damage to the port (Photo by Chief Hira). Bottom: Shinchi train station lies in ruin (Photo by Kuha455405)

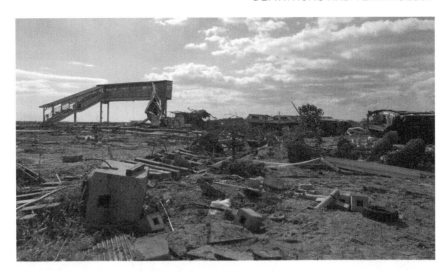

Figure 1.5–1.6 (Continued)

when the previously discussed definitions are considered, this event caused a serious disruption to community life which threatened or caused death or injury. Controlling and dealing with the problem required an investigation and measures which were beyond the normal capacity of the government and water authorities. For more on this disaster, read the final inquiry report dated December 1998 available at URL: https://www.dpc.nsw.gov.au/assets/dpc-nsw-gov-au/publications/Sydney-Water-Inquiry-listing-427/5cb60e9942/Fifth-Report-Final-Report-Volume-2-December-1998.pdf

The Global Financial Crisis 2008

The Global Financial Crisis of 2008. Again, it may not meet the immediate (media) definition of a disaster (cyclone, tsunami, or earthquake), but when you consider the extensive impact on community infrastructure and on the health and wellbeing of people then it probably does meet the disaster definition. What impact would it have had on health and wellbeing of the poorest in society? The ongoing consequences for this vulnerable group may last a generation.

Other disasters

Consider also the impact of Foot and Mouth diseases outbreaks not only on the economy but on food supplies. Consider how Epidemics such as polio (1938 and 1953) (see Figure 1.7), influenza (1844, 1919, 1957 and 1968) and COVID-19 have had a massive impact on the health and wellbeing of people and required responses well beyond that traditionally associated with the provision of health services. Critical health infrastructure is required to support the community throughout these events, yet as COVID-19 has clearly shown, they are also subject to the effects of the event either physical damage or staff absences which reduce their capacity to respond. Critical infrastructure, such as hospitals, can also experience damage caused by earthquakes (see Figure 1.8).

Many of these events have not been conceptualised as 'disaster' even though they clearly meet the conceptual definitions outlined above.

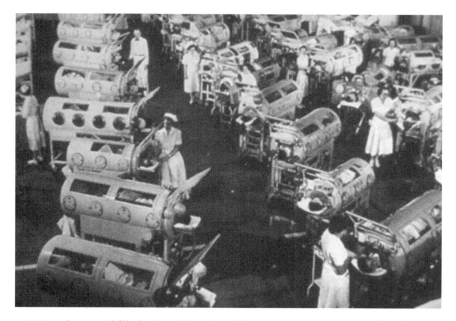

Figure 1.7 Iron lung ward filled with polio patients, Rancho Los Amigos Hospital, California (1953)

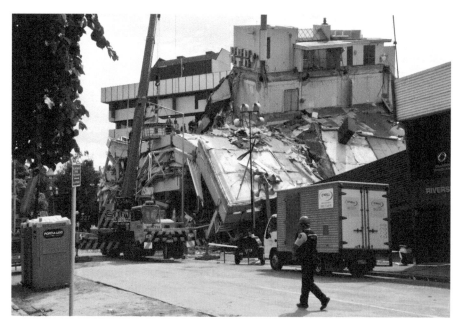

Figure 1.8 Pyne Gould building destroyed by earthquake, Christchurch New Zealand 2011 Photo by Gabriel Goh

Disasters typically impact all aspects of the community and require support from all response agencies. The very complexity that is integral to the systems that give us a remarkable standard of living also produces significant problems when a disaster strikes. Critical infrastructure such as electricity and transport networks are often damaged. This has a significant impact on a country's economy, and the ability of response agencies to access the whole community.

If these are the challenges disasters create, what then can be done about reducing the effects and increasing the adaptation across society and the economy? This all takes place with the context of ever-increasing complexity and interdependency in our society and economy. At an individual level and to an extent, organisational level, the safety paradox is relevant. The safer and more stable the environment, the greater the surprise when there is a major failure.

There are also differences in the community's reaction to different types of events. There is often outrage over non-natural events with extensive media coverage and government intervention. People tend to react differently to events where responsibility, whether real or implied, can easily be apportioned. They will also react differently to events that suggest a horrific experience for those involved. For example, a large number of deaths from one plane crash is given more attention than one death from a road traffic crash. The reality is more people die in car accidents than plane crashes. Boin et al. [30] asserted;

> The democratic context has changed over the past decades. Analysts agree, for instance, that citizens and politicians alike have become at once more fearful and less tolerant of major hazards to public health, safety and prosperity. The modern Western citizen has little patience for imperfections; he has come to fear glitches and has learned to see more of what he fears. In this culture of fear – sometimes referred to as the 'risk society' – the role of the modern mass media is crucial.

ACTIVITIES

1. With the information outlined above, develop a working definition of a disaster. Once done, consider all of the above examples and identify how they meet that definition. Briefly explain the rationale behind your definition.
2. Identify two different disasters and explain how they meet this definition.

KEY READINGS

1. Laakso, K., and Palomäki, J. The importance of a common understanding in emergency management. *Technological Forecasting & Social Change*, 2013. **80**(9): p. 1703–1713.
2. TFQCDM/WADEM. Health Disaster Management: Guidelines for Evaluation and Research in the "Utstein Style". Chapter 3: Overview and concepts. *Prehospital Disaster Medicine*, 2002. **17**(Suppl 3): p. 31–55.

3. Mayner, L., and Arbon, P. Defining disaster: The need for harmonisation of terminology. *Australasian Journal of Disaster and Trauma Studies*, 2015. **19**(Special issue): p. 21–25.
4. Çallşkan, C., and Üner, S. Disaster literacy and public health: A systematic review and integration of definitions and models. *Disaster Medicine and Public Health Preparedness*, 2021. **15**(4): p. 518–527. https://doi.org/10.1017/dmp.2020.100

References

1. Prince, S., *Catastrophe and social change*. 1920, New York (NY): Columbia University Press.
2. Fritz, C.E. and J. Mathewson, *Convergence behavior in disasters: Disaster study No. 9*. 1957, Washington (DC): National Academy of Sciences, National Research Council. p. 148.
3. Fritz, C.E., Disaster, in *Contemporary social problems*, R.K. Merton, and and R.A. Nisbet, Editors. 1961, New York (NY): Harcourt, Brace and World. p. 651–694.
4. Barker G. and Chapman D., *Man and society in disaster*. 1962, New York (NY): Basic Books.
5. Barton, A.H., *Communities in disaster: A sociological analysis of collective stress situations*. 1969, New York (NY): Double Day.
6. Dynes, R.R., *Organized behavior in disaster*. 1970, Lexington (MA): Heath Lexington Books.
7. Scanlon, T., Forward, in *What is a disaster?*, R. Perry and E. Qurantelli, Editors. 2005 (US): International Committee on Disasters.
8. Gilbert, C., Studying disaster: Changes in the main conceptual tools, in *What is a Disaster?*, E. Quarantelli, Editor. 1998, London (GB): Routledge. p. 21–30.
9. Al-Madhari, A. and A. Keller, Review of disaster definitions. *Prehospital and Disaster Medicine*, 1997. **12**(1): p. 17–21.
10. Centre for Research on the Epidemiology of Disasters. *CRED explanatory notes*. [cited 2022 16th September]; Available from: www.emdat.be/explanatory-notes.
11. United Nations Office for Disaster Risk Reduction. *Hazard definition & classification review technical report*. 2020.
12. International Committee of the Red Cross. *What is a disaster?* 2022 [cited 2022 16th September 2022]; Available from: https://www.ifrc.org/what-disaster.
13. United Nations High Commissioner for Refugees. *Coordination in complex emergencies*. 2022 [cited 2022 16th September]; Available from: https://www.unhcr.org/en-au/partners/partners/3ba88e7c6/coordination-complex-emergencies.html
14. United Nations General Assembly (UNGA). *Report of the open-ended intergovernmental expert working group on indicators and terminology relating to disaster risk reduction*. 2016. Geneva: United Nations Office for disaster Risk reduction. Available from: https://www.undrr.org/publication/report-open-ended-intergovernmental-expert-working-group-indicators-and-terminology
15. UN Office for Disaster Risk Reducation. *Hazard information profiles. Supplement to: UNDRR-ISC Hazard definition and classification review - Technical report*. 2021.
16. World Health Organisation. *WHO definition of health*. 2003 [Dec 14 2015]; Available from: http://www.who.int/about/definition/en/print.html.
17. Bradt, D.A., K. Abraham, and R. Franks, A strategic plan for disaster medicine in Australasia. *Emergency Medicine*, 2003. **15**(3): p. 271–282.
18. Sundnes, K.O. and M.L. Birnbaum, Health disaster management: Guidelines for evaluation and research in the Utstein style. *Prehospital and Disaster Medicine*, 2003. **17**(3): p. s1–s14.
19. Australian Institute of Health and Welfare. *Emergency department care, 2020–2021*. 2021; Available from: http://www.aihw.gov.au.
20. World Health Organization. *Fact sheet: Tuberculosis*. 2021; Available from: https://www.who.int/news-room/fact-sheets/detail/tuberculosis.
21. World Health Organisation. *Fact sheet: HIV/AIDS*. 2021; Available from: https://www.who.int/news-room/fact-sheets/detail/hiv-aids.
22. World Health Organisation. *Fact sheet: Obesity and overweight*. 2021; Available from: https://www.who.int/news-room/fact-sheets/detail/obesity-and-overweight.
23. World Health Organisation. *Public health for mass gatherings: Key considerations*. 2015; Available from: https://www.who.int/publications/i/item/public-health-for-mass-gatherings-key-considerations.

24. World Association for Disaster and Emergency Medicine. *Mass gatherings.* 2022; Available from: https://wadem.org/sigs/mass-gathering/.

25. Lomaglio, L., et al., Mass casualty incident: Definitions and current reality, in *WSES handbook of mass casualties incidents management.* 2020, Switzerland: Springer. p. 1–10.

26. Below, R., A. Wirtz, and D. Guha-Sapir. *Working paper: Disaster category classification and peril terminology for operational purposes.* 2009; Available from: https://www.cred.be/node/564.

27. Horlick-Jones, T. and G. Peters, Measuring disaster trends part one: Some observations on the Bradford fatality scale, in *Risk Management.* Gerald Mars, David T. H. Weir, Editors. 2000. London: Routledge. p. 23–27. ISBN978042928251.

28. Wald, D.J., et al. Earthquake impact scale. *Natural Hazards Review*, 2011. **12**: 125–139.

29. Kreps, G.A. and T.E. Drabek, Disasters as non-routine social problems--2. *International Journal of Mass Emergencies and Disasters*, 1996. **14**(2): p. 129–153.

30. Boin, A., E. Stern, and B. Sundelius, *The politics of crisis management: Public leadership under pressure.* 2016, Cambridge (GB): Cambridge University Press.

2

Disaster trends and impact

Benjamin Ryan and Richard Franklin

INTRODUCTION AND OBJECTIVE

Chapter 1 discussed the definition of disasters and explored how disasters may be considered in a social construct. In other words, is it a disaster if it does not affect people? Therefore, our understanding of the history of disasters is largely constrained to the period of our records. However, there is sufficient evidence within recorded history to enable us to understand the nature and trends of disasters and their impacts on humans.

There is a broad belief that disasters are increasing, but is this perception real or is it a product of increased awareness and reporting? Are disasters increasing in frequency or severity, or are they having more impact? More broadly, are the indirect impacts greater than we previously thought? What does the future hold in terms of disaster trends?

The aim of this chapter is to examine the trends in disasters in an historical context and to identify the factors that influence their occurrence and impact. By understanding the causation and impacts of disasters we may be better placed to identify ways in which disasters may be anticipated, averted, or moderated and their impacts reduced on all aspects of society.

On completion of this chapter, you should be able to:

1. Identify and discuss historical perspectives.
2. Describe the factors influencing the trends in disasters and their severity.
3. Identify and evaluate future risks.
4. Explain the impact disasters have on all aspects of society including human health and wellbeing, community, and the economy.

HISTORICAL PERSPECTIVES

Naming the worst disasters of all time depends on the criteria used, meaning the results are subjective and open to debate. What defines the worst? Is it death toll, the extent of damage, economic cost both direct and indirect, and what time frame is used? Due to the complexity in identifying the worst disasters, death toll has been used in Table 2.1. A combination of sources was used to identify the 15 worst disasters using this category [1–3].

 DOI: 10.4324/9781032626604-3

Table 2.1 Ten worst disasters by death toll (including disease outbreaks) in history [1–3]

	Year	*Disaster*	*Death Toll*
1	1877–1977	Smallpox pandemic	500 million
2	1347–1350	Bubonic plague (black death)	75–200 million
3	1918–1919	Spanish flu	35–75 million
4	1981-present	HIV/AIDS pandemic	32 million
5	1959–1961	Chinese famine	20 million
6	1855–1960	Third plague pandemic	>15 million
7	1769–1773	Indian famine	> 10 million
8	1876–1879	Drought, China	> 9 million
9	2019-present	COVID-19 pandemic	> 6 million
10	1931	China floods	4 million

In total, these disasters have resulted in more than 700 million deaths. Although this does not consider indirect costs it provides good insight into what has historically occurred.

What makes the events in Table 2.1 significant is not just the total body count, but also the different nature of their impact. Compare these events with the 55 million people who die each year around the world [4], which includes 18 million from Cardiovascular Diseases (6.8 million considered premature, under 70 years), 4.4 million injuries, 1.5 million Tuberculosis, and 627,000 Malaria [5]. In contrast, the lower end estimate of the 1918–19 pandemic deaths was 35 million and accounted for 2% of the world's population at that time. Meanwhile, during COVID-19 around 6 million deaths from March 2019 to the end of 2021 was 0.06% of the world's population. Considering these factors, another measure beyond deaths must be considered which includes economic damages. The worst disasters in terms of economic damages are listed in Table 2.2 [6].

Earthquakes result in largest economic losses around the globe. This is closely followed by storms (hurricanes) and floods. Overall, storms have been the most prevalent cause of damage and are the sole hazard for which the attributed portion towards disasters is continually increasing [8]. Economically vulnerable populations and nations will be hardest hit as they cannot endure long-term business closures, lockdowns, or other measures stifling the long-term function of society in a disease outbreak or disaster situation [9]. Also, most countries lack the ability to maintain a full nationwide relief operation [9]. Understanding this data, historical context, and the indirect impacts is vital to ensure disaster health and risk management strategies reflect both whole of society's needs and future disaster trends.

DISASTER TRENDS

The Centre for Research on the Epidemiology of Disasters (CRED) was established in 1973 to monitor worldwide trends in disasters and their impact [10]. It became a WHO collaborating centre in 1980 and launched the Emergency Events Database (EM-DAT) in 1988 to rationalise decision-making for disaster preparedness, providing an objective base for vulnerability assessment and priority setting [11]. CRED works in collaboration with many international organisations and agencies such as the United Nations Department of Humanitarian Affairs, European Union Humanitarian Office, International Federation of

Table 2.2 Ten worst disasters by economic damage (1980–2019) [7]

	Year	Disaster	Economic Losses (US$Billion)
1	2011	Earthquake, Tsunami (Japan)	210
2	2005	Hurricane Katrina (United States)	125
3	1995	Kobe earthquake (Japan)	100
4	2017	Hurricane Harvey (United States)	85
5	2008	Sichuan earthquake (China)	85
6	2012	Hurricane Sandy (Canada, Caribbean, and United States)	68.5
7	2017	Hurricane Ima (Caribbean and United States)	67
8	2017	Hurricane Maria (Caribbean)	63
9	1994	Northbridge Earthquake (United States)	44
10	2011	Flooding (Thailand)	43

the Red Cross and Red Crescent, and the Office of Foreign Disaster Assistance. EM-DAT contains essential consistent core data on the occurrence and effects of disasters since 1900 [12]. Examine the CRED website http://www.cred.be/.

According to EM-DAT, the number of disasters reported across the globe has been increasing since the 1980s. Between 1980 and 1999 there were 7,796 disasters reported, which increased to 13,895 from 2000 to 2020 (Table 2.3). Of the 21,691 disasters during this period, 62% (13,420) were due to natural disasters. This includes 4,776 natural disasters from 1980 to 1999 and 8,644 between 2000 and 2020, an 81% increase. The natural disasters with the most events in this 40-year period were hydrological (5,497) followed by meteorological (4,199), biological (1,461), geophysical (1,237), and climatological (1,025). The other 38% of disasters included technological (8,259) and 12 complex. For technological there were 3,015 disasters between 1980 and 1999 with 5,244 from 2000 to 2020. Technology includes transport, industrial, explosion, collapse, fire, and other events.

Improved reporting and recording of disasters can explain some of the increase, however, a combination of climate-related disasters and poorly planned development has increased disaster risk [13]. For example, storms and floods accounted for 63% of all natural disasters from 1980 to 2020 (Table 2.3), More specifically, floods accounted for 29% (1,389) of all natural disasters from 1980 to 1999 and this increased to 40% (3,459) between 2000 and 2020. Natural disasters have affected more than 7.4 billion people since 1980 and technological events around 4.1 million.

High-income countries have the greatest economic losses from natural disasters. Countries in this category account for 67% of economic losses compared to 24% for high-middle income, 8% for low-middle, and 1% for low-income countries [14]. No continent in the world has been spared, however, Asia has experienced the greatest impact of all disaster types. For example, Asia accounts for 86% of flood- and storm-related disasters, and for geophysical 62% of all events, 85% of the people affected, and 78% economic damages [15]. Low-income countries account for 23% of total disaster deaths despite accounting for less than 10% of the world's population [14].

The death rates from disasters have been decreasing but the number of people affected has increased. This can be contributed to multi-hazard early warning systems

Table 2.3 Natural disasters 1980–2020 [11]

Type and Percentage of Natural Disasters	Occurrence	Deaths	Injured	Total Affected
Animal incident – 0.01%	1	12	0	5
Drought – 4.58%	615	581,693	32	2,356,491,641
Earthquake/Tsunami – 7.50%	1,006	884,668	1,952,288	177,739,752
Epidemic – 10.22%	1,372	247,142	2,442,327	25,304,294
Extra-terrestrial – 0.01%	1	0	1,491	301,491
Extreme temperature – 4.23%	567	186,924	2,050,876	103,634,913
Flood – 36.13%	4,848	257,838	1,233,984	3,585,144,564
Insect infestation – 0.66%	88	0	0	2,802,200
Landslide – 4.84%	649	33,118	10,933	10,545,897
Mass movement (dry) – 0.30%	40	2,293	368	23,987
Storm – 27.06%	3,632	458,714	708,223	1,133,948,838
Volcanic activity – 1.42%	191	26,577	21,626	8,489,350
Wildfire – 3.06%	410	2,835	10,935	17,230,763
Total	13,420	2,681,814	8,433,083	7,421,657,695

and improved disaster risk management strategies [8]. For example, deaths have fallen decade by decade, the 1970s and 1980s reported an average of 170 related deaths per day, in the 1990s this was 90 related deaths per day, and then in the 2010s it was 40 related deaths per day [8]. In contrast, the number of people affected by disasters, including injuries and disruption of livelihoods, especially in agriculture, and the associated economic damage is increasing with an average of 200 million people per year being affected by disasters [14].

It would appear disasters are being managed better and the death toll reducing due to improved awareness, preparedness including risk reduction strategies and response management. However, are these impacts a true indicator of disasters' impact on all aspects of society? Should the effectiveness of the response and recovery be measured by direct deaths, indirect deaths from other causes, overall disease burden in the following years or the impact of the response on all aspects of society (i.e., employment, education, relationships, etc)?

The need for a holistic consideration has been outlined by the Global Preparedness Monitoring Board in their 2020 annual report. For example, COVID-19 border restrictions and lockdowns slowed agricultural production, increased food insecurity worldwide, pushed close to 100 million people into extreme poverty, interrupted access to treatment and care, and school closures may have a US$10 trillion earning loss over time for the younger generation [16]. Understanding disaster impacts and the consequences of selected mitigation measures within different development, economic, and social constructs is required to tailor preparedness, response, and recovery actions to meet community capabilities and needs.

So, returning to the fundamental question; are disasters increasing, and if so, why?

Chapter 1 provided a range of perspectives on the definition of disaster. There are a number of factors that may impact on the rate of reported disasters or the perception that disasters are having an increased impact. These include increased reporting, population

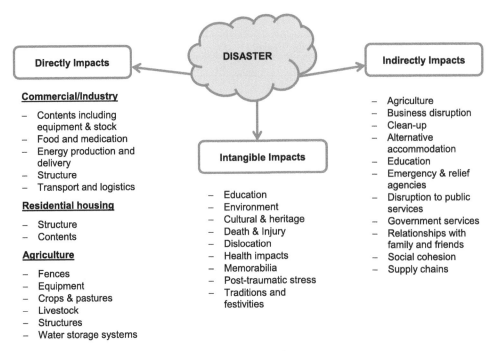

Figure 2.1 Disaster impacts – direct, intangible, and indirect

Source: Adapted from Bureau of Transport Economics 2001, Economic costs of natural disasters in Australia, Report 103, Canberra

density, mass transportation, dependence on technologies, and climate change. Other factors include military (or terrorist) conflict, however, without seeking to engage in the political aspects of this debate, in comparison with the global conflicts of the 20th Century, we are probably living in one of the safest times in history. Military conflicts are not considered disasters for the purposes of disaster management. Finally, vulnerability of the world's economic systems increases disaster risk because a financial collapse has flow-on effects such as reducing access to essential infrastructure including health services, especially for the most vulnerable populations.

THE IMPACTS OF DISASTERS

The impact of disasters is dependent on the type, size, and scale of the incident, as well as the composition and economic standing of the population affected. There is no predictable and scientific relationship between the hazard and its impact. Often the impact is highly variable. Inexplicably, a bushfire will engulf well-protected houses while sparing others. The impact of any particular building collapse (or the collective impact of many occurring in an earthquake) will often depend on the particular use of the building at a particular time. For example, a collapsing school building may cause massive loss of life during school hours but have little effect outside of those hours (Figure 2.1).

The impact of disasters can be considered in terms of health impacts, economic costs, and social consequences.

Health impacts

The health consequences of disasters are not necessarily direct or predictable. Deaths resulting from a building collapse in an earthquake or flood are clear. Less clear, are the impacts resulting from the economic consequences of a disaster and its impact on life-sustaining public health services. This limits clarity of understanding of the disaster's effects. While the number of people drowning in floodwaters can be counted, will we ever know the number of people who die of chronic diseases because they cannot afford or access life-sustaining medications after losing their employment.

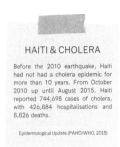

HAITI & CHOLERA

Before the 2010 earthquake, Haiti had not had a cholera epidemic for more than 10 years. From October 2010 up until August 2015, Haiti reported 744,698 cases of cholera, with 426,884 hospitalisations and 8,826 deaths.

Epidemiological Update (PAHO/WHO, 2015)

Health consequences can span the full range from minor distress through to death. Often the focus is on those killed without understanding the range of injuries survivors can suffer. On average, for every death there will be a similar number who are critically injured. Many times, that number will suffer sufficient injuries that warrant hospitalisation. Many more will be injured to some extent but not warrant hospitalisation. The ratio between these is dependent on the nature of the event. For example, an aircraft crash may have many deaths and few injuries, while a pandemic may have few deaths and many ill. The public focus is often on the deaths, whilst the focus of health systems will be on those requiring treatment. Permanent injuries arising from disasters can leave a lifelong legacy.

Understanding the complexity of relationships to mortality and morbidity in the days and years after a disaster is necessary to ensure strategies are tailored to the consequences. There is a need to continue treatment and care for all diseases to avoid preventable deaths. For example, the disruptions to treatment and care during the response to COVID-19 could result in an increase of deaths from HIV (10%), tuberculosis (20%), and malaria (36%) over the next five years [17]. The impact on loss of life years in locations with a high burden of these diseases is expected to be at the same magnitude at COVID-19 [17]. Also, cancer screening programs were disrupted in many locations during the pandemic response, resulting in delayed diagnosis and potentially significant increases in the numbers of avoidable cancer deaths [18].

An understanding of the complexity of these relationships is critical to the development of effective and resilient disaster management processes. For example, the strategies to manage drowning (search and rescue) are completely different to those required to manage the long-term consequences of malnutrition resulting from economic deprivation and destruction of livelihoods following a disaster. Finally, disasters can be detrimental to both physical and mental health. The physical impacts are generally obvious and directly related to the nature of the event (e.g., trauma, burns, and respiratory problems). The mental health impacts are often subtler and range from understandable and normal reactions to horrendous events or loss, through to severe Post Traumatic Stress Disorder (PTSD). The psychosocial impact of disasters is discussed in detail in Chapter 12.

There is also a relationship between the physical injuries and the mental health consequences. Consider the position of someone who has lost their livelihood due to a long-term injury. They are likely to suffer depression and anxiety, which can in turn have physical health consequences. In addition to the effects on the health of individuals and the community, there may be significant damage to the infrastructure required for health service provision. Or to the infrastructure that supports the health system (e.g., gas, electricity, communication, and transport networks).

Heatwave association versus casualty. Excess deaths, vulnerable die.

When access to public health infrastructure is disrupted for people with a chronic disease there is an increased risk of illness exacerbation or even death. For example, most adverse health impacts peak within six months following a hurricane, however, chronic diseases, including cardiovascular disease and mental disorders, continue to occur for years following [19]. These consequences for patients with chronic illnesses may be grouped into the following:

- *Loss of access to health systems* for patients with chronic and acute health needs such as those undergoing chemotherapy or dialysis.
- *Exacerbation of chronic health conditions* due to stress caused by a disaster. Consider the person with heart disease who must rapidly evacuate from a flash flood.
- The *loss of life-sustaining medications or infrastructure* for example, loss of power depriving people with sleep apnoea of access to breathing support.

Economic costs

The economic damage caused by disasters varies. The economic costs of disasters include both actual costs (with a value) and intangible costs. Infrastructure and capital assets such as equipment, housing, manufacturing, schools, roads, dams, and bridges are lost, and human capital can be depleted due to the loss of life, the loss of skilled workers, and the destruction of infrastructure that disrupts the pipeline from education to the workforce [20]. The extent of this damage may not be immediately apparent, for example, damage to building foundations through subsidence after a flood may be discovered months afterwards. A number of the major physical effects include:

- Loss of essential services including gas, electricity, water, hospitals, communication, transport, and sanitation systems.
- Damage to residential areas, possibly requiring evacuation or longer-term relocation.
- Loss of or reduced services from commercial facilities including banks, service stations, supermarkets, etc.
- Food security through the loss of crops and primary production will have an impact in the short-term and mid-term.
- Loss of educational and training facilities.
- Loss of entertainment and recreation facilities such as sporting clubs, cultural and entertainment venues, restaurants, and hotels may be damaged.
- Environmental detriments will include pollution, loss of flora and fauna, and the degradation of national parks.

The economic cost of disasters is extremely complex. For example, one dollar invested in disaster preparedness can prevent seven dollars' worth of disaster-related economic [21]. Japan's Tōhoku earthquake and tsunami caused the largest dollar impact since 1980 with an estimate of $210 billion [7]. Table 2.4 provides an example of indirect/direct costs in a major chemical accident at a factory. Indirect and direct costs are measured and allocated through routine accounting methods. Note that intangible costs are also an issue.

Table 2.4 The direct and indirect costs in a major chemical accident at a factory

Direct Costs	Indirect Costs
Medical costs	Lost earnings (including fringe benefits)
Private insurance and transfer programs (medical)	Reduced growth in new home construction
Overhead costs for workers' compensation, private insurance and transfer programs	Workplace training, restaffing, and disruption
Infrastructure and property damage	Time delays
Fatigue and potential chemical exposure to police and Fire Services	Health problems can present many years after the event
Direct costs to innocent third parties	Indirect costs to innocent third parties
	Resources moved to manage and clean up the incident

There is a direct association between the economic standing of a community and the impact and consequences of disasters. Disasters tend to impact disproportionately on the poorest countries with the frequency of disasters potentially reducing economic growth of the community.

Social consequences

Chapter 19 details many of the psychosocial impacts of disasters. Disasters can result in severe civil disruption and conflict. Mostly people do not panic, they generally respond in rational ways. People will act rapidly to protect their own life and safety, and at times this *survival instinct* is misinterpreted as *panic*. When lives are placed at risk either through ongoing exposure to a threat or through the loss of life-sustaining essential items, then people will do everything in their power to secure their own safety and that of their family. If the need for this support such as food, medicine, and income, is not recognised early in the response the situation could become rapidly complicated due to perceptions of injustice, potentially leading to civil unrest and conflict [22].

Often decision-makers need to balance protecting lives versus the need to enable community viability before, during, and after a crisis. For example, socially and economically vulnerable populations cannot endure long-term livelihood interruption given cash support limitations; capacity limits in addressing supply chain breaks during disasters; and other impacts on the ability to meet basic human needs [9].

Families may also become stressed as competing demands of work and family are further complicated by the need to respond and recover. Children may not be able to access their friends and education, or they may be required to help with the recovery. This *loss of childhood* can have lifelong consequences for children. Disasters can be the final straw for marginal businesses, particularly if business decisions have left them vulnerable. Loss of work and income adds to the stresses that result from disasters. This can have life-altering consequences.

The impact of disasters is often determined by the nature and extent of the hazard and the vulnerability of those affected. The concept of resilience may be considered to be the obverse of vulnerability. Vulnerability is a broad spectrum but encompasses the elderly, children, women, people suffering from a disability or chronic disease, the poor and the homeless and those incarcerated and unable to escape. The social dimensions of disasters are discussed in detail in Chapter 19.

ACTIVITIES

1. Make a list of the factors that you consider may influence the frequency of disasters.
2. Write a brief paragraph on whether you consider disasters are becoming more common and why you think this.
3. Consider a small rural town. What are the factors that influence the impact a disaster (e.g., a flood) would have on the town and its people?
4. Write notes on how poverty contributes to the vulnerability of people in disasters and other crisis situations.

KEY READINGS

Sendai Framework https://www.undrr.org

The Sphere Handbook: Humanitarian Charter and Minimum Standards in Humanitarian Response https://spherestandards.org/handbook

Health emergency and disaster risk management framework https://apps.who.int/iris/handle/10665/326106

CRED Crunch 66- Disasters Year in Review 2021 https://cred.be/sites/default/files/Cred-Crunch66.pdf

Worlds Apart to a World Prepared: Global Preparedness Monitoring Board report 2021 https://www.gpmb.org/annual-reports/annual-report-2021

References

1. Disasterium. *10 Worst natural disasters of all time*. 2015 [December 6, 2021]; Available from: http://www.disasterium.com/10-worst-natural-disasters-of-all-time/.
2. Public Health Online. *History's worst global pandemics*. 2021 [December 6, 2021]; Available from: https://www.publichealthonline.org/worst-global-pandemics-in-history/.
3. Statistics and Data. *The 10 natural disasters that caused the most deaths*. 2021 [December 6, 2021]; Available from: https://statisticsanddata.org/data/global-deaths-from-natural-disasters/.
4. World Health Organisation. *The top 10 causes of death*. 2020 [December 9, 2021]; Available from: https://www.who.int/news-room/fact-sheets/detail/the-top-10-causes-of-death.
5. World Health Organisation. *Fact sheets*. 2021 [December 6, 2021]; Available from: https://www.who.int/news-room/fact-sheets.
6. Statista. *The 10 biggest natural disasters worldwide by economic damage from 1980 to 2019*. 2021 [December 9, 2021]; Available from: https://www.statista.com/statistics/268126/biggest-natural-disasters-by-economic-damage-since-1980/.
7. Statista. *The 10 biggest natural disasters worldwide by economic damage from 1980 to July 2022*. 2022 [September 4, 2022]; Available from: https://www.statista.com/statistics/268126/biggest-natural-disasters-by-economic-damage-since-1980.
8. World Meteorological Organization. *WMO Atlas of mortality and economic losses from weather, climate and water extremes (1970–2019)*. 2021, Geneva (CH): World Meteorological Organization.
9. Ryan, B.J., et al., COVID-19 community stabilization and sustainability framework: An integration of the Maslow hierarchy of needs and social determinants of health. *Disaster Medicine and Public Health Preparedness*, 2020. **14**(5): p. 623–629.

10. Centre for Research on the Epidemiology of Disasters. *Over 40 years on the front lines.* 2015 [December 14, 2021]; Available from: https://www.cred.be/abou.
11. Centre for Research on the Epidemiology of Disasters. *Welcome to the EM-DAT.* 2021 [December 14, 2021]; Available from: https://www.emdat.be/.
12. Centre for Research on the Epidemiology of Disasters. *History.* 2021 [December 14, 2021]; Available from: https://www.emdat.be/history.
13. United Nations Office for Disaster Risk Reducation. *Poorly planned urban development.* 2021 [November 26, 2021]; Available from: https://www.preventionweb.net/understanding-disaster-risk/risk-drivers/poorly-planned-urban-development.
14. Centre for Research on the Epidemiology of Disasters. *Human cost of disasters: An overview of the last 20 years (2000–2019).* 2020. Brussels (BE): Centre for Research on the Epidemiology of Disasters (CRED) and UN Office for Disaster Risk Reduction.
15. Centre for Research on the Epidemiology of Disasters. *Economic losses, poverty & diasters: 1998–2017.* 2018, Brussels (BE): Centre for Research on the Epidemiology of Disasters and United Nations Office for Disaster Risk Reduction.
16. World Health Organisation. *A world in disorder. Global preparedness monitoring board annual report 2020.* 2020, Geneva (CH): World Health Organization.
17. Sands, P., HIV, tuberculosis, and malaria: How can the impact of COVID-19 be minimised? *The Lancet Global Health*, 2020. **8**(9): p. e1102–e1103.
18. Alkatout, I., et al., Has COVID-19 affected cancer screening programs? A systematic review. *Frontiers in Oncology*, 2021. May 17;**11**:p.675038. doi: 10.3389/fonc.2021.675038. PMID: 34079764; PMCID: PMC8165307
19. Waddell, S.L., et al., Perspectives on the health effects of hurricanes: A review and challenges. *International Journal of Environmental Research and Public Health*, 2021. **18**(5): p. 2756.
20. Deraniyagala, S., Economic recovery after natural disasters. *UN Chronicle*, 2016. **53**(1): p. 31–34.
21. World Meteorological Organization. *Natural hazards and disaster risk reduction.* 2022 [September 4, 2022]; Available from: https://public.wmo.int/en/our-mandate/focus-areas/natural-hazards-and-disaster-risk-reduction.
22. Nardulli, P.F., B. Peyton, and J. Bajjalieh, Climate change and civil unrest: The impact of rapid-onset disasters. *Journal of Conflict Resolution*, 2015. **59**(2): p. 310–335.

3
Concepts and principles

Nahuel Arenas-García and Vicenzo Bollettino[1]

INTRODUCTION AND OBJECTIVES

The aim of this chapter is to identify the basic concepts, principles, and practical application underpinning best practice in all aspects of disaster risk management and disaster risk reduction. The chapter briefly explores the evolution in thinking about disasters and disaster risk, and the current principles that underpin practice. On completion you should be able to:

1. Demonstrate an understanding of the evolution of thinking in the way disasters have been regarded.
2. Critically analyze the conceptual basis of disaster risk reduction and disaster management practice and the way those concepts are interrelated.
3. Identify, describe, and critically evaluate the principles that guide disaster risk reduction, disaster management systems, and their application to practice.

DISASTERS ARE NOT NATURAL: CONCEPTUAL EVOLUTION OF DISASTER MANAGEMENT AND DISASTER RISK REDUCTION

A disaster is defined as a serious disruption of the functioning of a community or a society at any scale due to hazardous events, of natural, anthropogenic (human-induced) or socio-natural origin, interacting with conditions of exposure, vulnerability and capacity, leading to human, material, economic and/or environmental losses and impacts [1]. While the immediate impacts of a disaster can be localized, its effects can be widespread and last for a long period of time [2].

Approaches to understanding and framing disasters have evolved over time. A series of significant disasters of natural origin in the 1960s and 1970s (including the 9.5 Valdivia earthquake in Chile in 1960, Bhola Cyclone in Bangladesh in 1970, and a number of famines following droughts affecting the Sahel, among others) led to an increased attention to the way disasters jeopardize development trajectories, impacting societies, communities,

DOI: 10.4324/9781032626604-4

and livelihoods, and absorbing significant amounts of resources that could otherwise be invested in growth and development.

In the 1970s and 1980s, many countries enhanced their emergency management capacity creating emergency management systems at the national level [3]. In 1984, Timberlake and Wijkman [4] were among the first to dispel the myth that disasters are *natural, instead pointing to social and economic vulnerabilities that contributed to the creating of a disaster*. The concept of 'natural disasters' persists until today, but the widescale rejection of its use has gained considerable traction in the last years. To make this distinction clear, consider a landslide in the middle of the Amazon tropical forest, in an area with no population; is that a disaster? There might be a certain loss of biodiversity, but this would be just a natural hazard in the strict sense. On the other hand, if the landslide sweeps across a community living downhill (perhaps because the land was cheap there or occupied, and norms regulating the use of land were not respected, perhaps due to corruption, or due to deforestation from logging along the hillsides etc.), it will cause significant damage to life and property, triggering a disaster. Further, the amount of damage will increase if the community has low access to public infrastructure (such as transportation for evacuation) and sub-standard physical infrastructure (such as highly vulnerable public housing). In contrast, if measures are put in place and capacities strengthened chances are that the landslide of the example above creates minimal or no losses and damages. Measures can include ensuring the community is knowledgeable about the risks they face, putting in place early warning systems (even simple ones such as someone alerting of the accumulation of water uphill) establishing evacuation routes and minimizing the exposure of infrastructure, among others. In other words, if we understand the risks we face and align our decisions to reduce them, we will contribute to building resilience.

In sum, hazards become disasters as a consequence of our decisions and development trajectories. Poverty, inequality, bad governance, limited access to basic services, etc. are all factors that contribute to making us more vulnerable. As we have seen in the example above, disaster risk cannot be explained solely by the triggering hazard, but as a function of hazard, exposure, vulnerability and capacity. Also, disasters affect people differently. For this reason, it is of critical importance to consider the views and impact of disasters on vulnerable groups – such as women and girls, children, the youth, older persons, people living with disabilities, indigenous populations, migrants, and other marginalized groups requiring special protection – when designing, implementing, and evaluating disaster risk reduction and disaster response activities.

The recognition that disasters are the materialization of pre-existing risk and exaggerated conditions has contributed to a shift in the focus of attention, from managing disasters to reducing risk. This has been reflected in the conceptual evolution behind global efforts to reduce disaster risk, from the International Decade for Natural Disaster Reduction in the 1990s to the set-up of the United Nations International Strategy for Disaster Reduction in 1999, the establishment of the Hyogo Framework for Action during the years 2005–2015 and its successor, the Sendai Framework for Disaster Risk Reduction 2015–2030.

UNDERSTANDING HAZARDS

Many types of hazards can contribute to disastrous consequences for our societies and communities. These hazards include natural hazards, some examples of which are listed around the seismic graph icon at the top in Figure 3.1; biological hazards, including

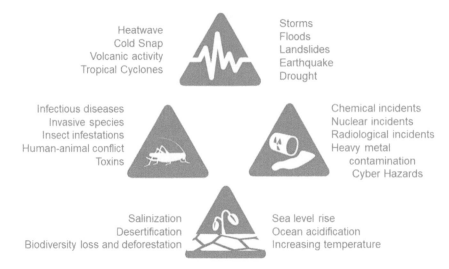

Figure 3.1 Hazard types (Adapted from UNDRR 2020 [5])

diseases and invasive species, listed on the left; and technological hazards, listed on the right of the graph [5].

Meteorological and hydrological hazards such as floods and tropical cyclones displace more people than any other natural hazard and encompass huge economic losses. Geophysical hazards such as earthquakes and tsunamis, on their part, kill more people than extreme weather events. Human activity is also responsible for severe loss of life (e.g., industrial pollution, infrastructure failure). Environmental degradation can exacerbate the impact of other hazards. For example, the destruction of coastal and marine ecosystems or deforestation can contribute to the damaging effects of storm surges and landslides. Technological hazards such as the recent chemical explosion in the port of Beirut (Lebanon) in 2020 or the Brumadinho (Brazil) tailing dam failures in 2019 can have devastating consequences. In fact, any of these types of events can trigger or compound other risks with damaging effects given the increasing complexity and interaction of our social and economic systems. In 2011, an earthquake and tsunami in Japan destroyed three nuclear reactors causing a major release of radioactivity. In addition, multiple-hazard scenarios are increasingly common.

Further, the continued degradation of the natural world (e.g., pollution of the air, water, or soil) means that environmental hazards will be on the rise, as is extreme and/or unseasonal weather. In the context of global climate change, hazards that can threaten

The single natural hazard approach to the study and management of disasters has been replaced by more complex approaches that recognize that multi-hazard scenarios are more common and can include the coexistence of various natural hazards or a combination of natural, technological and social hazards interacting at the same time and in the same place.

[6]

development also include slow-onset climate change-related hazards such as sea-level rise, increasing temperatures, biodiversity loss, deforestation, and soil salinization.

Furthermore, not all disasters are associated with major hazards of high severity (intensive risk). In fact, most disasters are the result of extensive risk: highly localized disasters that have a less pronounced impact but are recurrent in nature. For instance, localized, recurrent floods, storms or drought can take place undetected or unreported by national or international media, and yet erode the resilience of affected populations, particularly of the most vulnerable.

The interconnected nature of our world and the effects of climate change have become risk multipliers. As highlighted in the Global Risk Assessment Report [7], new risks and correlations are emerging in a way that we have not anticipated. Human, economic, and political systems are in an increasingly complex interaction with natural systems [7]. In fact, our current development models have an impact on the natural world that makes us more vulnerable. For instance, an increase in emerging infectious diseases and remerging infectious diseases has been observed globally [8]. Zoonotic diseases (transmitted between animals and humans), like the coronavirus that caused the 2020 pandemic, result from the complex interconnections and mutual dependencies between wildlife and people (e.g., through increasing urbanization of the world). That means that risk in one part of a system could trigger cascade effects and impact other dependent systems. COVID-19 has made evident how risks can cascade and have systemic impacts. A biological hazard that emerged in a Chinese city quickly travelled the world and impacted health, transportation, and education systems, disrupted social interactions and the global economy.

Climate change further threatens global stability through both an increase in the severity of weather-related events but also, importantly, through changing weather patterns across the globe. These shifts can lead to more pronounced flooding and more frequent and longer droughts thereby undermining livelihoods. The melting of arctic ice contributes to sea level rise, threatening the lives of hundreds of millions of people living in low-lying coastal regions around the world. These changes are leading to events that we have not previously seen and threaten to undermine both advances in development but also in disaster management and disaster risk reduction. The world has developed disaster management plans and practices and disaster risk reduction practices for a world that has now fundamentally changed. In short, our best practices are no longer fully fit for purpose in the world we now live and will live in for decades if not centuries to come.

Addressing disaster risk in complex systems: beyond hazard-by-hazard approaches

To effectively address disaster risk, we need both the methods and instruments to accurately calculate it and we need to understand underlying vulnerabilities within the human and ecological systems we live in. Linear risk models lack the precision and reliability to address the types of dynamic changes we are currently experiencing within global climate and environmental systems. According to Gordon and Williams [9], understanding a complex system is not enough to know the parts:

> It is necessary to understand the dynamic nature of the relationships between each of the parts. In a complex system, it is impossible to know all the parts at any point in time. The human body, a city traffic system, or a national public health system are examples of complex systems.

The level of complexity and non-linearity in systemic risk is associated with the degree of system interdependence. Interdependence implies that even the smallest manifestation of risk in one system may generate impacts in other systems. As system complexity and interdependence increases, the channels though which direct impacts are translated into direct impacts and wider effects are characterized by non-linearity and multiple feedback loops.

[10, 11]

'These risks are not necessarily obvious using traditional hazard-by-hazard risk assessments and revealing them requires an understanding of the degree of magnitude of failure across these systems that could suddenly or gradually exceed society's capacity to cope.' [12]

Risk needs to be understood considering its possible cascade effects across systems and its impacts across different scales.

As a consequence, disaster and emergency risk management is evolving to include systemic disaster risk and resilience to inform broader risk reduction efforts [12].

Preparedness measures need not only consider cross-systemic impacts but also impacts at different levels. It requires good coordination among national and local levels and, more importantly, capacities to absorb, respond to, and recover at the local level.

Moreover, preparedness measures need to be enhanced for different types of hazards. The COVID-19 pandemic showed us how a public health emergency could cause a large loss of life, creating the biggest global crisis in 50 years. The recently published report by the Independent Panel for Pandemic Preparedness and Response, established by the World Health Organization to review the global response to COVID-19, identified 'gaps and failings at every critical juncture of preparedness and response' [13].

UNDERSTANDING DISASTER MANAGEMENT

Disaster management encompasses a wide range of activities that take place prior to, during, and following a disaster event. It brings together a range of complementary concepts that contribute to our understanding of its complexity and scope. Disaster management refers to the organization, planning, and application of measures preparing for, responding to and recovering from disasters [2]. The goals of disaster management include: avoiding or reducing losses and damage from hazards; assuring prompt assistance to those affected, and achieving rapid and effective recovery, building back better, or in other words, taking advantage of the reconstruction process to enhance resilience, avoiding reconstructing pre-existing vulnerabilities. Failures in the design and implementation of a disaster management plan may result in loss and damage. The disaster management cycle is usually described as consisting of four phases: mitigation, preparedness, response, and recovery.

Mitigation refers to the lessening or minimizing of the adverse impacts of a hazardous event, acknowledging that these impacts cannot always be prevented fully but their scale or severity can be substantially lessened by various strategies and actions [2]. Examples of these measures are the development and enforcement of building codes, disaster-resilient infrastructure and public education and awareness, and avoiding building communities and structures that are in highly exposed places, such as flood zones. The concept of mitigation in disaster management should not be confused with the meaning of the term within climate change policy, which refers to the reduction of greenhouse gas emissions.

Preparedness refers, broadly, to the planning of the response. Preparedness measures can include planning (developing communication plans, evacuation routes), training (having disaster management officials as well as community leaders and others with a response role engage in disaster response exercises), and material investments in disaster management resources (first responder equipment, generators, go-bags) An efficient management of the emergency can only happen if sufficient anticipatory action is in place to build the capacities and knowledge of the different actors involved in the response. These may include developing a sound understanding of the risks, contingency planning with clear roles and responsibilities to facilitate coordination, logistic arrangements, etc.

Disaster response (sometimes called *disaster relief* or *disaster management*) is predominantly focused on immediate and short-term needs. It includes the actions taken directly before, during, or immediately after a disaster in order to save lives, reduce health impacts, ensure public safety, and meet the basic subsistence or lifeline needs of the people affected. *Emergency management* is also a term used interchangeably with disaster management, particularly in the context of biological and technological hazards and for health emergencies, although an emergency can relate to events that do not necessarily disrupt the functioning of a society [2].

The term *recovery* has also evolved, from its narrower conceptualization of returning back to normal, restoring livelihoods and health as well as economic, physical, social, cultural and environmental assets and activities of a disaster-affected community or society, to the broader 'building back better', which understands that the goal is not to reconstruct the conditions of exposure and vulnerability that led to the disaster in the first place but to further enhance resilience and foster sustainable development. Build back better has been defined by the United Nations [2] as:

> the use of the recovery, rehabilitation and reconstruction phases after a disaster to increase the resilience of nations and communities through integrating disaster risk reduction measures into the restoration of physical infrastructure and societal systems, and into the revitalization of livelihoods, economies and the environment.

Recovery efforts can also be an opportunity to 'build back better *and greener*', acknowledging the importance of protecting environmental assets.

CORE PRINCIPLES OF DISASTER MANAGEMENT

There is a wide diversity in the way national disaster response systems are structured and resourced around the world. Some systems are articulated around centralized and vertical structures while other systems integrate horizontal and decentralized operational arrangements. The level of professionalization of these systems and the mechanisms to integrate or coordinate with different stakeholders and across sectors also vary from country to country. However, there is a certain level of agreement around some of the core principles that underpin disaster management, which have developed across many countries through experience from both communities and organizations. FEMA [14], for instance, identifies eight principles to use to guide the development of doctrine of disaster response management, these include:

1. **Comprehensive** – disaster response managers consider and take into account all hazards, all phases, all stakeholders and all impacts relevant to disasters.
2. **Progressive** – disaster response managers anticipate future disasters and take preventive and preparatory measures to build disaster-resistant and disaster-resilient communities.
3. **Risk-driven** – disaster response managers use sound risk management principles (hazard identification, risk analysis, and impact analysis) in assigning priorities and resources.
4. **Integrated** – disaster response managers ensure unity of effort among all levels of government and all elements of a community.
5. **Collaborative** – disaster response managers create and sustain broad and sincere relationships among individuals and organizations to encourage trust, advocate a team atmosphere, build consensus, and facilitate communication.
6. **Coordinated** – disaster response managers synchronize the activities of all relevant stakeholders to achieve a common purpose.
7. **Flexible** – disaster response managers use creative and innovative approaches in solving disaster challenges.
8. **Professional** – disaster response managers value a science and knowledge-based approach based on education, training, experience, ethical practice, public stewardship, and continuous improvement.

For further explanation of the FEMA principles refer to *Principles of Emergency Management* (2007) available from: http://www.fema.gov/media-library/assets/documents/25063

DISASTER RISK REDUCTION

The shift of focus, from managing disasters to reducing disaster risk, translates into efforts oriented at preventing new disaster risks, reducing existing disaster risks that also strengthen resilience. Disaster risk reduction strategies and policies define goals and objectives across different timescales, with concrete targets, indicators and time frames. Disaster risk management, thus, can be understood as 'the application of disaster risk reduction policies and strategies to prevent new disaster risk, reduce existing disaster risk and manage residual risk, contributing to the strengthening of resilience and reduction of disaster losses' [15].

Disaster risk management encompasses *prospective*, *corrective*, and *compensatory* actions. The former addresses risk that may develop in the future and seeks to avoid the creation of new risk (e.g., disaster-resilient infrastructure). Corrective disaster risk management activities address existing identified risks, which need to be managed or reduced (e.g., retrofitting of critical infrastructure). Finally, compensatory disaster risk management involves a series of activities designed to strengthen the social and economic resilience of individuals and communities in the face of residual risks that cannot effectively be eliminated or reduced (e.g., enhancing preparedness capabilities, the availability of contingency funds or risk transfer mechanisms; Figure 3.2).

The global blueprint for addressing disaster risk is the Sendai Framework for Disaster Risk Reduction 2015–2030, whose expected outcome over the next 15 years is: 'the substantial reduction of disaster risk and losses in lives, livelihoods and health and in the economic, physical, social, cultural and environmental assets of persons, businesses, communities and countries'. The Sendai Framework has four priorities: (i) Understanding disaster risk; (ii) Strengthening disaster risk governance to manage risks; (iii) Investing in disaster risk reduction for resilience; and (iv) Enhancing disaster preparedness for effective disaster response and to 'build back better'.

For further details refer to the Sendai Framework for Disaster Risk Reduction 2015–2030 https://www.undrr.org/publication/sendai-framework-disaster-risk-reduction-2015-2030

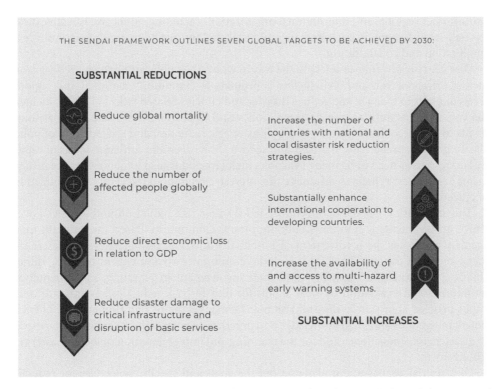

Figure 3.2 UNDRR seven global targets for disaster risk reduction (Adapted from United Nations Office for Disaster Risk Reduction. What is the Sendai Framework for Disaster Risk Reduction? [16])

The International Conference on the Implementation of the Health Aspects of the Sendai Framework for Disaster Risk Reduction 2015–2030 recommended seven measures to prevent and/or reduce the risk of health emergencies such as pandemics that have the potential for huge social and economic impact. The 'Bangkok Principles' place strengthened coordination at the heart of efforts to reduce risk from biological hazards. They call for an inter-operable, multi-sectoral approach to promote systematic cooperation, integration and, ultimately, coherence between disaster and health risk management. The 'Bangkok Principles' can be accessed here: https://www.preventionweb.net/publication/bangkok-principles-implementation-health-aspects-sendai-framework-disaster-risk"https://www.preventionweb.net/publication/bangkok-principles-implementation-health-aspects-sendai-framework-disaster-risk

GOVERNING DISASTER RISKS

Effective disaster management and disaster risk reduction rely on the efforts of many different stakeholders, including local and national government, specialized agencies (e.g., civil protection, police and fire services, public health agencies, etc.), private actors, civil society organizations, and the media among others. When national capacities are overwhelmed, it can also involve UN agencies, international non-governmental organizations, and/or other regional and international organizations including militaries. Effective disaster risk management is anchored in multi-stakeholder, multi-sectoral, and multi-level cooperation and collaboration.

Disaster risk governance refers to the way in which the public authorities, civil servants, media, private sector, and civil society coordinate at community, national and regional levels in order to manage and reduce disaster and climate-related risks [17]. This includes the system of institutions, mechanisms, policy and legal frameworks and other arrangements to guide, coordinate and oversee disaster risk reduction and related areas of policy [1]. To prevent, prepare for, manage, and recover from disasters sufficient levels of capacity and resources need to be made available. Inclusive and transparent governance mechanisms are the best vehicle to articulate the interests and uphold the rights and obligations of citizens.

The articulation between community-led disaster risk reduction and disaster governance arrangements is fundamentally important. Community-based disaster risk management promotes the involvement of potentially affected communities in disaster risk management at the local level. This includes community assessments of hazards, vulnerabilities, exposure and capacities, and their involvement in planning, implementation, monitoring and evaluation of local action for disaster risk reduction. Local and indigenous peoples' approach to disaster risk management is the recognition and use of traditional, indigenous and local knowledge and practices to complement scientific knowledge in disaster risk assessments, and for the planning and implementation of local disaster risk management.

Disaster risk management plans set out the goals and specific objectives for reducing disaster risks together with related actions to accomplish these objectives. They should be guided by the Sendai Framework for Disaster Risk Reduction 2015–2030, and considered and coordinated within relevant development plans, resource allocations and programme activities. National-level plans need to be specific to each level of administrative responsibility and adapted to the different social and geographical circumstances that are present. The timeframe and responsibilities for implementation and the sources of funding should be specified in the plan. Linkages to sustainable development and climate change adaptation plans should be made where possible.

The Sendai Framework underlines that the States retain primary responsibility for disaster risk reduction, although this responsibility is shared with all stakeholders. Reducing existing risk, preventing the creation of new risk, and building resilience requires a whole-of-society approach. The national and local governments, different sectors, civil society, the private sector, the science and technology community, the media and the academia, among others, are all required to effectively address risks.

Recognizing that most of investments in any given country come from the private sector, engaging the business community in reducing disaster risk is critical for the sustainability of investments, to ensure business and service continuity in the case of disaster, and ultimately for building resilience.

In many countries, particularly throughout Asia, militaries play a key role in disaster response and are often the most significant players in response to disasters that have broad national scope. They are often the only players with the logistics capacity and command and control facilities, experience, training, and numbers to be able to mount a large-scale disaster response.

The COVID-19 pandemic has shown the level of interconnectedness of human, economic, political, and environmental systems. A disaster can have significant impacts across different sectors, including health, education, housing, energy and agriculture among others. This means that disaster risk governance arrangements need also be multi-sectoral, in addition to multi-level and multi-stakeholder. Relying heavily on specialized emergency management organizations to govern risk will not be as effective as ensuring that all sectors, at all levels and with the contribution of all relevant stakeholders understand risk, address risk, and play their role in preparing, responding and recovering from disasters.

Good governance and effective risk management require developing the knowledge and skills necessary to identify and respond to disasters in an appropriate and inclusive way. It is an important aspect of any society, community or organization's survivability. While day-to-day operations can be managed through normal processes and plans, disasters such as cyclones, epidemics, floods, critical infrastructure failure, exotic animal disease outbreaks and many others require significant reorganization to deal with the situation. Extremely large disasters will require substantial scaling-up of organizational approaches, systems and processes to manage the response. A disaster can exceed the coping capacity of a community or society, therefore requiring external assistance. In a world of limited resources, effective disaster response planning and coordination among intervening parties is crucial to ensure the best prioritization and allocation of resources.

Finally, in this interconnected complex world, risk management becomes critical to ensure resilience and enable sustainable development. Global agendas, such as the Paris Agreement, the Sustainable Development Goals, the Sendai Framework for Disaster Risk Reduction, and the New Urban Agenda need to be implemented in tandem, with a whole-of-society approach.

CONCLUSION

When disasters occur, many organizations and stakeholders are required to become involved. Throughout all phases of the disaster response cycle, disaster managers work to improve the ability of individuals and groups to manage risks, mitigate and overcome disaster impacts. Problem-solving capacity is enhanced by utilizing comprehensive approaches that can collect, organize, and allocate information and resources, identify problems, determine objectives and priorities, and assign available resources. These arrangements are built through a regular process in which various agencies interact to identify risks and their cascading effects, develop plans and strategies to address them, enhance preparedness measures, establish coordination and collaboration mechanisms across all stakeholders, and if a disaster cannot be avoided, ensure a rapid response and recovery.

As the planet continues to warm, global population grows and the frequency and intensity of disasters increase, more people will be affected. As we have seen above, this requires a profound understanding of risk, a whole-of-society approach to prevent the creation of new risks and systemic approaches to address existing and residual risk. Effective risk governance requires close collaboration between public agencies and private actors, as well as a participatory and inclusive approach to ensure no one is left behind.

ACTIVITIES

1. Identify ways in which the global inter-connectedness can create new risks.
2. Consider how the principles of disaster risk reduction may be applied to the protection of a community against a pandemic.

KEY READINGS

1. *Sendai Framework for Disaster Risk Reduction 2015–2030.* https://www.undrr.org/publication/sendai-framework-disaster-risk-reduction-2015-2030
2. *The 'Bangkok Principles' on the Implementation of the Health Aspects of the Sendai Framework for Disaster Risk Reduction 2015–2030.* https://www.preventionweb.net/publication/bangkok-principles-implementation-health-aspects-sendai-framework-disaster-risk
3. Australian Institute for Disaster Resilience (2021). *Systemic Risk Handbook* https://knowledge.aidr.org.au/resources/handbook-disaster-risk/
4. FEMA (2007) *Principles of Emergency Management Supplement.* Accessed at http://training.fema.gov/hiedu/emprinciples.aspx

Note

1. With acknowledgment to previous authors, Brett Aimers and Linda Winn.

References

1. United Nations Office for Disaster Risk Reduction. *UNISDR terminology on disaster risk reduction.* United Nations Office of Disaster Risk Reduction. Geneva 2009. Available from: https://www.undrr.org/publication/2009-unisdr-terminology-disaster-risk-reduction
2. United Nations General Assembly (UNGA). *Report of the open-ended intergovernmental expert working group on indicators and terminology relating to disaster risk reduction.* 2016.
3. Rajabi, E., et al., The evolution of disaster risk management: Historical approach. *Disaster Medicine and Public Health Preparedness*, 2022. **16**(4): p. 1623–1627.
4. Timberlake, L., and A. Wijkman, *Natural disasters: Acts of God or acts of man?.* 1984, London (GB): An Earthscan Paperback: International Institute for Environment and Development & the Swedish Red Cross.
5. United Nations Office for Disaster Risk Reduction. *Integrating disaster risk reduction and climate change adaptation in the UN sustainable development cooperation framework: Guidance note on using climate and disaster risk management to help build resilient societies.* 2020, Geneva (CH): United Nations.
6. United Nations Office for Disaster Risk Reduction. *Regional assessment report on disaster risk in Latin America and the Caribbean.* 2021, Panama City (PA): United Nations.
7. United Nations Office for Disaster Risk Reduction. *Global risk assessment report (GAR).* 2019, Geneva (CH): United Nations.
8. McArthur, D.B., Emerging infectious diseases. *Nursing Clinics*, 2019. **54**(2): p. 297–311.
9. Gordon, M. and S. Williams. *What is the difference between complicated and complex systems... and why is it important in understanding the systemic nature of risk?* United Nations Office of Disaster Risk Reduction. Prevention Web 2020. Available from: https://www.preventionweb.net/news/what-difference-between-complicated-and-complex-systems-and-why-it-important-understanding
10. Renn, O., et al., Systemic risks from different perspectives. *Risk Analysis*, 2022. **42**(9): p. 1902–1920.

11. United Nations Development Program (UNDP). *The social construction of systemic risk: Towards and actionable framework for risk governance. Discussion paper.* 2021; Availablefrom: https://www.undrr.org/publication/social-construction-systemic-risk-towards-actionable-framework-risk-governance-0.

12. Australian Institute for Disaster Resilience (AIDR). *Systemic Disaster Risk Handbook.* Melbourne 2021. Available from: https://knowledge.aidr.org.au/resources/handbook-systemic-disaster-risk/

13. Independent Panel for Pandemic Preparedness and Response (IPPPR). *COVID-19: Make it the last pandemic. A summary.* 2021.

14. FEMA. *Principles of emergency management supplement.* 2007.

15. United Nations Office for Disaster Risk Reduction. *Terminology: Disaster risk management.* 2023 [cited 2023 February 27]; Available from: https://www.undrr.org/terminology/disaster-risk-management.

16. United Nations Office for Disaster Risk Reduction. *What is the sendai framework for disaster risk reduction?* 2015 [10th October 2022]; Available from: https://www.undrr.org/implementing-sendai-framework/what-sendai-framework.

17. United Nations Development Program (UNDP). *Disaster risk governance. Issue brief.* 2013, New York (NY): Crisis Prevention and Recovery.

Part 2
Key elements of disaster management

4

Disaster risk management frameworks

Jonathan Abrahams, Helen Foster, and Graeme McColl

INTRODUCTION AND OBJECTIVES

The complexity of disaster risk management requires a commensurate level of organisation to optimise the available collective and specific resources, performance and relationships of all those systems, institutions and individuals that have roles in managing risks within a particular community or jurisdiction. Disaster risk management involves far more than skilled managers who can organise and coordinate the application of resources to respond to an incident. Given this complexity, managers and many actors with wide-ranging competencies and access to resources are required to work together to achieve outcomes aimed at prevention, preparedness, readiness, response and recovery. Interconnected systems and structures that apply a set of frameworks enable managers and actors alike to fulfil the roles and responsibilities of their organisations in order to reduce risks and consequences and optimise health, social, economic, cultural and environmental outcomes for individuals and communities.

Local, national and international frameworks provide support or guidance for the development and maintenance of systems, structures, policies, practices and procedures. Frameworks are often issued by governments or other authorities to address an area of public policy and practice with the purpose of providing a common basis for assessments, planning and implementation by all actors within a jurisdiction or administrative area. They should be co-developed in consultation with a range of stakeholders including the actors who are responsible for their implementation and the people or populations who may be affected by their implementation. In some instances, the term "frameworks" may be used synonymously with structures.

The term "structures" connotes the organisation of actors, their roles, responsibilities and the linkages or relationships that form the systems that are necessary to achieve objective and expected outcomes. As part of the disaster health structures, special entities may be established to perform particular roles in disaster health: in terms of governance many of these centre on multi-actor coordination in the health sector or across sectors, for example, for policy coordination, event or incident management support, hospital management, community consultative mechanisms and monitoring bodies.

DOI: 10.4324/9781032626604-6

Systems may refer to all the capacities that need to be in place to manage the health risks and consequences of emergencies and disasters such as policies, strategies and legislation, human and financial resources, health infrastructure, health services and monitoring and evaluation. Systems may focus on a particular function or services such as mass casualty management; incident management; water, sanitation and hygiene (WASH) and primary health care. The term "systems" also refers to governance processes, standard operating procedures and data management systems that organisations use. Such frameworks, systems and structures must be independent of specific individuals and collaborative in nature. Any management task requires all actors working in synergy to facilitate effective solutions to manage risks in a particular context.

The aim of this chapter is to identify key frameworks, systems and structures to support the management of health risks and consequences of disasters and to identify the roles and responsibilities of the key organisations and individuals involved.

On completion of this chapter, you should:

1. Understand international and national frameworks that could guide or support systems, structures, roles and responsibilities in your jurisdiction.
2. Become familiar with the systems and structures, relevant to your jurisdiction, including the roles and responsibilities of key actors.
3. Understand the factors that influence the establishment, operations and effectiveness of those systems, structures and frameworks.
4. Be able to identify the activities required to ensure the systems and structures are rapidly mobilised and effective.

DISASTER HEALTH FRAMEWORKS

The main influences on disaster health frameworks have emanated from: multisectoral emergency and disaster management, which have tended to focus on risks associated with natural and technological hazards; approaches to epidemic preparedness and response for biological hazards/infectious disease; and the international humanitarian system for emergencies involving displaced and refugee populations. Some countries or jurisdictions have agreed comprehensive all-hazards frameworks that are applied to the management of many, if not all types of risks, while other jurisdictions may have parallel frameworks for different types of health risks. Recent trends have led to more convergent frameworks that advocate for common approaches across these dimensions at national and local levels and at the global levels, for example, the Sendai Framework for Disaster Risk Reduction 2015–2030 [1] and the WHO Health Emergency and Disaster Risk Management Framework at the global level [2].

Frameworks have evolved over the decades and continue to do so due to changes in policy (e.g., when governments or their priorities change), practice (e.g., when new methods are proven effective), evidence (e.g., when new information is confirmed) and risks (e.g., when the natural and social environment changes). Frameworks may address dimensions of disaster risk management with respect to hazards (e.g., natural, biological, technological or societal), vulnerabilities (e.g., related to socio-economic status, disability, gender), prevention, preparedness, response or recovery or a particular function (e.g., policy, strategy, planning, health emergency operations centres, monitoring and evaluation).

Frameworks that address "resilience" vary in their focus from those centred on recovery and the "bouncing back" after a disaster to those that take a more holistic approach to the ability of societies to "prevent, resist, absorb, adapt, respond and recover positively when faced with a wide range of risks…". These have gained traction in recent years and have been applied to the development of more resilient communities, countries, health systems, health care facilities and other organisations, such as the United Nations Common Guidance on Helping Build Resilient Societies [3].

The scope and purpose of national and sub-national frameworks vary among countries depending on the risk profiles, governance, systems, policies and practices of the country or jurisdiction. The governance structure of countries and the designation of responsibilities across administrative levels determine how governments or agencies issue policy and planning frameworks. They are expected to be implemented or operationalised by all actors through coordinated action and adaptation of the frameworks to their roles and the risk context in which they operate. Therefore, key success factors for the effective implementation of frameworks include the level of acceptance and ownership of the frameworks by the implementing actors, which is facilitated by their participation in the development of the frameworks; leadership, advocacy and communication; and the availability of resources to support implementation. Incentives may also be available for successful implementation while penalties may be applied for non-compliance or low levels of implementation.

While frameworks issued by central governments may be characterised as examples of a "top-down" approach, the ongoing transformation of disaster risk management is founded on strengthening community leadership and participation, that is, the community-centred approach, which underlies the statement that "all disasters are local". Local implementation often requires the technical and operational support from financial, material and human resources from outside of the local area or from district, subnational or central levels of the health, disaster management or other systems, and sometimes international support is needed.

Therefore, national and subnational frameworks support cooperation in and across administrative levels and sectors within countries, while global and regional frameworks, for example, those issued by the United Nations and its agencies (e.g., World Health Organization, UN Office for Disaster Risk Reduction), regional bodies such as the Association of South East Asian Nations (ASEAN), international development banks (e.g., World Bank, Asian Development Bank) and other international entities, support international assistance and cooperation across national borders and among countries. Key international frameworks such as the Sendai Framework for Disaster Risk Reduction 2015–2030 and the International Health Regulations (2005) are described later in this chapter.

DISASTER HEALTH RISK MANAGEMENT SYSTEMS

Disaster health risk management systems provide for scalable arrangements to address the different dimensions of disaster risk. They are in accord with the respective roles and responsibilities of organisations, agencies and other actors in health and other sectors (1) in their day-to-day work with an emphasis on proactive measures that improve health, nutrition and immunisation status of individuals and populations, and managing smaller-scale incidents, and (2) for preparedness, response to and recovery from larger-scale emergencies and disasters that both build on the day-to-day actions and include measures to address increased risks and demands on societal systems.

- Routine/day-to-day work
  - hazard prevention, vulnerability reduction, exposure reduction, for example, water, sanitation and hygiene promotion (WASH); immunisation; nutrition; other primary care; disease surveillance; management of non-communicable diseases (NCDs); mental health; resilient health-related infrastructure
  - preparedness and response to smaller-scale events (e.g., traffic crashes, localised outbreaks)

- Preparedness, response to and recovery from larger-scale emergencies and disasters:
  - Preparedness: for example, multi-hazard early warning systems, disease early warning systems, emergency response planning, exercise simulations
  - Response: epidemic investigation, contact tracking and tracing, isolation, quarantine, medical care (pre-hospital, health care facility), health care (essential health care functions), psychosocial support
  - Recovery: management of ongoing and longer-term consequence for physical and mental health and well-being, restoration of health services, rehabilitation, integration of risk reduction practices

For example:

The WHO Health Emergency and Disaster Risk Management Framework [2] describes 10 components covering around 200 functions to effectively manage the risks of emergencies and disasters. These components with some indicative functions are:

1. Policies, strategies and legislation – health and multisectoral capacity development strategies
2. Planning and coordination – coordination mechanisms, planning for prevention, preparedness, response and recovery, exercises
3. Human resources – workforce development, training, safety and security
4. Financial resources – regular budget, contingency funding
5. Information and knowledge management – risk assessments, early warning, research
6. Risk communications – media engagement, risk communication
7. Health Infrastructure & Logistics – emergency kits, safe hospitals, stockpiles
8. Health and Related Services –
   a) Health-care services
   b) Specialised services and measures for specific hazards
   c) Public health measures (including immunisation)
9. Community EDRM Capacities – local health workforce participation, individual and community action
10. Monitoring and evaluation – after action reviews, national and international reporting of health impacts and capacities

NATIONAL DISASTER HEALTH RISK MANAGEMENT SYSTEMS

The organisation of each country's systems for managing the health risks of emergencies and disasters will reflect the country's governance and the distribution of roles and responsibilities across administrative levels and sectors. The key influences on national disaster health systems in a given country are usually the organisation of (1) the national disaster management systems and (2) the national health systems, in particular the way in which the risks of disease outbreaks are managed. The level of convergence of these systems for managing risks of all types of emergencies and disasters varies across countries: some countries may use similar arrangements for the management of disease outbreaks as are used for other types of emergencies and disaster; in some other countries the epidemic preparedness and response systems exist in parallel to the disaster management systems; in many countries there is a combination of these systems.

Systems and the respective frameworks and the structures that govern them have evolved over time. In order to maintain currency, it is important for managers and other actors to ascertain the extant frameworks and arrangements and if necessary to determine whether there are any other emerging changes under consideration.

NATIONAL MULTISECTORAL DISASTER RISK MANAGEMENT SYSTEMS

It is not possible to detail the national disaster management systems for all countries, as there are incredible variety and often diverse arrangements across and within individual countries. However, there are similarities in the governance of those disaster management systems in that they are likely to include:

- A legal framework that describes different types of law (subject to the country's legal system), which may include acts and statutes (enacted by a legislative body), common law (made by the judiciary) and regulatory arrangements (issued by agencies).
- Policies and/or strategic frameworks issued by governments.
- Guidelines issued by governments to implement policy. These may include emergency response planning frameworks.
- Structures including governance bodies and actors whose authority, roles and responsibilities within a given jurisdiction may be described in respective legal frameworks, policies and guidelines.

DISASTER RISK MANAGEMENT COORDINATION MECHANISMS AND ORGANISATIONAL STRUCTURES

Systems to manage the risks and consequences of emergencies and disasters require the capability to facilitate the collaboration and cooperation of all key actors, which is provided by organisational structures and coordination mechanisms. They are established within and across levels of administration, functional areas or sectors and within organisations to achieve outcomes in areas such as policy development, capacity development, planning, operational management and monitoring, reporting and evaluation.

These structures including the governance bodies and the way in which actors are organised (e.g., in hierarchies or matrices) and allocated responsibilities are specific to individual countries and to their political and constitutional arrangements.

As a general rule, they include a whole-of-government coordinating committee usually led by the President, Premier or Chief Minister and comprising Ministers; a head of agency level committee to advise Ministers; subcommittees by functional area (such as health) and technical advisory structures. Any or all of these structures may include representatives from a wide range of stakeholders including public, private and civil society sectors, academia and citizens. These arrangements are often replicated at sub-national and local administrative levels. Structures are also in place to coordinate across the various administrative levels on strategic, tactical and operational matters. Bodies or task forces may be established to address specific issues across and within administrative levels, such as disaster funding arrangements, risk assessments, recovery from a disaster or the management of specific events such as the COVID-19 pandemic.

Systems or structures are established for managing the response to events, ranging from incidents to disasters. Incident management systems provide for scalable arrangements among agencies for a multi-agency response and within organisations to manage incidents for which they are the lead agency (e.g., ambulance services provide pre-hospital emergency patient care, fire services respond to building fires, police services uphold law and order). Private sector organisations also adopt incident management systems. Companies may establish a Memorandum of Understanding with other organisations to provide support during emergencies or disasters. For example, a residential care facility may agree to take another facility's residents if a situation required evacuation. Incident management systems are described in Chapters 16 and 17.

As the complexity of the event increases, the systems and structures must be able to cater for a multi-agency, multi-jurisdictional responses; this may include international support or assistance (see Chapter 17). Emergency response structures (governance and coordination committees) and the systems supporting those structures, such as Coordination Centres, comprise multiple organisations (e.g., response agencies) that bring to the collaborative effort not only those normal responsibilities but also the ability to scale up to meet extraordinary challenges and to alter their operations to provide mutual aid and support. Each administrative level of the disaster management system should have coordination structures that are fully scalable depending on the severity and nature of the event. These structures should link the forward command/coordination operations centre close to the location(s) of the incident through to district and state then to national level with the strategic focus increasing at the state and national levels.

In many countries, a hierarchical escalation system applies to disaster health response where one level can seek assistance from adjacent areas or escalate to the next level, for example, local to district to state/provincial and national levels or even international level. For example, the response to COVID-19, because of the complexity of the risks and consequences, required wide spread assistance from many Government departments, agencies and community service providers.

The roles and responsibilities associated with the strategic, tactical and operational levels must be recognised and accepted by all actors. In the case of COVID-19 response in New Zealand, the roll out of vaccination and contact tracing were operational roles, the planning for those roles to function was conducted at the tactical level, and best practice and resource decisions were made at the strategic level.

Every day frontline response can then be expanded to recognise the escalation, complexity and urgency of any situation that requires an organised multi-faceted disaster management response arrangement. To ensure maximum efficiency and effectiveness, existing frameworks, systems and structures should be utilised where possible.

However, frameworks, systems and structures for large-scale emergency situations may differ from routine structure and the priorities of the organisations involved. Planning for response management and the creation of special purpose response teams should be part of routine planning and preparedness and acceptance across all agencies. The response management teams are similar to the task force approach taken towards planning and preparation for major events.

The systems and structures in turn also need to fit within a broader environment defining, for example, why those systems and structures exist; what they are trying to achieve;

the roles and responsibilities of those involved; the social, economic and environmental context; and a description of the risks and priorities. This is encapsulated in a strategy, whether at an organisational or government level. Once developed, a strategy is supported by plans, for example, an implementation plan, emergency operations plans, that include the systems and structures needed and the specific actions to be undertaken. It is worth emphasising again that these systems and structures must ensure connections are made across prevention, preparedness, response and recovery. A key factor for success is engagement and acceptance of the organisation's senior executive and all relevant stakeholders.

International systems, frameworks and structures

Many risks and associated events have localised effects; however, some escalate in terms of sub-national, national, regional and global risks, effects and interests, and the roles of countries and organisations in providing international assistance. While there are many examples of bilateral cooperation between countries, most international assistance flows to lower income countries whose populations are often suffer greater impacts from emergencies and disasters. This was demonstrated during the COVID-19 pandemic when risks, impacts and interest spread rapidly and was sustained across the world with disproportional effects in terms of impacts and inequitable access to vaccines within and between countries. Mechanisms such as the Access to COVID-19 Tools (ACT) Accelerator (https://www.who.int/initiatives/act-accelerator) were established by WHO and partners to support the global effort to develop tools and to address the equitable distribution of tests, treatments and vaccines.

International arrangements related to disaster risk management, health and resilience are complex. They may take many forms related to the relationships that countries have with one another, such as bilateral cooperation that is often facilitated by the international development portfolios in central governments and technical cooperation through line ministries; through regional groupings (e.g., ASEAN, the Economic Committee of West African States (ECOWAS) and the Pacific Community) and with international organisations such as the United Nations system and international non-government organisations. Countries collaborate directly and through multilateral organisations by sharing information on risks such as regional disease surveillance systems or climate outlook forums, providing physical assistance, undertaking joint capacity development including learning and exercises and offering financial assistance. International development banks, such as the World Bank, contribute financial assistance in the form of loans and grants that assist countries with risk management, including prevention, preparedness and recovery, for example, through the Global Facility for Disaster Reduction and Recovery (GFDRR).

Thus it is important that disaster managers at country level are aware of the international governance structures, the roles and responsibilities of leading international authorities and organisations and the national protocols for the provision and reception of international assistance.

The UN System consists of programmes, funds, specialised agencies and the UN organisation, which includes the General Assembly, the Security Council and the UN Secretariat. Many of the UN programmes and agencies have some roles to play in different aspects disaster management including:

- UN Office for the Coordination of Humanitarian Assistance which "brings together humanitarian actors to ensure a coherence response to emergencies"

- UN Development Programme, the UN's development agency, whose role includes building resilience to sustain progress towards the achievement of the Sustainable Development Goals
- UN High Commissioner for Refugees (UNHCR) that provides support to refugees and other displaced and stateless people
- UN Office for Disaster Risk Reduction (UNDRR) that "brings governments, partners and communities to together to reduce disaster risk and losses and to ensure a safer, sustainable future"

The Sendai Framework for Disaster Risk Reduction 2015–2030 was endorsed by the United Nations General Assembly following extensive negotiations by UN Member States that concluded at the 2015 Third UN World Conference for Disaster Risk Reduction. The expected outcome of the Sendai Framework is *the substantial reduction of disaster risk and losses in lives, livelihoods and health and in the economic, physical, social, cultural and environmental assets of persons, businesses, communities and countries.*

It builds on the progress made by countries under the *Hyogo Framework for Action 2005–2015: Building the Resilience of Nations and Communities to Disasters.* Notably the explicit inclusion of health in the outcome is supported by 38 references to health in the Sendai Framework compared to only three in the Hyogo Framework.

The Sendai Framework is structured around 13 guiding principles, 7 targets and 4 priority areas comprising many priority actions at national and local levels supported by actions at the regional and global levels. These priority areas are:

1. Understanding disaster risk
2. Strengthening disaster risk governance to manage disaster risk
3. Investing in disaster risk reduction for resilience
4. Enhancing disaster preparedness for effective response and to "Build Back Better" in recovery, rehabilitation and reconstruction

The Inter-Agency Standing Committee (IASC)

The Inter-Agency Standing Committee (https://interagencystandingcommittee.org/iasc), established in 1991, fosters inter-agency coordination and cooperation between the UN and non-UN partners on policies, strategic priorities and resource mobilisation for a unified response to crises. At the country level, the international humanitarian assistance is structured around the IASC Cluster system under the leadership of the Humanitarian Coordinator.

The international organisations, including the cluster systems, provide standards for the involvement of international assistance, for example, Emergency Medical Teams, and provide assistance to the national authorities for management of international organisations and individuals wanting to provide assistance often on a voluntary basis. In both national and international scenarios, experienced and well-resourced volunteer organisations contribute to response and other activities. On the other hand, the health response to the 2010 Haiti earthquake highlighted the problems disruptive, uncooperative and uncoordinated volunteers can cause [4]. National authorities should have protocols, standards and conditions for organisations and individuals, including volunteers, to enter the country and provide support. These organisations must fit with and accept the framework under which any response is managed.

In addition to the UN, regional organisations, such as the European Union, ASEAN and the Pacific Community, have established cross-national systems to support risk reduction, disaster preparedness and response coordination. There are key international strategies and programmes underway to try and regularise the provision of international assistance, and this is covered in detail in Chapter 17.

The International Health Regulations (IHR) (2005) is an international legal framework that defines countries' rights and obligations in managing public health events that have the potential to cross borders and require that all countries have the ability to detect, assess, report and respond to public health events [5]. The IHR Emergency Committee have provided advice to the Director General WHO on recommendations to countries on the management of "public health emergencies of international concerns" (PHEICs) such as the COVID-19 pandemic, the 2014 outbreak of Ebola in Western Africa, the 2015–2016 Zika virus epidemic and 2018–2020 Kivu Ebola epidemic. A UN Crisis Management Team, chaired by WHO, was established in the early stages of the COVID-19 pandemic to provide coherence across the UN entities including harmonisation of communication. Many UN actors participated including the existing coordination fora for the UN System (Development Coordination Office, UN OCHA).

Non-government organisations (NGOs) and civil society organisations (CSOs)

There are a vast range of international NGOs and CSOs and it is not possible to identify or list them all. We include here examples of international organisations, networks and professional associations that support the range of roles played by those agencies and actors in disaster risk management.

- The International Federation of Red Cross and Red Crescent Societies is formed by the respective national societies and plays a prominent role in strengthening national capacities and in international responses by providing people, resources and equipment.
- The International Committee of the Red Cross (ICRC) (https://www.icrc.org/) is an independent, neutral organisation that helping people affected by conflict and armed violence around the world and promotes the rules of war based on the Geneva Conventions of 1949.
- The International Council of Voluntary Agencies – ICVA (https://www.icvanetwork. org/) is a global network of almost 140 non-governmental organisations focused on policy and practice in humanitarian action
- Global Network of Civil Society Organisations for Disaster Reduction (GNDR) (https:// www.gndr.org/) is network of more than 1200 civil society organisations in 120 countries working together to strengthen CSO capacities for community resilience.
- The International Emergency Management Society (TIEMS) is a non-profit NGO that provides opportunities for the exchange of information and innovation in disaster management.
- The International Association of Emergency Managers (IAEM) aims to provide members with the opportunities to exchange information and network to advance the profession of emergency management.
- The World Association for Disaster and Emergency Medicine (WADEM) is a multidisciplinary professional association whose mission is the global improvement of pre-hospital and emergency health care, public health, and disaster health and preparedness.

- Médecins Sans Frontières (MSF) is an international and independent organisation that delivers "emergency medical aid to people affected by armed conflict, epidemics and disasters, and exclusion from health care".

Private sector organisations

A key component of disaster management is building collaborative partnerships between communities, government agencies and business within the community across the phases of prevention, preparedness, response and recovery to engage their full capacity.

Businesses provide essential functions to support community resilience. They are part of the community fabric, and their core business is contributing to the prosperity of their community. Utilising the capabilities of business in disasters is integral to further building community resilience, to bolster critical resources required in the event of severe to catastrophic disasters and to integrate them further in disaster management through the adoption of a whole-of-community approach.

Volunteers that are part of private sector organisations, government and non-government organisations as well as international- and national-based organisations are extensive and, when activated, are required to work within the framework under which any response is managed.

The importance of stakeholders

Coordination arrangements are often encapsulated in a strategy or a plan, whether at an organisational or government level. In developing the strategy at these levels, it is necessary to identify with whom, intra-organisationally or inter-organisationally, the organisation will need to communicate, that is, who the stakeholders will be. Stakeholder engagement is necessary to ensure effective policy implementation, communications and collaboration. Stakeholder engagement is the systematic identification of stakeholders, analysis, planning and implementation of actions designed to influence stakeholders. A stakeholder engagement plan identifies the needs and resources of key stakeholder groups, and partners play a vital role in addressing those needs and coordinating resources.

These stakeholders may be internal, to include executive management, department heads or other personnel. Or, they may be external, ranging from other organisations to suppliers, first responders and to the community at large. Not all stakeholders have the same interests, power or roles in disaster risk management or an incident; and therefore communication can be diverse.

It is important not to wait until the disruptive event to meet the many internal and external stakeholders for disaster risk management, whether in an emergency or in planning or capacity development. Engaging early and keeping them engaged is important as their involvement (or lack of) can have an impact on system-wide coordination and organisational or community resilience.

Engagement with stakeholders can be based on their perceived importance in disaster risk management. The more important the stakeholder, the more reason to develop relationships with the stakeholder, especially prior to an event occurring. Once identified, stakeholder primary functions can be included in a stakeholder management plan that details stakeholders and their specific roles during each of the disaster management stages. An indicative table of stakeholders and their potential roles is at Table 4.1.

Table 4.1 Disaster management stakeholder engagement plan – indicative only

Disaster stakeholder engagement plan

Level	Stakeholder, organisation, group	Prevention	Preparedness	Response	Recovery
International	International agencies	Guidelines, standards Increased awareness of disaster risk prevention	Risk monitoring Capacity development for emergency response	International coordination Mobilisation and delivery of aid and support	Support for recovery. Risk-informed development
National	National government disaster management committees and agencies	National building codes. National policies, frameworks, systems and funding for disaster prevention, resilient physical, social infrastructure	National disaster planning, exercises, capacity development, funding and weather services	National coordination. Damage assessment. Disaster declarations. Emergency response and resources. and relief programmes and resources	Recovery coordination Individual relief payments Recovery resources for rebuilding
State, territory, district, municipality	State, territory, district, municipality disaster management committees	Programmes to prevent creation of risk Risk-informed development Resilient physical and social infrastructure	State and local preparedness, including planning, training and exercises Community briefings regarding preparatory activities Early warning systems	Coordination of response to of events Assistance to communities for evacuations. Relief centres for displaced persons	Area-specific recovery processes including financial assistance

(Continued)

Table 4.1 (Continued)

Disaster stakeholder engagement plan

Non-government organisations	Local representatives	Relationships with communities. Vulnerability reduction and risk preventive measures	NGO planning and exercises, ongoing training and management of staff, volunteers and communities	Support and assistance to communities. Coordination with national, state and local authorities	Assistance to communities for recovery of people's health and well-being, restoration of personal assets
Community – organisations, groups	Local leaders, civil society organisations, businesses	Partnerships between communities and stakeholders, for risk prevention. Actions to prevent risks – e.g., small businesses. Community disaster awareness campaign	Organisational and business continuity planning, training and exercises. Assistance to community for preparedness	Community leadership. Local assistance to community including businesses. Mobilisation of external support to community	Small business recovery. Leadership and coordination economic and social recovery
Community – individuals	Community members and groups/individuals	Self-awareness of risks. Action to reduce hazard, vulnerability and exposure of self and property. Build social capital	Preparation for events. Act upon early warnings	Appropriate response for self, household and support to community	Provide support to displaced persons and work with the community recovery efforts

CASE STUDY 4.1 HURRICANE KATRINA

The historic Hurricane Katrina, a Category 4 hurricane, made landfall in Mississippi, on August 29, 2005, causing large-scale devastation along the Gulf Coast, leaving more than 1,800 people dead, displacing families to all 50 states and resulting in billions in losses to infrastructure and the economy.

Much of this damage caused by Katrina was likely unavoidable. Katrina was a huge, Category 3 hurricane when it hit Louisiana and Mississippi, and it hit areas including New Orleans that were largely below sea level and therefore vulnerable to flooding. But many of the issues were worsened if not caused by a government response that was unable to deal with the storm before, during and after it made landfall.

About 1.3 million people left southeast Louisiana and 400,000 evacuated from New Orleans itself, culminating in one of the largest evacuations in US history. As the storm battered the region, tens of thousands of people remained in the city not necessarily by choice, but rather because they were too poor to afford a car or bus fare to leave.

Those who stayed evacuated to an overcrowded convention centre and Superdome and were not adequately supplied with drinking water or food. The Red Cross set up shelters, but they were not enough. The Federal Emergency Management Agency (FEMA) slowly became aware that their response efforts were not adequate. The local government of New Orleans, despite setting up a command centre in a downtown New Orleans hotel ballroom, remained dysfunctional and lacked essential communication with both the state and federal governments. Each blamed the other and yet competed to do better. Meanwhile people continued to die on rooftops and not receive food and water. Though FEMA provided "record levels of support" to storm victims, emergency responders and state authorities, investigators found it was hampered by untrained staff, unreliable communication systems and poor coordination in delivering aid.

From a health perspective, the entire city's medical care system was destroyed. The hospitals were closed. Patients could not find their doctors, as offices were closed and many of the doctors themselves lost their homes. Jobs were lost and employees were lost to the employers even if the business could be reopened. Medical records were lost in the rubble and floods, and many patients who showed up in clinics did not know their medications. Pharmacies were closed and if re-opening had to discard their supplies because the medications had spoiled in the heat and new deliveries were not coming quickly. Laboratories were also not available to process blood tests, and delivery trucks were unavailable to send the samples elsewhere.

The federal government's response to the extensive and disruptive impacts of Hurricane Katrina faced criticism, which caused a significant re-evaluation of the execution of federal disaster response efforts and resource allocation. Much of this damage was likely unavoidable in the face of a storm as strong as Hurricane Katrina but the harms could have been at least mitigated by better government preparation and a stronger response, based on the many reports that have reviewed disaster prevention, preparedness, response to and recovery from Hurricane Katrina [6].

ACTIVITIES

1. What would be the advantages and disadvantages of applying existing formal organisational structures in society to the structure required for managing the risks of emergencies or disasters?
2. The chapter advocates that "frameworks, systems and structures must be independent of specific individuals and collaborative in nature". Analyse this proposition and provide a critique. Do you agree or disagree?
3. What have been some of the challenges associated with the management of the COVID-19 pandemic and how could these challenges be overcome?

KEY READINGS

1. World Health Organization. *Health emergency and disaster risk management framework*. Geneva: World Health Organization; 2019. Available from: https://apps.who.int/iris/bitstream/handle/10665/326106/9789241516181-eng.pdf
2. United Nations. United Nations Common Guidance on Helping Build Resilient Societies, New York: United Nations; 2020. Available from: https://unsdg.un.org/sites/default/files/2021-09/UN-Resilience-Guidance-Final-Sept.pdf
3. United Nations. *Transforming our world: The 2030 Agenda for Sustainable Development*; 2015. Available from: https://sdgs.un.org/2030agenda.
4. Nowell, B., T. Steelman, A.-L.K. Velez, and Z. Yang, The structure of effective governance of disaster response networks: Insights from the field. *The American Review of Public Administration*, 2018. **48**(7): p. 699–715.

References

1. United Nations. *Sendai framework for disaster risk reduction 2015–2030*. Geneva: United Nations; 2015. Available from: https://www.undrr.org/publication/sendai-framework-disaster-risk-reduction-2015-2030
2. World Health Organization. *Health emergency and disaster risk management framework*. Geneva: World Health Organization; 2019. Available from: https://apps.who.int/iris/bitstream/handle/10665/326106/9789241516181-eng.pdf
3. United Nations. *United Nations common guidance on helping build resilient societies*. New York: United Nations; 2020. Available from: https://unsdg.un.org/sites/default/files/2021-09/UN-Resilience-Guidance-Final-Sept.pdf
4. Pan American Health Organization. *Health response to the earthquake in Haiti: January 2010*. Washington, DC: PAHO; 2011. Available from: https://www.paho.org/disasters/dmdocuments/HealthResponseHaitiEarthq.pdf
5. World Health Organization. *International health regulations* (2005), 3rd ed. World Health Organization. 2016. Available from: https://apps.who.int/iris/handle/10665/246107
6. United States. Executive Office of the President & United States. Assistant to the President for Homeland Security and Counterterrorism. *The federal response to Hurricane Katrina: Lessons learned*. Washington, DC: White House; 2006. Available from: https://www.govinfo.gov/content/pkg/GOVPUB-PREX-PURL-LPS67263/pdf/GOVPUB-PREX-PURL-LPS67263.pdf

5

Risk and its management

Mike Tarrant and Carl Gibson

INTRODUCTION AND OBJECTIVES

The aim of this chapter is to outline concepts of uncertainty and risk and the principles and practice of risk management in the context of disaster health management. On completion of this chapter you should:

1. Have a detailed understanding of disaster health-related risk and the application of risk management as a means of achieving societal, community and organisational objectives in the context of disasters; and
2. Have an understanding of some of the techniques for making decisions about dealing with disaster health-related risk.

In Chapter 1, we identified that understanding risk and having capabilities to manage risk are essential parts of disaster management. This contributes to the effective allocation and mobilisation of scarce resources, and their continuing fitness-for-purpose. Risk is present in all aspects of disaster management and is associated with both the strategic and operating environments. This includes the threats and hazards that will be faced; the decisions and actions that will need to be taken; and the behaviours of those affected by and involved in responding to and recovering from a disaster.

Risk is so pervasive that to ignore it will at best guarantee suboptimal management of the disaster, more likely this would lead to disaster-affected people suffering needlessly, agencies and individuals suffering harm, precious resources and time being wasted, and confidence in the response and recovery being lost. To be better aware of risk, and to be more capable of dealing with risk requires a fundamental understanding of uncertainty, and how 'risk' is constructed in the face of such uncertainty.

WHAT IS RISK?

A widely accepted definition of risk is 'the effect of uncertainty on objectives' (International Standards, ISO 31000 2018). In the disaster context these may be the objectives of decision-makers, disaster managers, constituent institutions and providers, frontline workers, affected communities, individuals, or society at large. But what does this really

DOI: 10.4324/9781032626604-7

mean? We live in an uncertain world, where uncertainty can be present in many forms. Any type of disaster is characterised by high uncertainty, which can arise as a result of:

- *High levels of complexity*: in a disaster there are a myriad of systems and subsystems that are affected by the disaster, emerge because of the disaster, or are mobilised in response to it. These systems and subsystems have multiple different interactions and interdependencies that will be largely unknown, and many of which may only become apparent long after the disaster has finished.
- *High levels of novelty*: there will be situations and problems that could occur that decision-makers and responders will not have encountered before, be unfamiliar with, and have little understanding of how they could evolve over time.
- *High levels of ambiguity*: the limited data and information that will be accessed may be quite validly interpreted in multiple different and conflicting ways. The true meaning will remain obscured until additional information is made available, which may never happen.
- *High levels of volatility*: frequent, sudden and unexpected change in the strategic and operating contexts and high turbulence: intense bursts of change that may be destructive.

Whilst these characteristics all contribute to high levels of uncertainty during a disaster, it also needs to be recognised that in addition to the above cause of aleatory uncertainty (arising from the change in our environment), epistemic uncertainty, generated by our own and shared incomplete knowledge or ignorance, may also be present [1, 2].

Slovic [3] makes the point that while danger is real there is no such thing as 'real risk' or 'objective risk'. Risk is a judgement about how objectives are affected by a situation. To put it simply, hazards are *facts* and risk is a *conclusion* about how a hazard may affect you, your organisation, community, network or society at large. In other words, risk is a *social construct* about how we foresee the different types of uncertainty affecting how we and others pursue our purpose and intent (our objectives). All of this contributes to our understanding and uncertainty about the disaster context, about the problems that need to be solved, about the relative merits of different options that may be used to resolve those problems. Simply, risk is a way of encapsulating our uncertainty about the situation, the decisions we must make, and the actions that need to be taken, and risk management provides us with the means of reducing the uncertainty and acting on the remaining uncertainty.

THE IMPORTANCE OF RISK IN DISASTER HEALTH MANAGEMENT

It is convenient to think of risk in terms of potential losses and benefits that could occur over some future timeframe, arising as a result of the decisions we make and the actions we take, or the non-decisions and non-action we allow to occur. By not considering and dealing with risk, we may therefore fail to reduce harm that occurs, permit otherwise avoidable additional harm to emerge, and fail to capitalise on beneficial opportunities. Risk management therefore allows us to understand and prioritise actions to deal with this potential harm and benefit, in relation to:

- Making decisions about what sources of risk and their potential interactions with individuals, communities, and other organisations will need to be managed.
- The vulnerabilities and susceptibilities of individuals, communities and other organisations to interactions with these risk sources, thus creating risk.

- Making decisions about the best options for prevention, exploitation, and preparedness for these risks.
- Making decisions about risks that emerge during disaster health response and recovery activities.

In identifying and defining risk in disaster health management, it is important to continually reflect back on which actors are affected by and are involved in the disaster, and how these actors' objectives may be affected by health-related issues that arise in the lead up to, during, and in the recovery from the disaster. It is also important to specifically consider how broader issues may affect the specific health-related objectives of the various actors. These actors could include:

- Communities affected directly by the disaster.
- Other communities and institutions that may suffer collateral impacts, for example through
  - an overwhelming or collapse of the health system,
  - the translocation of directly affected populations,
  - the purposeful redirection of resources away from initially unaffected populations to those in or fleeing from the disaster zone,
  - those subsequently exposed to disaster contagion effects, for example: emerging public health issues such as increase in infectious diseases, local collapse of financial systems, social unrest, failure of localised government support services, etc.
- Organisations and individuals formally and informally involved in and supporting emergency and disaster management efforts.
- The broader civil society that may be affected indirectly by economic and service provision impacts. For example, during the COVID-19 pandemic, broad sections of society (such as many rural areas) had little or no exposure to infection but were still adversely affected by public health measures.

Following a disaster, the indirect economic and social impacts are usually higher than the direct impacts of the disaster. Immediate economic loss, such as damage to infrastructure, loss of productivity, and an inability to work are often offset by insurance and disaster relief payments. Whilst these short-term effects may be quickly recoverable, longer-term impacts such as the increased inequality, migration of populations, movement away of industry and transfer of jobs out of the affected areas can have devastating long-lasting impacts on communities.

Similarly, the indirect effects on the health system are usually far higher than the direct impacts. For example, long-term underfunding of the public health and hospital systems in some jurisdictions also meant that they were ill-prepared for the disruption driven by the reaction to the pandemic. Consequently, a whole range of 'non-essential' health services had to be suspended, creating severe long-term harm. For example, the suspension of cancer screening services and health promotions (such as skin cancer prevention) on multiple occasions during the pandemic has established the high risk of significant numbers of late and undiagnosed cancers and delayed treatment. As a result of which, it is almost certain that there will be a surge in preventable cancer deaths [4, 5] in the following years.

Therefore, during a disaster, a major focus should be on dealing with the direct and indirect impacts of a disrupted health system both on disaster-affected communities, and on the broader population. In doing so, the long-term health impacts resulting from the disruptions of other societal systems (such as economic, infrastructure, civil cohesion, etc.) and requirements for their management should not be ignored.

Even the way that risk management is approached can diminish or amplify adverse health risk. Historically, very significant resources have been allocated to hazard analysis and assessment but very little to how will risk reduction will be achieved and how adverse outcomes will be addressed.

RISK MANAGEMENT AND DISASTER MANAGEMENT

Risk management is defined in the ISO 31000 as: '*The culture, processes and structures that are directed towards realizing potential opportunities whilst managing adverse effects*'. This definition makes the point that risk management is an integral element of any purposeful activity and where the outcome is about maximising gains and minimising loss.

An historical perspective

Initially, this risk management was largely focused on hazard analysis and technical risk analysis, which had been popularised in hazardous industries such as nuclear power plants large dams and petrochemical industries in the late 1980s and 1990s [6–8]. This was part of a transition from looking at hazards in isolation, to seeing hazards as a source of risk. It was also during this time period that early risk assessment tools were introduced into disaster planning and preparedness [9, 10].

However, the adoption of risk management during this time was challenging. The work on risk in the environmental field from the 1970s to the 1990s provided a very unhelpful development in separating risk assessment and risk management. In this model the scientists did the risk assessment and handed the answer to the policy people to manage the risk. A dichotomy that still persists today in many government bodies.

The development of comprehensive disaster management (PPRR) enabled thinking about approaches beyond response and relief. The use of risk management was crucial in providing a common conceptual framework and language for disaster management to engage more widely across the economy and society. This type of risk management was initially called 'disaster risk management' and is still practised as a traditional linear approach as articulated in the National Emergency Risk Assessment Guidelines (2020). However, there is growing reticence about the usefulness of such approaches in the highly uncertain and complex context of the dynamics of a disaster.

Disasters: a different risk focus

The critical point about risk management is that it is a systematic process to ensure scarce resources are best allocated for an entity (an individual, organisation or system) to deal with the uncertainty associated with achieving its purpose and objectives. For example, although the details of how risk management is applied in a small rural health clinic compared to a large tertiary hospital will be different, the core concepts and principles remain the same.

Disasters are viewed as non-routine and highly novel social problems [11, 12], requiring that closely aligned fields such as disaster and disruption-related risk management especially focus on the non-routine part of the risk spectrum (Figure 5.1), where predictably is low or non-existent. The presence of such non-routine risk and the need to manage

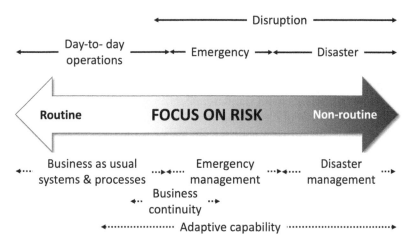

Figure 5.1 The risk spectrum

it force an entity to adopt non-routine decision-making and practices (e.g., emergency response, disaster management, etc.), in order to minimise adverse and maximise beneficial outcomes. By doing so, disaster management helps society, at the micro and macro levels, prevent or reduce the potential adverse outcomes described by these risks, as well as improving beneficial opportunities. Under this broad disaster management umbrella these risk treatments can be as varied as preparedness (such as capability development), risk prevention/mitigation (such as land use planning and improvement), establishment of contingencies (for example with strategic and operational continuity), emergency response, crisis management, and a whole range of disaster response, relief, and recovery activities.

This is a very flexible approach that can be used in any context because it is defined by the need of the part of the system that has to run in a non-routine way. For example, a storm in a remote rural community may require the local system to move to non-routine operation whereas in a large urban area this situation could be managed through normal processes. It should also be remembered that 'disaster' is not an absolute concept. It is really a function of the rate and magnitude of change and the affected entities' capability to cope with that change.

Now in the 21st Century, the need to manage risk is widely recognised as a key facet of all aspects of disaster management and is featured prominently in the Sendai Framework and many other disaster-related publications. Today, many organisations include risk management principles and practices in their disaster preparedness and disaster response capabilities, although there is still no universally accepted approach, especially so in disaster health management. However, many organisations have adopted the methodology described in the international risk management standard ISO31000, originally developed in and then readopted by Australia (Australian Standards, 2018).

One hangover from the focus on hazards led to the assumption that all risk can be objectively quantified and calculated, with risk often expressed in equations such as risk = consequence × probability. This is a faulty concept, but has prevailed as an attempt to give some sort of quasi-scientific status to decision-making. This gross simplification/trivialisation is very unhelpful in trying to deal with the complexity, uncertainty, and ambiguity associated with very low probability – high consequence situations. It is now broadly recognised that such linear risk management thinking and methodologies struggle as uncertainty, complexity, and volatility increase, exactly those situations faced during a disaster. Accordingly, with the experience of failures in risk management during a number of prominent disasters, including the COVID-19 pandemic, a more flexible risk management approach has been developed by the authors of this Chapter and subsequently adopted as a new risk management standard: AS/NZS 5050 (int): 2020.

Although the application of risk management within disaster management is becoming increasingly recognised as a highly skilled technical area, that very professionalisation has created problems for the non-professionals' acknowledgement of risk.

RESPONSIBILITY FOR MANAGING RISK

A theme which is often discussed in disaster management is that there is a lack of community and organisational responsibility in managing risk. Why don't people see the disaster-related risks the way that 'experts do' and invest time and resources in making themselves 'safe'?

If there is an expectation by disaster management agencies of significant changes in behaviour by individuals then, risk assessment and/or risk management will have to move beyond the idea that risk is something that is independent of minds and cultures, waiting to be measured. Unless an approach is developed that moves beyond technical assessments, we are doomed to be met with either apathy or occasional aggression by the public when attempting to engage them in managing risk.

The public have an expectation that 'experts' deal with objective facts and statistics and have all of the answers. However, much of risk management within disaster management is not probabilistic and owes more to interpretation of perceived patterns within situations interpreted through a lens of prior experiences. Subjectivity permeates low probability/high consequence risk assessments because of the very high levels of uncertainty and complexity. Risk assessments rely on very limited data and so significant judgements are required at every step of the process. The likelihood of a disaster occurring in any one place is very uncertain and estimating the consequences is equally problematic because of the range of variables, including issues such as unknown interdependencies and interactions.

This makes for a difficult and often confusing conversation when trying to explain disaster risk and treatment requirements to non-experts, and can result in important risk information being ignored or misinterpreted. This is particularly true for comparative work where judgements have to be made about allocating resources, and where decision-making may not make the rational choices based upon the risk information. At the core of this issue is the common reliance on expected utility theory. It is generally assumed that people will follow rational rules, in order to maximise benefits, if they have sufficient information and time to consider the consequences of different paths [13]. Whilst it is essential to have a sound scientific perspective, this is not sufficient. Individuals rarely make decisions and act entirely rationally; they are subject to a range of cognitive and emotional biases and heuristics that make them potentially non-rational actors. For the disaster risk analyst, the context and boundaries of the problem may be very different to that understood by community groups. The perceived non-rational behaviour of communities may well be a function of them framing the issue differently. This is especially true when they are faced with the unfamiliar, unexperienced, and often fear-inducing risk associated with disasters.

The 'objectivist' approach to risk is too limited a perspective on which to deal with complex policy problems such as disasters [14]. If a goal of public policy is active participation by the public and organisations in managing risk, then a richer understanding of the influence of the social contexts (in which ideas or beliefs about risk are constructed) is required.

SOLVING TRADITIONAL PROBLEMS: THE EMERGENCE OF RESILIENCE CONCEPTS

Some of the recent work on resilience and disasters has been a reaction to the limitations of simple Cartesian-Newtonian (cause and effect) approaches to risk management and management in general. Kettl [15] has observed that the number of cross-cutting problems governments have to deal with is increasing and this is placing ever-increasing challenges for function-based government departments. In other words, social problems do not stop at government department boundaries. Health outcomes are more than just the activities of the Health Department especially in disasters.

Instead of the traditional focus of risk assessment and plan-based treatment of a near-infinite range of potential risk, it is often better to take a different approach. Alternative approaches seek to better understand the nature of a complex problem (sensemaking), rather than leaping straight in risk analysis by rote. Once sense has been made about the problem, the vulnerability of various actors can be considered in the context of that problem and will lead to a more explorative and speculative understanding of risk. Risk treatment then becomes focussed on addressing these vulnerabilities, and in building agile and adaptive capacity to change that can deal with new problems and vulnerabilities as they emerge.

DISASTER HEALTH RISK MANAGEMENT PROCESS

The internationally recognised risk management standard (ISO 3100:2018) works well across a broad range of risk, but can be problematic in dealing with certain types of non-routine situations, especially those associated with high consequence/low (or non-estimable) likelihood. Accordingly, this linear approach has been adapted to provide a more flexible non-linear methodology (AS/NZS 5050 (int): 2020) specifically for disruption-related (and disaster-related) risk (Standards Australia, 2020). A further development of this approach is described below in Figure 5.2.

The disaster health-related risk management process is an iterative cycle which is supported by continuous monitoring and review, and by communication and consultation with stakeholders and independent advisors as appropriate. Unlike traditional linear risk management processes which conduct activities in a step-by-step process, this updated methodology recognises that some activities will occur simultaneously at some points during the process, and will be sequential at other times. Thus, while exploring and establishing the context, a great deal of insight may be gained about individual risks (risk identification), about the nature and interrelationships of these risks (risk analysis), and of their importance (risk evaluation). As we move through the cycle, the emphasis shifts from the context to a more concerted effort to further identify and understand these risks, until such a point that informed decisions can be made to modify (treat) the priority risks. As more insight is gained through moving through the cycle, it may become apparent that further information is required from earlier activities. For example, during evaluation, if there is insufficient understanding to prioritise the risks, then the process revisits and conducts a deeper analysis.

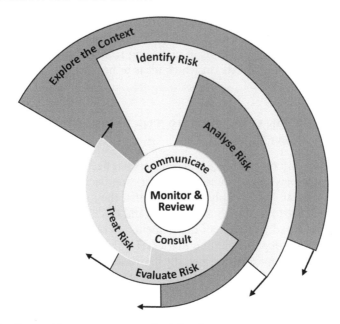

Figure 5.2 Non-linear risk management methodology[1]

Although the risk management process is best undertaken through these nested cyclical activities, it is simpler to describe each of the activities separately, below.

EXPLORING THE CONTEXT

Defining the scope and boundaries

Exploring and understanding the context involves understanding the broad strategic and operating contexts within which disaster could occur, and then defining the scope which establishes the boundaries within which the risk management process will be undertaken. This also includes those aspects of the context that may be specifically excluded, or need to be dealt with under a separate risk assessment.

Understanding and establishing the context includes:

- Identifying the potential or actual disaster scenarios and prevailing conditions that could occur, taking account of past disaster history.
- Examining in further detail the physical, natural, social, political, economic, technological, and cultural aspects of the context in which the disaster(s) may occur or has occurred.
- Identifying key stakeholders affected by or involved in the potential or actual disaster, and other individuals and organisations that may hold actionable information.
- Determining the capabilities and constraints of communities and organisations affected by the disaster.
- Defining the capabilities and constraints of the organisations contributing to the management of disaster-related risk and of managing the disaster more broadly.
- Clarifying and allocating roles, responsibilities, and other resourcing for the risk management process.

- Selecting and customising the risk management process and methodologies to meet the needs of the specific context. This will include deciding on the criteria by which risk will be assessed, evaluated, and prioritised.

UNDERSTANDING RISK: RISK IDENTIFICATION AND ANALYSIS

Hazard identification and mapping

Risk arises from an interaction between hazards and the vulnerabilities of actors (individuals, communities and organisations: both those affected by the disaster and those managing the disaster), depending on the context. Identifying and mapping of these sources of risk is a key aspect of understanding risk. Hazards are characterised by varying levels of predictability and different levels of hazard exposure which are influenced by a multitude of factors such as: type of the event, the geographical location, season of occurrence, behaviours of other actors, etc. Identification requires a systematic and comprehensive '*all hazards*' approach to ensure that all disaster-related hazards are considered.

Hazards will have a range of effects and patterns on different societal levels and functions. These effects may change over the duration of a disaster and have direct and indirect impacts that degrade existing functionality and exacerbate already failing systems, including:

- Degrade the capability and performance of health systems, facilities, and services, including health care (including special needs such as chronic conditions), public health, and other surveillance systems.
- Degrade disaster management capability.
- Impair infrastructure and the provision of essential services, such as water, food, sanitation, and shelter.
- Disruption of economic, social and governmental mechanisms and services.
- Increase the displacement of populations, placing additional stress on infrastructure and services, through overcrowding and unsanitary conditions, increased exposure to communicable disease, etc.

Specifically, the human health effects of hazards may include increased:

- Death and injury.
- Population displacement.
- Higher incidences and severity of communicable and non-communicable diseases.
- Increased cases and severity of disability and impairment.
- Elevated psychological and social behavioural disorders.
- Increased nutritional deficiency.
- Increased population morbidities as a result of poverty, stress, poor diet, etc.

Vulnerability mapping and assessment

Comprehensive vulnerability mapping and assessment are essential to achieve a robust risk assessment. Vulnerability is an expression of the population's or organisation's susceptibility to hazards and threats and includes their capacity to anticipate, cope with, resist and recover from adverse impacts.

Specific criteria that should be considered in vulnerability assessment include determining those vulnerabilities that:

- Are inherent to the 'system', arising as a result of design errors and omissions, invalid operating assumptions, faulty development or mobilisation of the system.
- Arise over time, as a result of unintentional and deliberate decisions, improper activities, inadequate governance and oversight, or the accumulation of normal 'wear and tear' of the system.
- Emerge as a consequence of the impacts of a disaster, or because of the consequences of trying to manage the disaster.

The potential interactions of hazards and threats with system and actor vulnerabilities establishes the presence of risk.

IDENTIFYING AND ANALYSING RISK

Identifying risk involves, at its simplest, determining how the actors and hazards could interact, how these risks could interact with other risks, and the range of consequences arising from those interactions (with consideration of vulnerability). These identified risks are then described in a rich narrative manner that facilitates shared sensemaking about the risk. Such a description could describe:

- The potential event (the different ways in which these hazards and vulnerabilities could interact).
- The range of impacts (the direct and indirect consequences arising from those interactions).
- The effect of controls (procedural, engineering, governance, decision-making, behavioural, etc.) on these interactions and impacts.

The same hazard may pose very different risks, at different levels, to different systems (communities, organisations, etc.) as vulnerability varies [16]. Hazards may combine in different ways to amplify the effects of vulnerability, which in turn may also combine to create highly complex risks. Describing risk is best based on input from both experts and community/organisational representatives. Different participants will likely have very different views on risk driven by prior experience, knowledge, biases, and heuristics.

In describing risk, a substantial practical problem often arises, where there is a very large number of hazards, vulnerabilities and consequences making subsequent analysis a daunting if not near impossible task. A systematic way to limit the number of possible interactions under consideration needs to be adopted. Risk scenarios provide a useful technique to deal with this problem, particularly when combined with an initial low-intensity screening analysis and prioritisation, through which highly implausible and inconsequential risks can be excluded from more detailed analysis.

A risk scenario is a sample of described potential interactions between hazard and vulnerability that generate risk.

The key steps in developing a risk scenario are:
i. Review the range of hazards identified and confirm their potential occurrence and based on this, prioritise the hazards and select a number of hazards to match the available analytical resources and time availability.
ii. For the prioritised list of hazards establish an intensity range and select a limited representative sample of intensities. For example, select upper limit of the intensity range, the reasonably expected intensity and the lower limit of the intensity range. Sensitivity analysis can be applied to ensure that selected samples are representative.
iii. Once these have been established it is then possible to define and describe the resulting consequences by referring to the vulnerability analysis.

Traditional risk analysis has been largely based on generating a risk rating by estimating the consequences associated with the risk and the likelihood of the described scenario occurring (with those consequences). However, with risk assessment in the disaster context, likelihood is often difficult if not impossible to estimate in any meaningful way. In such circumstances, judgements about the importance of risk need to be based on other factors in addition to the potential consequence, which may include:

- The speed of onset of the changing conditions and consequences described by the risk.
- The duration over which the consequences may be experienced.
- The ability of the system to cope with the potential consequences.
- The extent of contagion (the dispersion and distribution of consequences) over time.
- The criticality of systems that may be affected should the situation described by the risk occur.
- The level, cost, and time required to recover from the expected consequences
- The potential for the interaction and consequences to create new vulnerabilities.
- The level of fear and shock that may arise as the consequences are felt.
- The degree of interdependencies of the risk with other risks.

Professional judgement then needs to be exercised in combining this range of factors to provide a deeper picture of the absolute and relative importance of each risk
Evaluate the risks
The outcome from this part of the process is to determine the need for and prioritise the importance of risks for modification of the risk, which will ultimately guide the allocation of resources towards treatment of those risks. Decisions about the treatment of risk involve balancing acceptability and tolerance for exposure to the risk and consequences against the feasibility of modifying the risk to an acceptable level or state.
Treat the risk
Treating the risk involves modifying the conditions that gave rise to the risk source, its means of interaction with the system, and the vulnerabilities of the system itself. Usually this involves developing a range of modification options and selecting the best suite of options that will achieve the objectives for managing the risk. This suite of options should consider different mechanisms that would allow:

- Avoiding the risk (e.g., banning a chemical., relocating an at-risk population, etc.).
- Changing the likelihood (e.g., land use planning, disease control, etc.).
- Changing the consequences (e.g., warning systems, contingencies, etc.).
- Sharing the risk with another party (e.g., insurance, partnership arrangements, etc.).

Judgement is informed by using an acceptable cost-benefit approach (which considers tangible and intangible costs and benefits, including the level of harm reduction that could be achieved) and should reflect the values and perceptions of the community, organisation and key stakeholders to ensure the activities are acceptable and credible.

Some suitable criteria to evaluate treatment options might be:

- Can we afford them and are they cost-effective?
- What is the full life cycle cost?
- Is there continuity of effects?
- Do we have the authority to undertake them?
- Are there any additional benefits?
- Are there synergies with other treatment options?
- Will new risks be generated?
- How practical is the option?
- How easy is it to implement?

The selected options are then documented into an actionable plan which considers:

- Why the actions for modifying risk were selected?
- Who will be accountable and responsible for implementing the plan?
- What resources are needed?
- Schedule and timing for mobilisation and implementation.
- Reporting, monitoring, and assurance requirements.

Monitoring and reviewing the process

A very important part of the risk management process is to ensure that any change in the disaster context (including in the situation, the actors and disaster management capabilities and activities), that may have occurred are reflected in the outcomes of the process. Regular monitoring and review are an integral part of the risk management process to ensure that risk continues to be modified in line with risk management and disaster management objectives, with available resources, and with the needs of the community or organisation. It also helps to ensure that the risk treatment continues to be relevant to a changing context.

Some key areas to be considered are:

- New evidence or research.
- The degree to which treatments and mobilised controls for modifying risk are working as intended.
- The emergence of new risks or changes in the nature of risks already identified.
- Changes to existing or the emergence of new vulnerabilities.

COMMUNICATION AND CONSULTATION

High complexity, uncertainty and novelty of disaster-related risk mean that effective communication and consultation are critical to the risk management processes, establishing an adequate understanding about risk with stakeholders, and where necessary changing stakeholder behaviours. Each stakeholder or stakeholder group may have very different knowledge, understanding, and views on the risks they face. Effective risk management requires the sharing of information and perspectives on risk with the goal of achieving a better allocation of scarce resources to enhance community wellbeing. This is particularly the case when dealing with low-probability high-consequence risk, which is not amenable to typical statistical analysis. In most cases risk treatment will depend on the willingness of stakeholders to commit time or financial resources to managing risk.

Risk assessment is a critical process in building understanding and a commitment to act. While the technical aspects of risk assessment are essential, effective communication and consultation underpins every aspect of the process. Even when risks can be managed through very direct treatments such as legislation and regulation, their effectiveness still largely depends on stakeholder support and acceptance.

CONCLUSION

Risk management makes a very important contribution to the field of disaster management. It provides a recognised and repeatable methodology which is used very widely in all aspects of society and the economy. Risk management provides an excellent opportunity to not only guide more effective disaster management but also provide a common approach to allocating scarce resources.

ACTIVITIES

1. In your own words explain the difference between a risk and a hazard.
2. Explain why communication and consultation are so important to decision-making under uncertainty.
3. Identify a disaster-related risk to your community or organisation. How might the risk be reduced, evaluate options, and decide on a course of action? Try using the evaluation criteria used in the chapter.

KEY READINGS

A range of risk management-related handbooks can be downloaded for free from Australian Government websites.

Australian Institute for Disaster Resilience (2021). *Systemic Risk Handbook* https://knowledge.aidr.org.au/resources/handbook-disaster-risk/

Land use Planning for Disaster https://knowledge.aidr.org.au/resources/handbook-land-use-planning/

Note

1. Copyright Executive Impact Consulting 2020, and Gibson and Tarrant (2020), subsequently adopted by AS/NZS 5050 (int): 2020 managing disruption-related risk. Reproduced with permission of the copyright holder.

References

1. van Asselt, M.B.A. and E. Vos, The precautionary principle and the uncertainty paradox. *Journal of Risk Research*, 2006. **9**(4): p. 313–336.
2. Patt, A. and S. Dessai, Communicating uncertainty: Lessons learned and suggestions for climate change assessment. *Comptes Rendus Geoscience*, 2005. **337**(4): p. 425–441.
3. Slovic, P., Trust, emotion, sex, politics, and science: Surveying the risk-assessment battlefield. *Risk Analysis*, 1999. **19**: p. 689–701.
4. Maringe, C., et al., The impact of the COVID-19 pandemic on cancer deaths due to delays in diagnosis in England, UK: A national, population-based, modelling study. *The Lancet Oncology*, 2020. **21**(8): p. 1023–1034.
5. McFarling, U.L. *The COVID cancer effect*. Scientific American, 2021.
6. Angus, D., Application of a risk management approach in a Queensland disaster management context. *The Australian Journal of Emergency Management*, 1997. **12**(1): p. 31–34.
7. Salter, J., Towards a better disaster management methodology. *The Australian Journal of Emergency Management*, 1995. **10**(4): p. 8–16.
8. Vogel, C., Disaster management in South Africa. *South African Journal of Science*, 1998. **94**(3): p. 98–100.
9. Nakabayashi, I. Urban planning based on disaster risk assessment, in *Disaster management in metropolitan areas for the 21st century, Proceedings of the IDNDR Aichi/Nagoya International Conference*. 1994.
10. Quarantelli, E.L., Implications for programmes and policies from future disaster trends. *Risk Management*, 1999. **1**: p. 9–19.
11. Kreps, G.A., Disaster as systemic event and social catalyst: A clarification of subject matter. *International Journal of Mass Emergencies & Disasters*, 1995. **13**(3): p. 255–284.
12. Spence, P.R. and K.A. Lachlan, Disasters, crises, and unique populations: Suggestions for survey research. *New Directions for Evaluation*, 2010. **2010**(126): p. 95–106.
13. Renn, O., S. Krimsky, and D. Golding, *Social theories of risk*. Westport: Praeger, 1992.
14. Beck, U., S. Lash, and B. Wynne, *Risk society: Towards a new modernity*. Vol. 17. 1992, London (UK): Sage.
15. Kettl, D.F., *The future of public administration report of the Special NASPAA/American Political Science Association Task Force*. 2003.
16. Cannon, T., *Reducing people's vulnerability to natural hazards. Communities and resilience, Research paper No. 2008/34, United Nations University, UNU-WIDER*. World Institute for Development Economics Research, 2008.

6

Business continuity management (BCM)

David Parsons[1]

INTRODUCTION

All organisations are potentially at risk of disruption as a result of incidents. Healthcare organisations like other emergency services may face the additional challenge of surging service delivery operations to meet increases in demand caused by an incident, while at the same time managing disruptions to internal processes resulting from the incident. This challenge leads to the implementation of business continuity plans (BCPs) to maintain service continuity while deploying incident response plans.

Healthcare organisations are subject to disruption risks including direct physical damage, restricted resources (including personnel and supplies), loss of critical infrastructure (including water, gas, electricity and internet) and restricted access. To ensure continuity of services at all times, these risks must be managed through the application of business continuity management (BCM) principles and processes.

The aim of this chapter is to examine the principles and practices of good *BCM*. At the end of this chapter, you should be able to

1. Clearly define BCM and its components
2. Identify and understand the steps to develop and maintain a BCP for a healthcare organisation

BUSINESS CONTINUITY – ITS APPLICATION

The ISO: 22301 international standard for Business Continuity Management Systems (BCMS) – Requirements is considered to be the best framework for managing business continuity in an organisation. This chapter draws on the business continuity process as outlined in the international standard. Business continuity is defined as:

'*capability of the organisation to continue delivery of products or services at acceptable predefined levels following a disruptive incident*' [ISO 22301:2012, Terms and Definitions, p. 2]

A BCP is defined as:

'*documented procedures that guide organisations to respond, recover, resume and restore to a pre-defined level of operation following disruption*' [ISO 22301:2012, Terms and Definitions, Pg. 2]

DOI: 10.4324/9781032626604-8

BCPs typically address, but are not limited to, the following seven types of major disruptive events or incidents:

1. Loss of people
2. Denial of access to facilities
3. Loss of technology
4. Failure of suppliers
5. Failure of internal or external dependencies
6. Loss of telecommunications facility
7. Failure of special requirements specific to a function of the business

When invoked, BCPs focus on the consequences of a major disruption or incident, not the cause of the disruption. For example, a flood, fire or police exclusion zone due to criminal activity or terrorist attack could cause denial of access to facilities. The impact that needs to be addressed by the BCP is not being able to access the facility, not the actual flood, fire or police exclusion zone.

It is important to make the distinction between operational robustness and business continuity.

Figure 6.1 is a typical business continuity continuum and depicts the range of responses that may occur on any given incident. The level of response is governed by the nature and impact of the incident.

The impact of incidents can vary significantly. Minor incidents may disrupt an organisation, but the impact can be readily addressed through pre-defined procedures or operating arrangements. Whilst this may be considered business continuity in the sense that there are documented procedures that guide the organisation to absorb the impact of the disruption and to continue to operate using alternate means, this is in fact incident management.

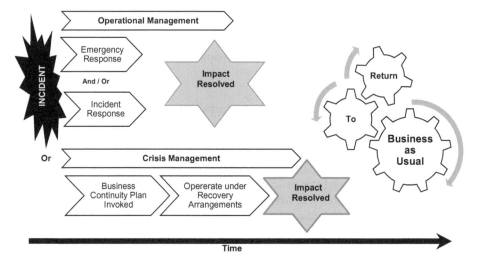

Figure 6.1 Business continuity continuum

Examples of incident management in a hospital environment include:

- Disruption to electricity supplies
- Loss of parts of a hospital complex due to fire or water ingress
- Extended disruption to potable water supplies
- Unexpected patient surge

BCPs may involve operating out of different premises/locations and reducing the range of functions performed to the most critical/bare minimum or redirecting functions to be performed by other teams in the organisation operating from different locations not affected by the disruption.

Operating under the invocation of BCM is considered short-term until the return to business as usual (BAU). Examples of business continuity activation in a healthcare environment include:

- Disruption to medical gas supplies
- Air conditioning failure
- Disruption to staff rostering systems
- Failure of communications systems
- Disruption to catering services
- Disruption to electronic patient records

BUSINESS CONTINUITY PROCESS OVERVIEW

The principles of setting up and managing a BCMS as outlined in ISO 22301:2012, also apply in the context of the healthcare environment. This standard emphasises the importance of:

1. Understanding the organisation's needs and the necessity for establishing BCM policy and objectives,
2. *Implementing and operating controls and measures for managing an organisation's overall capability to manage disruptive incidents,*
3. *Monitoring and reviewing the performance and effectiveness of the BCMS, and*
4. *Continual improvement based on objective measurement.*

[ISO 22301:2012, Introduction, p. 5]

CONTEXT OF THE ORGANISATION

When developing and implementing a BCP that will enable an organisation to recover from a disruption, it is necessary to establish the context of how the organisation operates and the environment in which it operates. This requires an understanding of the organisation's functions, activities, products and services, supply chains, partnerships and relationships with interested parties, and the legal and regulatory context in which it operates. Furthermore, it requires a comprehensive understanding of the links between the business continuity policies and procedures and the organisation's objectives and risk management strategies.

The organisation must identify all internal and external issues that may have the potential to impede its ability to achieve its objectives. Criteria must be established for the level

Table 6.1 Defining the context of a healthcare organisation

Define	*Examples*
Core functions and services	Obstetrics
	Outpatients
	Emergency department
	Mental health etc.
Key resources required to operate	Electricity
	Water
	Sanitation
	Communications systems
	Patient records
	Catering
	Security etc.
Regulations standards and legal obligations	Healthcare accreditation
	Patient confidentiality
Dependencies on key suppliers or service providers	Electricity
	Medical gases
	Laundry services
	Catering
Governance structure	Regulatory requirements
	Board of Directors
	Other healthcare providers

of risk the organisation can accept and still maintain services before crucial action is required e.g., evacuation, removal of services [ISO 22301:2012]. Table 6.1 provides some examples a healthcare facility would need to consider when developing a BCP.

LEADERSHIP AND COMMITMENT

One of the greatest enablers for implementing an effective BCMS within an organisation is executive sponsorship. Executive support legitimises the process, makes it a priority in the organisation and combats complacency.

Examples of how leadership and commitment to business continuity are demonstrated include, but not limited to ensuring:

- Responsibility is defined with the appropriate level of authority and accountability across the organisation e.g., an executive owner identified and incorporated into managers performance agreements
- Policy and objectives align with strategic direction and form part of the governance structure e.g., integrated into business plans and reporting
- Fully integrated with the organisation's processes e.g., requirements for business continuity included in contracts, building design and staff training

- Resources needed are available
- Communication regarding the importance of and compliance with the BCMS is cascaded down through the organisation
- Provide direction and support for all staff ensuing commitment to the BCMS
- Monitor the effectiveness of the BCMS ensuring objectives are met
- Actively engage in testing and exercising the BCMS
- Audit and review BCMS regularly
- Promote continual improvement [ISO 22301:2012].

POLICY AND OBJECTIVES

The above information is generally captured in the BCMS policy. The BCM policy must be appropriate for the purpose of the organisation and provide a framework for the objectives the BCMS must achieve [ISO 22301:2012]. The policy should define, but are not limited to:

- Definition of the type of disruptive events/incidents that are considered in and out of scope of the BCP e.g., in scope – patient call system failure/out of scope – pandemic
- Reference to applicable standards or regulatory/legal requirements e.g., healthcare accreditation standards
- Resources, roles and responsibilities to achieve the objectives e.g., BCM executive owner, business continuity planner, business area managers
- How objectives will be measured e.g., milestones and targets for plan completion and testing
- BCMS monitoring and reporting

RESOURCES/EDUCATION AND AWARENESS/KNOWLEDGE MANAGEMENT

There are various models for resourcing BCM within an organisation. Larger organisations have a team that manages the BCMS and are supported by staff across the organisation that may have the responsibility to manage the BCP for their functional area. Smaller organisations may allocate all responsibilities to one person or make it a part role with another position in the organisation.

It is common to embed responsibility for BCM across the organisation with managers being responsible for their functional area. Consequently, it is very important to ensure that the following elements are in place:

- Job descriptions that formally define the BCM role and responsibility and allocation of time to perform this role when shared with other responsibilities
- Training delivery program including, but not limited to
  - Risk management fundamentals
  - Conducting a business impact assessment
  - Developing and maintaining a BCP
  - Testing a BCP/conducting exercises
- Competency development on, but not limited to, written and oral communication skills, influencing skills

- A robust documenting and auditing process to ensure all BCPs and training are formally managed and maintained including, but not limited to,
  - Being kept up-to-date
  - Version control
  - Formal approval
  - Change tracking
  - Controlled distribution

OPERATIONAL PLANNING AND CONTROL

ISO 22313:2012 BCMS – guidance comprises five key elements in the business continuity cycle, Figure 6.2 [1].

Operational planning and control are essentially programme management and control of the business continuity process within the organisation. This includes defining the methodology, implementation plan and programme management to ensure the BCMS meets the organisation's objectives.

Business risk assessment and impact analysis

The BCM cycle starts with conducting a risk assessment. The risk assessment identifies the sources of risk (hazards and threats) and determines the likelihood of occurrence and consequence to the business. This information is used to inform risk mitigation/treatment actions or the most appropriate recovery strategy should the risk occur.

The risk assessment is the business impact analysis (BIA). This allows the organisation to identify the functions or processes including dependencies, internal and external resources and suppliers that support its key products or services as well as the impact over time of not performing these functions or processes.

The BIA also allows the organisation to define the timeframe within which these functions or processes must be restored before the impact of them not being available would be unacceptable. This is referred to as the *recovery time objective* (RTO) [2][2] and *maximum acceptable outage* (MAO; Table 6.2) [2].[3]

Decisions as to the level of investment in mitigation/treatment actions or recovery strategies are driven by the level of *risk appetite*. A low appetite for risk means that a greater

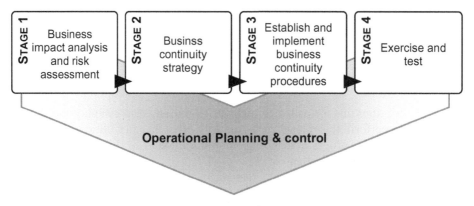

Elements of business continuity management

Figure 6.2 Elements of business continuity management

Table 6.2 Provides an example of suitable headings for a BIA

Business function	Impacts				Highest impact	MAO	Internal short-term workarounds	Comments
	1–4 hours	1 Day	2–7 days	2–4 weeks				

CASE STUDY 6.1 – 2019–2020 AUSTRALIA BUSHFIRES

The 2019–2020 bushfires season in Australia was the worst on record. Over 24 million hectares were burnt. Tragically, 33 people died and extensive smoke coverage across much of eastern Australia may have caused many more deaths. Over 3,000 homes were destroyed. Estimates of the national financial impacts are over $10 billion. The health care system was significantly impacted by supply chain and utility services disruptions. The Royal Commission into Natural Disaster Arrangements conducted by the Australian Government noted:

- "road closures had consequences for other sectors as it made it difficult to resupply towns with water, food, fuel and medical supplies"
- "internet and power failed we had no means of communicating with the outside world, [nor] could we receive information on the status of the fires",
- "the lack of electricity also meant no mobile phone coverage, no water, no petrol"
- "The interconnectedness of systems in society causes cascading consequences in emergencies"

Source: Royal Commission into Natural Disaster Arrangements. Australian Government. 2020 https:/royalcommissions.gov.aau/natural-disasters

---

investment is made in mitigation and recovery. In a hospital setting it may be acceptable to lose the public cafeteria for an extended period, however a disruption to medical gases would not be acceptable for any duration.

When conducting a risk assessment consideration should be given to the through chain organisations the healthcare organisation depends on. The through chain includes suppliers to and those dependent on the health system [3]. Disruptions to through chain partners may have a significant impact on the healthcare organisation. Disruptions to suppliers such as medical gas, medical equipment, utilities, laundry services are important to consider. So too are those organisations who take products and patients from the healthcare organisation such as morgue facilities, patient transfer services and waste services. Healthcare organisations may choose to impose business continuity requirements on through chain organisations to reduce risk.

Business continuity strategy

The business continuity strategy defines the most appropriate way to reduce the impact of or recover from a disruption. It is directly informed by the outcome of the risk assessment and BIA including *risk appetite* and drives the level of investment the business continuity strategy requires.

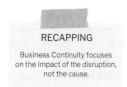

RECAPPING

Business Continuity focuses on the impact of the disruption, not the cause.

Consider the example quoted earlier of a denial of access to facilities due to a flood, fire or police exclusion zone. Business continuity strategies combined with a risk treatment may consider ensuring that critical facilities such as emergency power generators or data centres are not located in building basements due to the risk of flooding. Discussions could be held with police or fire authorities so they have a better understanding of your organisation's critical operations and the impact that an exclusion zone or fire response may have. This level of preparation and investment in building relationships and mutual understanding of key actions and priorities can significantly reduce the impact of a disruption.

Considerations for business continuity strategy involve decisions on whether to invest in protective treatments that may reduce the likelihood or duration of a disruption. Other strategies are to assume that the impact of the disruption falls outside of the level of investment for risk mitigation/treatments and that the function must be recovered or resumed using resources not impacted by the disruption, often from another location.

It is necessary to have a very clear understanding of the resources required to support the function. There is a distinction between the resources required when operating in BAU and the resources required under business continuity. Often decisions are made to only provide a subset of full functions or services when operating under business continuity arrangements, hence it is only these resources that need to be identified in a BCP. This includes, but not limited to staff, technology, physical facilities, specialised technologies or facilities, transportation, key suppliers and internal dependencies.

Examples of business continuity strategies in a healthcare context may include providing:

- Manually operated resuscitation equipment for electricity disruptions
- Portable gas bottles for medical gas disruption

Business continuity procedures

This relates to controlling the response to a disruptive incident. Business Continuity Teams work under the coordination of an organisation's Incident Management Team (IMT). The role of the IMT is to manage the overall incident. During a major disruption event, these teams work together to manage the recovery of the key functions of the organisation so they return to BAU.

BCPs are activated when a disruption to one or more business functions is expected to exceed the MAO for that function. The activation of a BCP may involve the activation of the organisation's IMT. An IMT may already be activated due to the hazard causing the disruption. Organisations with mature BCM processes may automatically invoke a BCP in response to a disruption with formal notification back to the IMT that business continuity has been activated for the impacted area of the business.

The key tool used is a BCP. The BCP addresses the following, but not limited to, key components:

- Description of the business function being addressed by the plan
- Defined roles and responsibilities and authority for people enacting the plan to recover the business function
- Resources required to recover the business function
- Procedures to follow in the event of a disruption including:
  - Engagement with the IMT
  - Contact details to determine the welfare of staff and patients

- Options and procedures to respond to the disruption and prioritised actions
- A communications plan for staff, management, internal and external dependencies and key suppliers
- Procedures to recover operations under business continuity arrangements and to return to BAU when appropriate

Exercising and testing

An important element of implementing a BCP is exercising and testing the BCP. This process is the key control measure to ensure that BCPs can be relied upon to recover from a disruption within the specified RTO. BCPs should be tested annually at a minimum. A variety of methods can be used for test including:

- *Desktop walk through* – BCP owners are presented with a scenario, and they walk through their plans to check that they appropriately address the scenario.
- *Facilities test* – special recovery facilities such as equipment at back up or recovery locations are tested. Sometimes equipment is stored at the location and needs to be set up when recovery is required. Facilities testing provides ideal training for staff and ensures the equipment is maintained, working properly and has up-to-date software.
- *Full recovery tests* – conducted when the *risk appetite* is such that partial testing such as the desktop walk throughs or facilities test is not deemed sufficient. Whilst a full recovery test ensures that all staff, stakeholders and equipment or facilities required for a recovery are fully tested, there is a level of disruption to the business. Full recovery tests involve actually implementing the BCP in full.

Many organisations conduct a combination of these tests so as to minimise disruption to the business and ensure all key stakeholders are involved in the process.

Performance evaluation and continuous improvement

As with any management process, the BCMS needs to be constantly monitored for efficiency and effectiveness and to identify opportunities for improvement. Characteristics of a performance evaluation and continuous improvement process may include, but are not limited to:

- Review of performance against a set of metrics such as:
  - Completing the development, review, and testing of BCPs within specified timeframes
  - Evidence of test results
  - Evidence of achieving recovery within RTOs
- Evidence of meeting compliance or legal obligations where appropriate
- Identification and implementation of opportunities for continuous improvement
- Independent review of performance metrics by senior management and internal or external audit
- Bi-annual updates of the BCM policy, framework and procedures

COORDINATING INCIDENTS

The response to a disruptive event in a healthcare organisation may require the implementation of BCPs for multiple business services and systems. The disruption could be caused by an event external to the healthcare organisation such as a flood or hurricane.

The healthcare organisation may be required to interact with the local community's disaster response agencies.

To effectively co-ordinate internal resources, a healthcare organisation requires a method of establishing a quick decision-making team. The team collects and assesses information, liaises with external agencies, decides course of action, and task business units in a coordinated manner. Where there is a requirement to work in an integrated way with community disaster responders, it is an advantage to use a response system they will understand such as the Incident Command System (ICS). The components and functions of the ICS are discussed in detail in Chapter 16.

CONCLUSION

This chapter has provided an overview of the nature and purpose of business continuity, when it is applied and how it interacts with the IMT. Business continuity is a professional discipline with formal accreditation offered by several institutions. Below is some recommended reading for those seeking to gain a better understanding of the discipline:

KEY READINGS

Standards

- ISO 22301 – Business Continuity Management Systems – Requirements
- ISO 22313 – Business Continuity Management Systems – Guidance

Organisations

- Business Continuity Institute Good Business Guide – *www.bci.org*

ACTIVITY

Consider a healthcare organisation with which you are familiar and identify strategies that could be used to maintain its services in the event of a major disaster.

Notes

1. With acknowledgement to previous author Peter Brouggy.
2. Period of time following an incident within which the product or service must be resumed, or activity must be resumed, or resources must be recovered.
3. Time it would take for adverse impacts, which might arise as a result of not providing a product/service or performing an activity, to become unacceptable.

References

1. ISO *ISO 22313:2012 Societal security-business continuity management systems-guidance* 2012.
2. The British Standards Institution. *ISO 22301 business continuity management.*
3. Parker, C.F., Complex negative events and the diffusion of crisis: Lessons from the 2010 and 2011 Icelandic volcanic ash cloud events. *Geografiska Annaler: Series A, Physical Geography*, 2015. **97**(1): p. 97–108.

7
Risk and crisis communication during health disasters

Amisha Mehta, Ingrid Larkin, Bob Jensen, and Robina Xavier

INTRODUCTION AND OBJECTIVES

From responding to a disease outbreak to the recall of a pharmaceutical product, communication plays an essential role in health disasters. Health disasters can emerge directly from events like pandemics or occur following organisational or natural disasters (e.g., heatwaves). Health disaster communication can be a contested space of many voices. Influenced by media, politicians, corporations, and faith-based groups, the way health organisations communicate prior to, during, and following health disasters is critical to public safety.

This chapter identifies concepts that guide good practice in risk and crisis communication. At the end of this chapter, you should be able to:

1. Value trust as the foundation for effective communication.
2. Outline the importance of identifying and maintaining relationships with stakeholders.
3. Understand the role of response agencies, community, and the media.
4. Apply risk and crisis communication message design strategies.
5. Understand the challenges and opportunities for health disaster communication.

TRUST AS THE FOUNDATION FOR EFFECTIVE HEALTH DISASTER COMMUNICATION

Trust is a critical for effective communication during health disasters. Trust is defined as:

> The willingness of a party to be vulnerable to the actions of another party based on the expectation that the other will perform a particular action important to the trustor, irrespective of the ability to monitor or control that other party.
>
> [1]

This definition reflects several key constructs that are critical to healthcare in general but become even more significant during crisis.

DOI: 10.4324/9781032626604-9

Studies of trust in government risk and crisis communication further consider the components or dimensions of trust. Specifically, these dimensions comprise competence, fairness, integrity, transparency, objectivity, honesty, empathy, commitment, and accountability [2]. During health disasters, organisational messages should reflect these dimensions. For example, a health department could signal transparency by inviting key stakeholders to participate in decision-making.

Ideally, organisations and communities have trust and social capital prior to health disasters. However, trust can be swiftly created [3] and should be formalised for long-term benefit [4]. A fundamental strategy to support such trust and social capital is community engagement [5]. A strong relationship among key parties before, during, and after disasters creates social capital, whereby enabling public relations and communication activities to achieve positive social outcomes [6]. There are multiple ways to engage communities and other stakeholders from deep integration into decision-making, to policy commitments, or public-facing activities such as the communication of information [7]. The value of long-term community relations programs is their ability to build community capability when disasters occur [8]. Engagement is a two-way process and organisation staff and leadership need to understand the concepts of active listening to help foster a strong relationship.

KEY COMMUNICATION STAKEHOLDERS IN HEALTH DISASTERS

Stakeholders are people or organisations with a stake or interest in an organisation and its actions. Stakeholder analysis can help identify and prioritise stakeholders and define strategies that support organisations [9]. During health disasters, there are several critical stakeholders including response agencies (e.g., government), community members, and media. Relationships with these stakeholders can be inter-related or path-dependent. For example, before an organisation communicates, it must have sufficient data, which may emerge from other response agencies. In infectious disease outbreaks, public information officers will often leverage existing relationships with subject matter experts to provide content about the disease and broaden engagement [10].

To appropriately identify stakeholders, an organisation could identify stakeholders by using lists such as this presented by Pereno and Eriksson [11]:

- National or international authorities
- Policy makers and advisers
- Public decision-makers
- Universities and research centres
- Non-government organisations
- Professional groups
- Pharmaceutical companies
- Health providers
- Patients
- Patient associations
- Community and community groups
- Media
- Allied health networks
- Related industries (e.g., component manufacturers).

Table 7.1 Framework for stakeholder analysis

Stakeholder	Interest	Knowledge	Urgency	Power
Patient	High – moderate - low/no	High – moderate - low/no	High – moderate - low/no	High – moderate - low/no
Government	High – moderate - low/no	High – moderate - low/no	High – moderate - low/no	High – moderate - low/no
Media	High – moderate - low/no	High – moderate - low/no	High – moderate - low/no	High – moderate - low/no

Source: Franco-Trigo et al., 2020 [9]

Following on from the identification of stakeholders, it is useful to evaluate these stakeholders. First, at an individual level, each stakeholder group comprises attributes that are general and particular to the disaster at hand. These attributes comprise interest level, knowledge or awareness of issue or disaster, urgency, and power or influence [9]. A framework to guide stakeholder analysis is provided in Table 7.1.

Second, it is useful to consider how stakeholders are connected to each other. Such a network-based view may highlight where multi-stakeholder groups can add pressure or enable the actions of the core organisation. Furthermore, some stakeholders may be able to communicate with greater conviction or impact and relevance than the core organisation, which may lead to collaborative responses. Overall, before an organisation engages in risk or crisis communication it is important to understand, define and prioritise, where possible with data, its stakeholders. Doing so will enable a stronger outcome for communication and operational actions.

COMMUNICATION WITHIN AND BETWEEN RESPONSE AGENCIES

Responding to health disasters often involves multiple response agencies such as regulators and government. For example, pandemic response organisations include governments, the World Health Organisation (WHO), pharmaceutical companies, hospitals, medical associations (e.g., Australian Medical Association), and regulators (e.g., Therapeutic Goods Administration, Australia). This sub-section covers the way information is shared among response agencies, the role of technology to capture actions, and communication frameworks that can structure within-agency decision-making.

Information sharing, communication modalities, and redundancy among response agencies

Cooperation and alignment are especially important in international health disasters. Often the WHO and its frameworks guide responses of individual country members. For example, the WHO's pandemic phases are aligned to the response strategies of individual nation states. However, past studies highlighted opportunities to ensure a common understanding of phases [12], the accurate depiction of threat to avoid public confusion [13]. Coordination within and between nation states is critically important as divergence in messaging across different levels of health authorities during the COVID-19 pandemic has also led to public confusion in countries such as the United States and Australia.

Logging of disaster communications including software applications

During health disasters, information moves quickly within and between response agencies. In addition, crisis decision-making teams operate on a roster system to manage fatigue and support optimal performance. These factors support the use of crisis management software applications like EMQnet (emqnet.com) from Dynamiq and Noggin (noggin.io). For example, EMQnet is designed to support organisational resilience and comprises platforms to train for and manage crises or disasters alongside ongoing risk management. It is used by multinational organisations to gather and record informational inputs from experts or those directly involved in the crisis to other decision-makers, communicate at speed to other critical stakeholders, and enable collaboration alongside individual task activity. Critically, the system records and retains information so that post-disaster reviews and learning can examine critical decision points to support professional practice.

Agency communication frameworks

As illustrated with EMQnet, a framework is useful to guide communication inputs. In health and emergency response settings, there are several frameworks that structure communication within and between clinical and response teams such as ISBAR and METHANE.

The ISBAR framework, endorsed by WHO, provides a standardised approach across different clinical events and can reduce power differences that may impact effective transfer of information [14].

The ISBAR framework comprises five elements:

I – Introduction
Who are you? What is your role? Where are you? Why are you communicating?
S – Situation
What is happening at the moment?
B – Background
What are the issues that led up to this situation?
A – Assessment
What do you believe the problem is?
R – Recommendation
What do you recommend to correct the situation?

In the United Kingdom, the Joint Emergency Services Interoperability Programme (JESIP) links emergency services providers so a multi-agency response is organised, structured and practised. JESIP is one group that uses the M/ETHANE framework as the common model to pass information between emergency responders and control rooms. There are seven elements to the M/ETHANE framework:

M – Major incident declared?
E – Exact location
T – Type of incident
H – Hazards present or suspected
A – Access – routes that are safe to use
N – Number, type, and severity of casualties

E – Emergency services present and required

For further information, see: https://www.jesip.org.uk/methane.

These frameworks share common elements including situational assessments and action steps. The adoption of ISBAR or METHANE could support inter- and intra-organisational communication by enabling the transfer of information in a consistent and structured way.

COMMUNICATION WITH THE COMMUNITY

Community as a key communication stakeholder

Health disasters affect communities directly and indirectly. They can bring uncertainty and variance in warning and response times, providing significant challenges to both responding organisations and other stakeholders. For health disasters with longer lead times, gaining and maintaining the attention and trust of community members is critical to their perception of, and response to the hazard [2, 15].

Communities comprise individuals and groups (e.g., households and community groups), and businesses. People in communities have diverse experiences, interests, and backgrounds. People will engage with and respond to risk information depending on their individual characteristics including demographics (e.g., age and gender), personality, self-efficacy, and past experiences [16, 17]. Understanding these individual differences, and tailoring communication to suit these differences is important prior to and in response to disasters [18]. In response to COVID-19, the Centers for Disease Control and Prevention (CDC) curated and updated regular guidance with information tailored to different audiences from employers and businesses to educators and school administrators, individuals, and healthcare professionals (see https://www.cdc.gov/coronavirus/2019-ncov/communication/guidance.html).

Community-led communication

Community members who become both the source and recipient of critical information during disasters more commonly model these experiences. Existing research shows that people found local sources or information more persuasive than media appeals [19]. At the same time, the accuracy of this information is critical and can contribute to misinformation. Understanding and working within the networks of communities is an important way to enhance relationships prior to health disasters.

MEDIA AS A KEY COMMUNICATION STAKEHOLDER

Understanding the dynamic landscape of media is essential for disaster managers. Both traditional and social media are an important source of information.

Traditional media

There are many types of traditional media, which broadly comprise print (e.g., newspapers) and broadcast mediums (e.g., television). In traditional media, information (i.e., either from a health department via media release) is evaluated by editors, producers, or journalists. This evaluation process is undertaken by experienced and trained professionals who commit to ethical codes. The process may result in a news story, or the decision to not publish or share information. This process is critical to building trust in the news story content and the credibility of the sources. It reflects an information verification process undertaken behind the scenes to assure the accuracy and trustworthiness of the content.

Journalists will first make a decision about whether to publish the content or not reflecting on the link between the story and news values such as deviance and social significance [20]. For example, news about deviant or unusual and infrequent events could be produced following pharmaceutical product recalls and news about social significance would be reflected by pandemics [20]. Within these broad categories, other news values include stories about people or organisations with prominence, power, or influence. Once newsworthiness has been determined, the journalist will determine the nature and angle of the story, its content, and the sources quoted. Where possible, journalists will provide two spokespeople to reflect balance in the story.

In addition, it is important to remember the differences between each type of medium. Generally, print and online news media can present detailed information. For example, this could include timelines of events and maps that plot the areas affected by smoke haze. While visuals are integrated into print and online news media, broadcast channels (e.g., television and radio) require specific visual content. Television requires access to or the provision of videos and/or spokespeople either from the organisation or affected stakeholders. Radio may not require visual content, but it certainly relies on the provision of "grabs" or short statements from organisational or affected stakeholders. Critically, in addition to broadcasting news material, television and radio stations also promote stories via digital media channels (e.g., Facebook and Twitter) to encourage more audiences to engage with the content.

Digital or social media platforms

Social media platforms such as Twitter, Facebook, and Reddit are integral channels during health disasters. For some audiences, they become the primary source of new or up-to-date information given the speed at which organisations can update social media content.

Social media takes on several functions for multiple users during disasters from signalling and detecting events, to working as a platform that connects multiple users to share information about disasters and recovery processes [21], and to gather information, share and observe emotions [22].

However, unlike traditional media, a social media post may not go through a verification process. For example, individual influencers or bloggers may have many followers, but may lack formal training in journalism and post content that may support self-interest, rather than public interest. As a result, digital and social media platforms may comprise verified and unverified content. Both sensationalism and unverified content can challenge the accuracy of risk information about disasters and bias the way people assess and respond to the risks they face.

The functions of social media in the response and post-event recovery stages are identified in Figure 7.1

Media effects and consumption

Media in traditional and digital forms produce different effects. Researchers identify that disaster media effects can range from creating awareness, shaping perceptions, and triggering mental and behavioural health reactions as well as perceptions of trust and distrust in organisations responsible for health disasters [21]. Some of these effects, such as shaping attitudes to maintain non-pharmaceutical interventions during pandemics, are

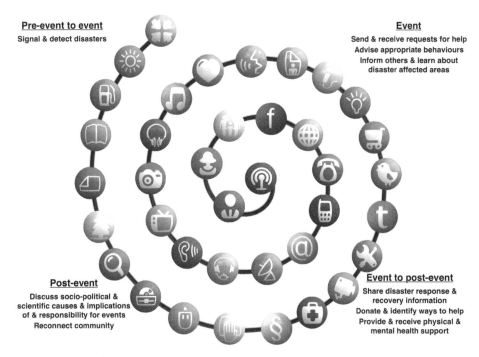

Pre-event to event
Signal & detect disasters

Event
Send & receive requests for help
Advise appropriate behaviours
Inform others & learn about
disaster affected areas

Post-event
Discuss socio-political &
scientific causes & implications
of & responsibility for events
Reconnect community

Event to post-event
Share disaster response &
recovery information
Donate & identify ways to help
Provide & receive physical &
mental health support

Figure 7.1 Functions of disaster social media – adapted from Houston et al. 2015 [23]

CASE STUDY 7.1 – MEDIA REPORTING OF HEALTH DISASTERS

As a public utility, water is critical to strong public health outcomes. Yet, even developed countries experience problems with the quality of water supplied. When water is contaminated or not fit for consumption, public health advisories are issued by authorities and often also through the media. For example, the CDC provides specific information to support advisories about the need to boil water (https://www.cdc.gov/healthywater/emergency/drinking/drinking-water-advisories/boil-water-advisory.html).

A study examined the extent to which CDC guidelines for boil water advisories were incorporated into local news media by comparing a CDC press release with 1,040 local news articles across 38 states in the US [25]. The news release comprised these elements: (a) who is impacted, (b) the cause of the impact, (c) how to sanitise water for consumption, and (d) the uses of boiled water (e.g., drinking and brushing teeth).

In comparison, although the majority of local news articles reflected the water system impacted, affected population, and cause of the boil water advisory, there were key failings. Only half of these articles included information about how water should be boiled and only 3% included the complete instructions for boiling water [25]. This finding highlights an opportunity to educate journalists about risk communication content and the importance of using multiple sources to communicate such advisories.

positive and intended. However, it is important to be ready to support the unintended effects of disaster media (e.g., anxiety).

Now more prevalent than ever are patterns of multiple media use or their convergence by individual users [24]. Through media convergence, people integrate information from multiple media, reflecting complex patterns of media use and understanding of news and sources [24]. For organisations responsible for communicating during health disasters, this means communication should be issued across multiple channels that are controlled by the organisation (e.g., health department Facebook page) as well as through others' pages (e.g., politician or key opinion leader Facebook page). Doing so helps people connect different information sources and also share information.

RISK AND CRISIS COMMUNICATION

Risk and crisis communication primarily occur at a time when people are vulnerable. In this context, an organisation's communication philosophy is as important as the message. Experts highlight the value of empathy:

"People (especially people who are upset) don't care what you know until they know that you care" (Sandman 2008, p.1) [26].

Rickard [27] defined two types of risk communication:

Pragmatic risk communication is a strategic, one- or two-way, and sometimes iterative process of sharing information, often, but not exclusively, with an intended outcome, such as limiting exposure to a given hazard; message, such as avoiding a geographic location; messenger, such as a government agency; and audience, such as a local community.

Constitutive risk communication is the act of communicating about risk, intentionally or unintentionally: (re)creates the definition of "risk" for a given social context, and suggests how we can, and/or should relate to it; contributes to identity and expertise (re)formation; and involves questions of trust, fairness, and power.

(p. 468)

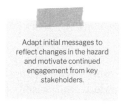

Adapt initial messages to reflect changes in the hazard and motivate continued engagement from key stakeholders.

Both types of risk communication can feature within campaigns or programs, yet, the urgency of the health disaster may naturally preference pragmatic risk communication. However, such risk communication should identify and tailor communication to suit an intended outcome such as creating awareness of the disaster and motivating protective action. In addition, the message is likely to need to adapt to changes presented by the disaster, for example, when an infectious disease outbreak crosses international borders.

The outcome and content of communication can be supported by three types of informational strategies: instructing, adjusting, and internalising [28]. *Instructing* information contains content to advise people about how to physically respond by noting specific and immediate behaviours. Instructional messages can comprise appeals that are direct and rational, threat/fear-driven, positive (to reward compliance), normative (to appeal to social consensus), or designed around behavioural inputs [29]. *Adjusting* information includes content that helps people psychologically cope with the event [28]. For example, this content could reassure community members about the presence of health services personnel. Finally, *internalising* information helps people formulate an image about the organisation [28] and is more commonly recognised in the public relations literature as an approach to help restore or improve the post-disaster image or reputation of emergency services organisations.

Risk communication message design and dissemination

There are many principles that guide the development of effective messages. Following from Sturges [28], Sellnow et al. [30] note that instructional messages should reflect these four components of the IDEA model:

- Internalisation: How am I and those I care about affected and to what degree?
- Explanation: What is happening, why, and what are officials doing in response to it?
- Action: What specific actions should I and those I care about take/not for self-protection?
- Distribution via variety of channels.

Ongoing risk communication should be clear, specific, accurate, certain, and consistent [31]. One challenge is to balance message content sufficiency with message length and the time frame of the disaster. It is important to recognise the potential for message habituation or fatigue.

Effective measures communicate content in clear, specific and accurate ways and maintain consistency

The tools and channels to disseminate messages should be selected to reach and engage different stakeholders. Organisations must fully consider the challenges of media convergence, multiple channels, balanced with the potential consequences for misinformation.

Crisis misinformation

Misinformation challenges organisations and especially during crises or disasters. Misinformation is defined as "explicitly false" information [32]. Crisis misinformation can include speculation, false information, misinterpreted information, and inconsistent information and arise from internal or external sources [33]. It has severe implications on trust in information and sources, protective actions, and organisational reputations [33].

Countering misinformation is a critical yet complex task, [33, 34] but there are several strategies organisations can use. In a public health crisis setting, Van der Meer and Jin [34] showed how corrective information (e.g., rebuttal or factual elaboration) that counters misinformation severity can change participants' attitudes about the crisis but does not motivate a change of behaviour. Crisis misinformation correction strategies could also re-assert the organisation as the authoritative voice for the crisis [33]. The prevalence of misinformation means communicators should be ready for it prior to disasters.

POST-DISASTER REVIEW

Following a disaster, an organisation should take the time to review disaster management and communication to identify areas of strength, and those in need of improvement. Ideally, this process should integrate different stakeholders to provide multiple viewpoints to highlight potential issues about the decisions or reactions of decision-makers internal to organisations as well as external issues such as a fall in public trust or confidence.

CHALLENGES AND OPPORTUNITIES

There are many challenges and opportunities in health disasters. Some of the key areas to consider during the planning and execution phases are:

- Avoid assumptions: It is best to not assume that all audiences interpret the message similarly. Individuals bring different lenses, biases, and experiences to information, leading to different interpretations and responses. Organisations can address this by using multiple channels, sources, and message frames.
- Create connections but expect non-compliance: Full compliance is ideal but rare. Some people may refuse vaccination [35], or fail to follow medical treatment, potentially risking their life. One way to communicate with diverse and disengaged audiences is to create connections with trusted opinion leaders who might add an alternative, but valuable perspective to the more traditional voices and arguments during disasters.
- Expect and respond to stress: Uncertainty and stress impact the decision-making of the community and of health communicators. Organisations must prepare for the impact of uncertainty and stress by designing messages and templates that reflect key message principles.

ACTIVITIES

Please read this short case study and answer questions to reinforce your learning. During a localised infectious disease outbreak, Townside Hospital was responsible for caring for a small town's patients. Together with the local Mayor, the Townside Hospital Chief Executive Officer (CEO) delivered daily media conferences to update the town about the outbreak, advise people about how to protect themselves from the outbreak (e.g., checking symptoms), and share the progress of affected citizens. Following one media conference, a post appeared on the town's Facebook page from a resident: *Townside Hospital is unsafe. There have been containment breaches and now my wife and children are unwell. The CEO should be fired and patients shifted for care to the out of our town to the major hospital in the city.*

- What else could daily media updates include?
- If you were working as the communication lead for Townside Hospital, what steps would you take to assess this post on the Facebook page?
- What are two ways you could respond to this post? Which one would you choose and why?
- What could you add to future daily media conferences in an attempt to mitigate this from happening again?

KEY READINGS

These papers are selected to enhance professional development in communication during health disasters.

1. This article provides key principles for message design during disasters including message principles: Sutton, J., E.S. Spiro, B. Johnson, S. Fitzhugh, B. Gibson, and C.T. Butts, Warning tweets: Serial transmission of messages during the warning phase

of a disaster event. *Information, Communication & Society*, 2014. 17(6): p. 765–787. https://doi.org/10.1080/1369118X.2013.862561

2. This article shares practical insights from public health communicators: Jin, Y., L. Austin, S. Vijaykumar, H. Jun, and G. Nowak, Communicating about infections disease threats: Insights from public health information officers. *Public Relations Review*, 2019. 45: p. 167–177. https://doi.org/10.1016/j.pubrev.2018.12.003

References

1. Mayer, R.C., J.H. Davis, and F.D. Schoorman, An integrative model of organizational trust. *Academy of Management Review*, 1995. 20(3): p. 709–734.
2. Liu, B.F. and A.M. Mehta, From the periphery and toward a centralized model for trust in government risk and disaster communication. *Journal of Risk Research*, 2021. 24(7): p. 853–869.
3. Mehta, A.M., A. Bruns, and J. Newton, Trust, but verify: Social media models for disaster management. *Disasters*, 2017. 41(3): p. 549–565.
4. Tschannen-Moran, M. and W.K. Hoy, A multidisciplinary analysis of the nature, meaning, and measurement of trust. *Review of Educational Research*, 2000. 70(4): p. 547–593.
5. Kang, M. and Y.E. Park, Exploring trust and distrust as conceptually and empirically distinct constructs: Association with symmetrical communication and public engagement across four pairings of trust and distrust. *Journal of Public Relations Research*, 2017. 29(2–3): p. 114–135.
6. Taylor, M. and M.L. Kent, Dialogic engagement: Clarifying foundational concepts. *Journal of Public Relations Research*, 2014. 26(5): p. 384–398.
7. Sloan, P., Redefining stakeholder engagement: From control to collaboration. *Journal of Corporate Citizenship*, 2009. (36): p. 25–40.
8. Heath, R.L. and M. Palenchar, Community relations and risk communication: A longitudinal study of the impact of emergency response messages. *Journal of Public Relations Research*, 2000. 12(2): p. 131–161.
9. Franco-Trigo, L., et al., Stakeholder analysis in health innovation planning processes: A systematic scoping review. *Health Policy*, 2020. 124(10): p. 1083–1099.
10. Jin, Y., et al., Communicating about infectious disease threats: Insights from public health information officers. *Public Relations Review*, 2019. 45(1): p. 167–177.
11. Pereno, A. and D. Eriksson, A multi-stakeholder perspective on sustainable healthcare: From 2030 onwards. *Futures*, 2020. 122: p. 102605.
12. Abeysinghe, S. and S. Abeysinghe, *Categorizing H1N1—the pandemic alert phases*. Pandemics, Science and Policy: H1N1 and the World Health Organization, 2015: p. 64–101.
13. Meymarian, M. and W. Parker, A next generation pandemic advisory system: Containing pandemic outbreaks though education and timely dissemination of information. *Journal of Homeland Security*, 2009: p. 1–17. https://parmey.com/wp-content/uploads/2009-Article_Pandemic_Planning.pdf
14. Burgess, A., et al., Teaching clinical handover with ISBAR. *BMC Medical Education*, 2020. 20(2): p. 1–8.
15. Laughery, K.R. and M.S. Wogalter, A three-stage model summarizes product warning and environmental sign research. *Safety Science*, 2014. 61: p. 3–10.
16. Cialdini, R.B. and N.J. Goldstein, Social influence: Compliance and conformity. *Annual Review of Psychology*, 2004. 55: p. 591–621.
17. Yang, Z.J., A.M. Aloe, and T.H. Feeley, Risk information seeking and processing model: A meta-analysis. *Journal of Communication*, 2014. 64(1): p. 20–41.
18. Strahan, K., J. Whittaker, and J. Handmer, Self-evacuation archetypes in Australian bushfire. *International Journal of Disaster Risk Reduction*, 2018. 27: p. 307–316.
19. Brenkert-Smith, H., et al., Social amplification of wildfire risk: The role of social interactions and information sources. *Risk Analysis*, 2013. 33(5): p. 800–817.
20. Shoemaker, P.J. and A.A. Cohen, *News around the world: Content, practitioners, and the public.* 2012, Routledge.
21. Houston, J.B., M.L. Spialek, and J. First, Disaster media effects: A systematic review and synthesis based on the differential susceptibility to media effects model. *Journal of Communication*, 2018. 68(4): p. 734–757.

22. Neubaum, G., et al., Psychosocial functions of social media usage in a disaster situation: A multi-methodological approach. *Computers in Human Behavior*, 2014. 34: p. 28–38.

23. Houston, J.B., et al., Social media and disasters: A functional framework for social media use in disaster planning, response, and research. *Disasters*, 2015. 39(1): p. 1–22.

24. Yuan, E., News consumption across multiple media platforms: A repertoire approach. *Information, Communication & Society*, 2011. 14(7): p. 998–1016.

25. O'Shay, S., et al., Boil water advisories as risk communication: Consistency between CDC guidelines and local news media articles. *Health Communication*, 2022. 37(2): p. 152–162.

26. Sandman, P., Handling explosive emotions demands five acts of empathy. *ISHN*, 2008. 42(1): p. 24–26.

27. Rickard, L.N., Pragmatic and (or) constitutive? On the foundations of contemporary risk communication research. *Risk Analysis*, 2021. 41(3): p. 466–479.

28. Sturges, D.L., Communicating through crisis: A strategy for organizational survival. *Management Communication Quarterly*, 1994. 7(3): p. 297–316.

29. Mehta, A.M., et al., Encouraging evacuation: The role of behavioural message inputs in bushfire warnings. *International Journal of Disaster Risk Reduction*, 2022. 67: p. 102673.

30. Sellnow, D.D., et al., The IDEA model as a best practice for effective instructional risk and crisis communication. *Communication Studies*, 2017. 68(5): p. 552–567.

31. Sutton, J., et al., Warning tweets: Serial transmission of messages during the warning phase of a disaster event. *Information, Communication & Society*, 2014. 17(6): p. 765–787.

32. Tan, A.S., C.-j. Lee, and J. Chae, Exposure to health (mis) information: Lagged effects on young adults' health behaviors and potential pathways. *Journal of Communication*, 2015. 65(4): p. 674–698.

33. Mehta, A.M., et al., A process view of crisis misinformation: How public relations professionals detect, manage, and evaluate crisis misinformation. *Public Relations Review*, 2021. 47(2): p. 102040.

34. Van der Meer, T.G. and Y. Jin, Seeking formula for misinformation treatment in public health crises: The effects of corrective information type and source. *Health Communication*, 2020. 35(5): p. 560–575.

35. Velan, B., et al., Major motives in non-acceptance of A/H1N1 flu vaccination: The weight of rational assessment. *Vaccine*, 2011. 29(6): p. 1173–1179.

8

Community engagement

Ghasem-Sam Toloo, Marie Fredriksen, and Stacey Pizzino

INTRODUCTION AND OBJECTIVES

One of the fundamental shifts that has occurred in disaster management over recent decades has been a change in emphasis from an almost complete focus on response agencies towards a more holistic approach that involves all aspects of community working in partnership to achieve improved whole-of-community outcomes. This greater involvement of the community directly permeates throughout the disaster management and risk reduction process.

The concepts that underpin this chapter are derived from those of disaster resilience and building a resilient community through engagement. Community engagement is important as it enhances resilience and long-term sustainability of the community by building trust and sharing the knowledge, experience, decision, and burden among the citizens and authorities.

On completion of this chapter, you should be able to:

1. Explain community engagement in disaster risk management.
2. Identify the factors that contribute to effective community engagement in disaster risk management.
3. Understand the significance of evaluating effective community engagement.

COMMUNITY ENGAGEMENT

It may be useful to clarify the concept of community within the disaster management context. Defining community and its characteristics can be complicated. Communities can be regarded as a source of strong values and spirit, of complex social units and systems operating within specific boundaries, often with a shared sense of identity, meaning, and common interests. Within the context of disaster management, the definition of community used throughout this chapter will be that of MacQueen et al. [1]

a group of people with diverse characteristics who are linked by social ties, share common perspectives, and engage in joint action in geographical locations or settings

DOI: 10.4324/9781032626604-10

This definition is also useful for our purpose as it encompasses the major characteristics that are important for engaging with heterogeneous communities in disaster management. This includes socio-demographic differences (e.g., age and gender), cultural diversity (e.g., ethnicity), and shared perspectives (e.g., religious). Effective disaster risk management should draw upon these characteristics to enable the participation of all community members, whereby leading to long-term resilience.

In this context, it is useful to define the concept. Brisbane Declaration [2] defined community engagement as:

A two-way process by which the aspirations, concerns, needs and values of citizens and communities are incorporated at all levels and in all sectors in policy development, planning, decision-making, service delivery and assessment; and by which governments and other business and civil society organisations involve citizens, clients, communities and other stakeholders in these processes.

In a more recent study, Johnston and colleagues [3] defined community engagement as:

A relational process that facilitates understanding and evaluation, involvement, exchange of information and opinions, about a concept, issue or project, with the aim of building social capital and enhancing social outcomes through decision-making.

While these definitions do not clarify the mechanisms of engagement, they emphasise the reciprocal responsibility and active participation and partnership in information sharing and decision-making relevant to the needs and values of the communities with the aim of improving the social outcomes. A notable distinction in the former definition is that it emphasises that communities are to be seen as stakeholders in the process, a valuable source of information on which disaster-planning authorities must capitalise.

COMMUNITY AS STAKEHOLDERS

Community engagement is closely linked to seeing people or citizens as stakeholders. The concept of stakeholders is equally difficult to define despite the constancy of reliance on *stakeholder engagement* as a cornerstone of modern management principles, particularly in disaster risk management. While literally meaning those "holding a stake in the outcome", some distinguish stakeholders from service providers or emergency responders, while others limit the use of the term to community representation. As mentioned above, community is a diffuse and movable concept, but regardless of how a community is defined, it is inevitably a composite of all its component parts. This includes its citizens, response organisations, government representatives, and officials.

One significant aspect of seeing community as stakeholders is shared decision-making. Community decision-making is not the same as individual decision-making. An individual can indeed weigh up the alternatives and make a best-case decision. However, decision-making processes at the community level are much more complex and are further aggravated by the intricate nature of communities. Additionally, individual and community priorities before an event may differ significantly after the event [4]. A broken piece of china seems far less important when someone has lost their home to fire or flood.

Collective decision-making may result in decisions that are combinations of elements from various perspectives that ultimately may not be favoured by all. To reduce conflict, it is important a common ground is reached to ensure decisions made provide the greatest good for the greatest number. For example, a part of the flood mitigation strategy in the Netherlands involves deliberately inundating some populated areas in order to prevent flooding in the wider community. The Dutch government carried out extensive consultation with landholders and whilst those who will be directly affected may prefer a different strategy, the cost-benefit analysis ensures the greatest good for the greatest number.[1] Community consultation was a critical part of the Dutch strategy. However, Kuziemsky and Varpio [5] warn that reaching common ground does not develop immediately. It requires an all-inclusive approach to engage with the community, and an interactive cycle of continual consultation, information exchange, networking, and collaboration.

COMMUNITY ENGAGEMENT AND DISASTER RISK MANAGEMENT

The Sendai Framework [6] emphasises the engagement of "all-of-society" and "all-of-State" institutions as guiding principles for disaster risk reduction, before-during-after an event:

> Disaster risk reduction requires an all-of-society engagement and partnership. It also requires empowerment and inclusive, accessible and non-discriminatory participation, paying special attention to people disproportionately affected by disasters, especially the poorest.

Similarly, the Sphere Project [7] makes it a core standard and priority to incorporate community participation and engagement in all humanitarian response activities, including water supply, sanitation and hygiene (WASH), food security and nutrition, shelter and settlement, and health. In a specific commitment, the Sphere emphasises that crisis-affected communities receive assistance appropriate to their needs, culture, and preferences. The assistance must correspond with assessed risks, on an ongoing basis, taking into account the vulnerabilities, capacities, skills, and knowledge of people requiring assistance and protection [7]. These are particularly important when planning suitable exit strategies, to ensure they will empower the crisis-affected communities and people to assume responsibility and ownership of the introduced programs for long-term recovery and resilience.

FACTORS AFFECTING COMMUNITY ENGAGEMENT

Socio-demographic characteristics and vulnerability

Disasters affect individuals, families, and communities in various ways. An important consideration for disaster management is the composition of the population in each area impacted by a disaster. Developing an understanding of the community/societal context is critical to understanding the impact of disasters and the potential for recovery. The key focus of disaster management involves meeting people's changing physical and social needs (food, shelter, safety, connections, income, info etc.) as well as their physical health and psychological needs. Disasters have a cumulative or compounding effect on community functioning, as the economic, physical, and mental health and wellbeing consequences interrelate.

Community engagement also helps to identify and inform the vulnerabilities of individuals and community groups that may require special consideration in all phases of the disaster management cycle. Vulnerability is the pre-event, inherent characteristics or qualities of a social system that creates the potential for harm. It is a function of the exposure (who or what is at risk) and sensitivity of the system (the degree to which people and places can be harmed), and is defined as

> the characteristics of a person or group and their situation that influence their capacity to anticipate, cope with, resist, and recover from the impact of a ... hazard
>
> [8]

Some socio-demographic characteristics that may impact on the vulnerability of communities in disasters include:

- Special needs groups
  The community affected by a disaster comprises individuals, groups and organisations with differing needs. Some may be directly affected, injured, deprived of access to normal supports or bereaved. Others may be indirectly affected either as responders or supporters. Some will be particularly vulnerable due to their special circumstances and needs such as children, elderly, women, people with physical/ intellectual disability or mental illness, those restrained (e.g., prisoners), alternate sexual orientation, and indigenous communities [9].

  These communities and groups can be easily excluded due to limited mobility or access to information, services, and support (financial, physical, emotional, and social). For instance, influenza pandemics and heatwaves often differentially impact on the elderly and children. Women are more vulnerable as they often fulfil a protective family function which complicates their ability to escape. In many societies, a woman's relative lack of education and economic capacity reduces their resilience even further. People with restricted mobility (e.g., disabled or imprisoned) may not be able to evacuate or escape. Residents in remote areas may not receive timely updates or appropriate support in preparing for and dealing with disasters. Disaster managers must engage with these communities to ensure they are included in all stages of disaster risk management.

- Communication barriers
  Community engagement should take into consideration language and educational differences within the community. Where different languages are spoken including sign language, or people with varying levels of literacy, multiple strategies for engagement are required to ensure the entire community can have the opportunity to be involved in the disaster management process. These may range from simple face-to-face contacts to multilingual information and educational resources and strategies or complex interactive exercises, computer programs, and games.

- Socio-economic status
  Lower socio-economic status is associated with higher vulnerability. The effect on these groups is more severe during disasters. Affluent communities have the ability to recover and "bounce back" quickly following a disaster. These communities generally will have individually and collectively prepared for and are able to adapt in the lead-up to a disaster. They possess a strong local community and a robust

and mostly trusted governance structure, with effective, well-trained essential service organisations, and a comparatively low level of social inequality [10]. By comparison, communities without a trusted governance structure and effective well-trained response organisations generally do not have the ability to *bounce back* as quickly [10]. Case studies of Cyclone Nargis, Burma and Cyclone Yasi, Australia provide a comparison of two countries with vastly different governance across the disaster management continuum of prevention, preparedness, response, and recovery (PPRR).

CASE STUDY 8.1 – CYCLONE NARGIS 2008, IRRAWADDY DELTA REGION, BURMA (MYANMAR)

The former government of Burma (a military junta) spent less than 2% of GDP on health and education combined, while military expenditure was 40% of GDP (1). Following Cyclone Nargis in 2008, the government was accused of crimes against humanity (2).

Warnings from the Indian Meteorological Department from 29 April 2008 that a cyclone would make landfall on the Irrawaddy Delta region were issued to the Burmese Department of Meteorology and Hydrology (3). Despite this, the then Burmese government failed to act, communities in the region were not advised, and no preparations were made (3). The cyclone made landfall on 2 May 2008 killing more than 150,000 people with a further 2.4 million people severely affected. Fifty per cent of the schools and 75% of the region's healthcare facilities were destroyed or damaged (1). Following the cyclone, the military regime prevented thousands of bilateral and international non-governmental humanitarian responders from entering the country. Furthermore, the government of the day failed to provide the basic necessities of life including food, water and shelter, restricted access to information, seized control of foreign aid, distributed aid based on ethnicity and religion, forcibly relocated survivors and confiscated land (4). A limited number of non-government organisations (NGOs) from within the region were granted access almost three weeks after the cyclone whereby enabling some assistance to be provided (2).

References

1. Willis, N. Natural disaster, national sovereignty and state negligence: An international law analysis of the denial of emergency relief after Cyclone Nargis in Myanmar (Burma). *University of Tasmania Law Review*, 2012. **31**(2):134–154.
2. Coppola, D. *Investigation of the political implications of disasters requiring international assistance.* 2011. Brisbane: Federal Management Agency and Emergency Management Institute.
3. Human Rights Watch. "I want to Help My Own People": State Control and Civil Society in Burma after Cyclone Nargis 2010 [February 9, 2016]. Available from: https://www.hrw.org/report/2010/04/28/i-want-help-my-own-people/state-control-and-civil-society-burma-after-cyclone.
4. Haacke, J. Myanmar, the responsibility to protect, and the need for practical assistance. *Global Responsibility to Protect*, 2009. **1**(2):156–184.

CASE STUDY 8.2 – CYCLONE YASI 2011, FAR NORTH QLD – AUSTRALIA

Australia has a democratically elected system of Federal, State, and Local governments. Throughout 2011–2015, Australia's spending on health was 9.4% GDP (1), education was 4.9% GDP (2), while military expenditure was 1.8% GDP (3). Australian states maintain comprehensive, all-hazards disaster management arrangements with extensive consultation between governments and communities in all aspects of PPRR.

On 3 February 2011, north Queensland was hit by category five cyclone Yasi. Cyclone warnings and information on cyclone preparations were widely distributed through a variety of mediums and continually updated (4). Prior to the cyclone, additional emergency services personnel and critical infrastructure technicians were positioned close to the region out of the impact zone so they could respond rapidly once the immediate threat had passed. Thirty thousand people, including patients from Cairns Base and Private Hospitals and dialysis patients were evacuated prior to cyclone Yasi making landfall (5). The official death toll from cyclone Yasi was one (6). Following the cyclone, response was swift, power and other essential services were restored quickly to most areas, and within four days, 70 of the evacuated patients had been repatriated back to Cairns (5). The remaining renal patients were repatriated within two weeks after the cyclone made landfall (5).

References

1. The World Bank. Health expenditure, total (% of GDP) [Internet]. 2015 [February 9, 2016]. Available from: http://data.worldbank.org/indicator/SH.XPD.TOTL.ZS.
2. The World Bank. Government expenditure on education as % of GDP (%) 2015 [February 9, 2016]. Available from: http://data.worldbank.org/indicator/SE.XPD.TOTL.GD.ZS
3. The World Bank. Military expenditure % of GDP 2015 [February 9, 2016]. Available from: http://data.worldbank.org/indicator/MS.MIL.XPND.GD.ZS.
4. Olsson, E.K. Crisis communication in public organisations: Dimensions of crisis communication revisited. *Journal of Contingencies and Crisis Management*. 2014. **22**(2):113–125.
5. Johnson, D.W., B. Hayes, N.A. Gray, C. Hawley, J. Hole, and M. Mantha, Renal services disaster planning: Lessons learnt from the 2011 Queensland floods and North Queensland cyclone experiences. *Nephrology*. 2013. **18**(1): p. 41–46.
6. Guha-Sapir, D., R. Below, and P.H. Hoyois, *EM-DAT: The CRED/OFDA International Disaster Database Brussels*, Belgium: Université Catholique de Louvain; [March 19, 2023]. Available from: www.emdat.be

- Cultural differences
    Well-established communities will often have knowledge of and experience with disasters. Generational knowledge handed down through stories and rituals in many indigenous communities is valuable to PPRR. However some beliefs or practices, e.g., fatalistic ideas or belief in metaphysical powers may impede effective PPRR. It

is important disaster managers acknowledge and work with all religious, cultural, and ethnic beliefs and practices. Engaging with communities as stakeholders fosters connectedness, a sense of coherence and belonging, and strengthens and empowers them to build resilience [11].

- Mass population movement
  Displaced communities, similar to the large movements of refugees across Europe, Africa, and the Middle East throughout 2015, are particularly vulnerable. In addition to socio-cultural differences, they may suffer increased incidence of health conditions including mental illness associated with exposure to traumatic events. Despite their vulnerability, these communities may also possess survival experience and knowledge, which can assist disaster managers. This is particularly significant when a large influx of refugees may place extra pressure on the host communities' resources allocated for disaster management activities. Given the infrequency and unpredictability of natural disasters, this may potentially shift funding away from disaster management programs. To strengthen resilience, it is imperative host communities ensure these populations are fully engaged in the disaster risk management process.

  In summary, it is important to understand the qualitative nature of communities and how these qualities may vary not only over time as a consequence of broader social and economic changes, but also when communities are placed under stress. As Marsh [12] warns, communities are not static and any destabilisation can severely impede their ability to *bounce back*.

Social capital

The concept of social capital is a core component of community engagement and resilience. Cheers et al. [13] define social capital as

> …a measure of the communal trust, cooperation, and reciprocity components of community capacity. Social capital is a community asset that can be accumulated, but when it is low it can reduce the strength of local social fields, including the community field, and be a barrier to the development of community activities and structures.

Poortinga [14] described the factors that contribute to social capital as: bonding and bridging strategies, social cohesion, civic participation, socio-economic relationships, and political efficacy. Townshend et al. [15] found a significant positive correlation between social cohesion and resilience in a community's ability to *bounce back* following disaster. However, social cohesion reduces when marginalisation increases. Figure 8.1 depicts Jenson [16] constituent dimensions of social cohesion and the factors that reduce social cohesion within a community.

Leadership and governance

Societal changes and historical trends have influenced the way many communities are governed. Governments can no longer be expected to be the sole agent responsible for protecting their citizens from the consequences of disasters. Governance structures need to be set up in a way that fosters participation and decision-making throughout

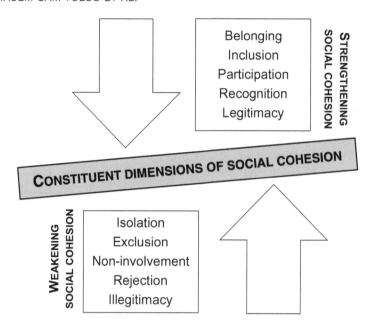

Figure 8.1 Dimensions of social cohesion – adapted from Jenson [16]

the community. An all-inclusive comprehensive approach to PPRR requires a shift from top-down to bottom-up decision-making processes. However, the success of this hinges on the leaders' ability to engage with the community. Leaders who do not have the trust or respect of their constituents will not be effective in building sustainable community resilience.

COMMUNITY ENGAGEMENT PRINCIPLES AND MECHANISMS

As the number of disasters increase and the population grows, the need to ensure sufficient funds to keep the community safe places added pressure on both government organisations and NGOs. Now more than ever it is important individuals and the community in which they live have the capacity to be actively involved in all aspects of disaster risk management and to learn how to be resilient. This has led to the need to develop *appropriate* programs to effectively engage communities in this process. Cox and Hamlen [17] state these programs must be flexible, location-based and context-specific with up-to-date assessment tools i.e. disaster plans and hazard risk assessments. The principles underpinning these programs include:

1. Strong partnerships between local leaders (e.g., community champions, influencers, brokers), response agencies, and authorities [18].
2. Sharing information and understanding the needs and perspectives [19]
   • Develop awareness and common ground [20–22]
3. Effective participation, building involvement and connected networks [19]
   • Community engagement must foster shared knowledge and connectedness [14, 23–25].

4. Consultation with and inclusion of all communities [19]
   - Integrative process which will involve, support, and empower the entire community [17].
   - Procedures responsive to the individual, contextual, and cultural factors [17].
   - Ensure unifying messages and involvement of all faith and non-faith organisations [26].
5. Collaboration and partnering with communities [19]
   - Community-led action [18] and incentives.
   - Engage with, and acknowledge the role of community organisations, groups, and volunteer networks [27].
6. Capacity-building skills and empowering individuals and communities [19]
   - Understanding the current level of community resilience at all stages of disaster risk management to reduce risk, but also to enhance the community's agency through actions that "lead to social transformative capacity" and "power to foster change" [28]
7. Building on existing assets and resources [19]
   - Adequate financial and human resources with a supporting legal framework [17].
   - Provide opportunities for innovative thinking and developing appropriate goals for collaborative initiatives [29, 30].
   - Infrastructure to support community resilience (i.e., evacuation centre). [18]

Fundamental to community engagement is research. It is through research and working with communities that we will be able to identify and validate the needs, priorities, vulnerabilities, capacities, and the impacts "on the ground" of the disaster risk reduction programs and activities on those who live with and are affected by crises. For instance, a recent study in Northland, New Zealand, found that flood maps were not easily accessible or comprehensible to the participants, hence giving them a false sense of security [31]. The study highlighted the need for enhanced communication and engagement between the local communities and authorities to integrate community knowledge and experience with the current risk communication plans.

Such research takes many forms and face many challenges. As Few and colleagues state [32], community engagement research takes many forms

> from conventional elicitation of responses to externally-generated questions to more collaborative, co-production processes. In essence, co-production refers to the collaborative production of knowledge between stakeholders – typically, in this field, between risk researchers (seen as the conventional producers of knowledge) and those who either live with risk or are charged with managing risk.
>
> [32]

To achieve resilient communities through the principles outlined above, robust methods and mechanisms are required. These include [33, 34]:

1. *Public consultation* is used to elicit community views and perspectives on a range of issues, through social and market research techniques (e.g., opinion polls, surveys, workshops, focus groups).
2. *Direct involvement* in decision-making through formal and informal deliberative processes (e.g., local councils and social forums).

3. *Target groups engagement*, e.g., faith, ethnicity, disability, elderly, LGBTIQA (lesbians, gays, bisexuals, transgenders, intersexes, queers, and allies). Community champions, respected leaders, and elders can utilise their authority to encourage their communities to engage in disaster risk management.
4. *Community assets utilisation* recognises and capitalises on community assets and resources both physical and human to maximise control over, and benefit from them.
5. *Education* including training, employment, and personal development to build and support skills and confidence of community members.
6. *Service delivery mechanisms* mobilise the community to respond to gaps in public service provision or local needs (e.g., environmental clean-ups, transport, and emergency support). Volunteerism plays an important role in this process. They can be formal government and NGOs (e.g., State Emergency Services and Surf Life Saving in Australia), or informal [35] (e.g., Brisbane's Mud Army in 2011 – refer chapter 19)

In practice however, organisations may need to adopt a mixed model approach to effectively engage communities. Furthermore, the part that traditional and modern mass media including electronic social forums (e.g., Facebook and Twitter) play in the disaster risk management process is considerable. This has been discussed in detail in Chapter 7.

Community engagement is not an easy task, it requires continuity and currency and involves challenges at all stages of the risk management. Given the fluid nature of many disasters, it may not be possible to fully prepare and plan in advance, or to respond and recover as quickly and efficiently as expected or desired. Also, communities change both naturally and as a consequence of disasters, as do the type, frequency and intensity of disasters. Therefore, it is important to continually monitor changes, evaluate the programs' effectiveness, and revise, improve and update as required.

Evaluation of community engagement is *"a process of assessment used to generate information about the way in which an activity or program of activities is undertaken (process) and the results of the activity or program (outcomes)"* [36]. It draws upon social sciences research and methodology [37, 38] and involves development of a conceptual framework, devising and testing data collection instruments, collecting and analysing data, and interpreting, sharing, reporting and responding to findings [39]. Evaluation is an opportunity to validate disaster risk reduction and management strategies. It should promote inclusive debriefing with the aim of identifying both successful and unsuccessful practices, identifying *lessons to be learnt*. It should also promote further engagement by involving the communities in the process.

Due to the complex nature of communities, human behaviour, and disasters, evaluating community engagement programs is an ongoing, reiterative and costly process. It requires context-trained and experienced evaluation researchers [40]. Figure 8.2 demonstrates the process for strengthening community resilience (adapted from White et al. [41])

ACTIVITY

Identify a community with which you are familiar.

1. How would you describe it?
2. Who are the key informal leaders of the community?
3. Are there people within the community who are particularly vulnerable?

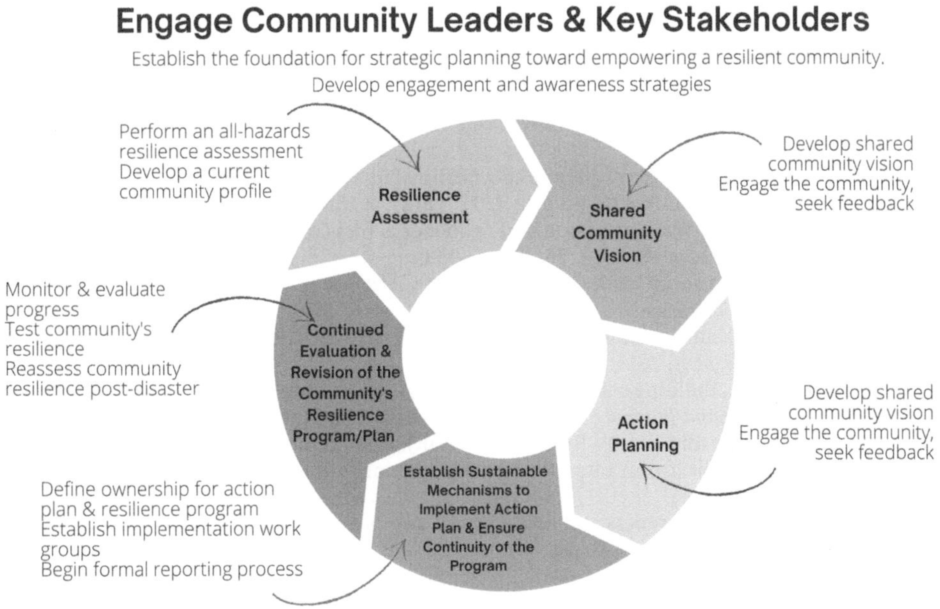

Engage Community Leaders & Key Stakeholders

Establish the foundation for strategic planning toward empowering a resilient community.
Develop engagement and awareness strategies

Perform an all-hazards resilience assessment
Develop a current community profile

Resilience Assessment

Shared Community Vision

Develop shared community vision
Engage the community, seek feedback

Monitor & evaluate progress
Test community's resilience
Reassess community resilience post-disaster

Continued Evaluation & Revision of the Community's Resilience Program/Plan

Action Planning

Develop shared community vision
Engage the community, seek feedback

Define ownership for action plan & resilience program
Establish implementation work groups
Begin formal reporting process

Establish Sustainable Mechanisms to Implement Action Plan & Ensure Continuity of the Program

Figure 8.2 Process for strengthening community resilience (adapted from White et al. [41])

Note

1. For more information visit https://www.technologyreview.com/2014/10/16/249972/sharing-flood-mitigation-strategies-with-at-risk-countries/.

References

1. MacQueen, K.M., et al., What is community? An evidence-based definition for participatory public health. *American Journal of Public Health*, 2001. **91**(12): p. 1929–1938.
2. United Nations. *Brisbane Declaration on Community Engagement*. 2005, Brisbane, Australia. Available from: https://cdn2.hubspot.net/hubfs/2619477/brisbane_declaration.pdf.
3. Johnston, K.A., et al., *Episodic and relational community engagement: Implications for social impact and social license*, in *The handbook of communication engagement*, 2018: p. 169–185. https://doi.org/10.1002/9781119167600.ch12
4. Cox, J., Louis Anthony, Community resilience and decision theory challenges for catastrophic events. *Risk Analysis: An International Journal*, 2012. **32**(11): p. 1919–1934.
5. Kuziemsky, C.E. and L. Varpio. *Describing the clinical communication space through a model of common ground: 'you don't know what you don't know'*. in *AMIA annual symposium proceedings*. 2010, Washington DC: American Medical Informatics Association.
6. United Nations, *Sendai framework for disaster risk reduction 2015–2030*. 2015, Geneva: United Nations.
7. Sphere Association, *The Sphere handbook*, in *Humanitarian charter and minimum standards in humanitarian response*. 2018, Geneva: Sphere Association.
8. Wisner, B., et al., *At risk: Natural hazards, people's vulnerability and disasters*. 2004, England: Psychology Press.
9. Australian Institute for Disaster Resilience, *Health and disaster management handbook*. 2019, Canberra: Commonwealth of Australia.
10. Walters, P., The problem of community resilience in two flooded cities: Dhaka 1998 and Brisbane 2011. *Habitat International*, 2015. **50**: p. 51–56.

11. Morgan A, Ziglio E. Revitalising the evidence base for public health: an assets model. *Promot Educ.* 2007; Suppl 2:17–22. doi: 10.1177/10253823070140020701x. PMID: 17685075.
12. Marsh, G. and P. Buckle, Community: The concept of community in the risk and emergency management context. *Australian Journal of Emergency Management*, 2001. **16**(1): p. 5–7.
13. Cheers, B., R. Darracott, and B. Lonne, *Social care practice in rural communities.* 2007, Sydney: Federation Press.
14. Poortinga, W., Community resilience and health: The role of bonding, bridging, and linking aspects of social capital. *Health & Place*, 2012. **18**(2): p. 286–295.
15. Townshend, I., et al., Social cohesion and resilience across communities that have experienced a disaster. *Natural Hazards*, 2015. **76**: p. 913–938.
16. Jenson, J., *Mapping social cohesion: The state of Canadian research.* 1998, Ottawa: Canadian Policy Research Networks.
17. Cox, R.S. and M. Hamlen, Community disaster resilience and the rural resilience index. *American Behavioral Scientist*, 2015. **59**(2): p. 220–237.
18. Thornley, L., et al., Building community resilience: Learning from the Canterbury earthquakes. *Kotuitui: New Zealand Journal of Social Sciences Online*, 2015. **10**(1): p. 23–35.
19. Australian Institute for Disaster Resilience (AIDR). *Community Engagement for Disaster Resilience.* 2020; Available from: https://knowledge.aidr.org.au/resources/handbook-community-engagement/.
20. Carroll, J.M., et al., Awareness and teamwork in computer-supported collaborations. *Interacting with Computers*, 2006. **18**(1): p. 21–46.
21. Carroll, J.M., et al., Beyond being aware. *Information and Organization*, 2009. **19**(3): p. 162–185.
22. O'Sullivan, T.L., et al., The EnRiCH community resilience framework for high-risk populations. *PLoS Currents*, 2014. **6**.
23. Norris, F.H., et al., Community resilience as a metaphor, theory, set of capacities, and strategy for disaster readiness. *American Journal of Community Psychology*, 2008. **41**: p. 127–150.
24. Chandra, A., et al., Building community resilience to disasters: A way forward to enhance national health security. *Rand Health Quarterly*, 2011. **1**(1). https://www.ncbi.nlm.nih.gov/pmc/articles/PMC4945213/
25. Edwards, F.L., *All hazards, whole community: Creating resiliency*, in *Disaster resiliency*. 2013, New York, NY, Routledge. p. 43–69.
26. Joakim, E.P. and R.S. White, Exploring the impact of religious beliefs, leadership, and networks on response and recovery of disaster-affected populations: A case study from Indonesia. *Journal of Contemporary Religion*, 2015. **30**(2): p. 193–212.
27. Abara, W., et al., Engaging a chemical disaster community: Lessons from Graniteville. *International Journal of Environmental Research and Public Health*, 2014. **11**(6): p. 5684–5697.
28. Manyena, S.B. and S. Gordon, Bridging the concepts of resilience, fragility and stabilisation. *Disaster Prevention and Management*, 2015. **24**(1): p. 38–52.
29. Robinson, L.W. and F. Berkes, Multi-level participation for building adaptive capacity: Formal agency-community interactions in northern Kenya. *Global Environmental Change*, 2011. **21**(4): p. 1185–1194.
30. McKnight, J., *Asset mapping in communities*, in *Health assets in a global context: Theory, methods, action*, Morgan A and Ziglio E, Editors. 2010, New York: Springer, p. 59–76.
31. Auliagisni, W., S. Wilkinson, and M. Elkharboutly, Using community-based flood maps to explain flood hazards in Northland, New Zealand. *Progress in Disaster Science*, 2022. **14**: p. 100229.
32. Few, R., et al., Working with communities on disaster risk research: Reflections from cross-disciplinary practice. *International Journal of Disaster Risk Reduction*, 2022. **70**: p. 102815.
33. Australian Emergency Management Institute, *Australian Emergency Handbook 6: Community Engagement Framework.* 2013, Canberra: Commonwealth of Australia.
34. Hashagen, S., *Models of community engagement.* 2002, Glasgow: Scottish Community Development Centre.
35. Bekkers, R., *Volunteerism*, in *International Encyclopaedia of the Social Science.*, W. Darity Jr, Editor. 2008, Detroit: Macmillan Reference USA.
36. Johnson, A.L., *Engaging Queenslanders: Evaluating community engagement.* 2004, Queensland: Department Communities.

37. Argyrous, G. and S. Rahman, *A monitoring and evaluation framework for disaster recovery programs.* 2016, Carlton South: The Australia and New Zealand School of Government.
38. AUSAID. *The logical framework approach.* 2005; Available from: https://vdocument.in/ausaid-2005-the-logical-framework-approach.html.
39. Stern, E., *Evaluation research methods.* 4th ed. 2004, London: SAGE Publications.
40. Sundnes, K.O. and M.L. Birnbaum, Health disaster management: Guidelines for evaluation and research in the Utstein style. *Prehospital and Disaster Medicine*, 2003. **17**(Supplement 3): p. 31–55.
41. White, R.K., et al., A practical approach to building resilience in America's communities. *American Behavioral Scientist*, 2015. **59**(2): p. 200–219.

9

Legal and ethical aspects of disaster management

Fiona McDonald, Michael Eburn, and Erin Smith

INTRODUCTION

Law and ethics have an important role to play in emergency management. In addition to coordinating functions, legal frameworks at the international, national, and sub-national levels provide a framework establishing who can lawfully act, what can and cannot be lawfully done, and the manner in which actions should be taken. Law also plays an important role in specifying that in the midst of an emergency situation, the vulnerable should be protected, and human rights respected. With a foundation of respect for the dignity of individuals and communities, law is as equally important as ethics and morality to inform decision-making around what should be done and the way it should be done.

This chapter introduces key elements of the legal framework at the international and domestic levels, followed by an introduction into some of the most significant ethical issues in the management of disasters and public health emergencies for health professionals. On completion of this chapter, you should have an understanding of:

1. The principles of domestic and international law as it pertains to disaster management and public health emergencies.
2. The instruments and covenants that support and guide an international response to disasters or public health emergencies.
3. The ethical challenges and professional responsibilities of response agencies and their staff.

INTERNATIONAL LAW ARRANGEMENTS

While disasters and public health emergencies have the capacity to cross national borders, there is no single comprehensive international treaty directly addressing how the international community could or should respond to disasters, although there is in respect of public health emergencies involving infectious diseases. The major obstacle to this is the concept of national sovereignty – that a nation state should govern itself without interference from other nations or international bodies. The international legal framework for

 DOI: 10.4324/9781032626604-11

disaster management is therefore fragmented with a variety of relevant hard (legally binding law such as covenants) and soft laws (quasi-legal instruments that are not legally binding, or which are only weakly binding), for example, United Nations (UN) resolutions that are directly or indirectly relevant, as well as multi- and bi-lateral agreements between nation states and within or between non-government organisations (NGOs). General human rights instruments, such as the International Covenant on Civil and Political Rights (ICCPR) (1966a) and the International Covenant on Economic, Social and Cultural Rights (ICESCR) (1966b), for example, the right to food and water, will also be relevant in disaster contexts. Some of the most significant instruments for disaster management are discussed below.

INTERNATIONAL LAW

There is no single comprehensive international treaty directly addressing how the international community could or should respond to disasters that cross borders.

Prevention – The main strategic framework for disaster reduction and mitigation is the Sendai Framework for Disaster Risk Reduction 2015–2030 (UN, 2015). This framework aims to encourage the integration of disaster risk considerations (including risk reduction strategies) into emergency preparedness, response and recovery planning and policy, and to develop and strengthen capacity.

Coordination – There are many actors in international disaster management ranging from UN Agencies, regional organisations, nation states, private companies, and NGOs. Effective coordination is therefore important but difficult to achieve.

United Nations – The 1991 the UN General Assembly passed a resolution (UN, 1991) to strengthen its role in coordinating disaster response efforts of the international community. With the aim of improving coordination, the UN created the Inter-Agency Standing Committee (IASC) and the position of the Emergency Relief Coordinator. ISAC is comprised of representatives from the UN, the International Organisation for Migration (IOM), the Red Cross, and various NGO consortia.

Regional and bilateral agreements – There are several regional and bilateral agreements between national states that aim to improve cooperation and smooth barriers to a regional or bilateral response to a disaster (e.g., the ASEAN – Agreement on Disaster Management and Emergency Response, 2005).

NGOs – The 1997 Seville Agreement (ICRC, 1997) specifies which arm of the Red Cross movement becomes the lead Red Cross agency in disasters. NGOs may also coordinate their operations and share information through the creation of networks, such as the Asian Disaster Reduction and Response Network (ADRRN).

Operations – entry and exit – Ensuring international aid and personnel can rapidly reach areas and people affected by disasters, and can operate with relative impunity (e.g., doctors can provide medical care without a license to practice in the host country) is another priority to enable international disaster management. Bi- and multi-lateral agreements usually specify rules in respect to the entry, exit and operation of organisations and their employees within disaster areas, as well as relief supplies needed to carry out their functions. International Conventions apply in respect of UN agencies (e.g., the Convention on the Safety of UN and Associated Personnel) and other international or regional organisations (UN, 1994). The UN General Assembly has also adopted a resolution (UN, 2003) urging states to reduce customs and administrative procedures related to the use of air space, and the entry, transit, stay, and exit of international search and rescue teams and their animals, equipment, and materials.

Human rights – In addition to general human rights protections accorded by the Covenants (UN, 1966a, 1996b), several international instruments focus on maintaining and promoting human rights in a disaster context. The Convention on the Rights of Persons with Disabilities (UN, 2006) Article 11 specifically addresses the obligations of states to provide for the protection and safety of persons with a disability in situations of risk. This includes humanitarian emergencies and natural disasters. The need for states to protect vulnerable people including the disabled, the elderly, women, and children in a disaster context is also explicit in the Guiding Principles on Internal Displacement (GPID) (1998) (UN High Commissioner for Refugees, 2004) and the IASC Guidelines (2011) for the protection of persons in natural disasters (ICRC, 1997). The IASC Guidelines recommend that displaced persons (including women and disabled persons) should be involved in the design and management of camps and food distribution systems. Key principles in the GPID stipulate:

- Principle 6.2 – people should only be displaced if evacuation is required to maintain the safety or health.
- Principle 7.2 – displaced people should, to the greatest extent possible, be provided with accommodation, nutrition, health services (see also principle 19.1) and hygiene and families should not be separated.
- Principle 18 – people should be provided with clean drinking water and clothing.
- Principle 23 – education should be provided as soon as conditions permit.

There are clauses in most human rights instruments that allow limitations to be imposed on some human rights for the duration of a period of a major emergency, for example, Article 4 of the ICCPR (1966a). The Siracusa Principles were developed by the American Association of the International Commission of Jurists (1985) to guide the use of limitation clauses. In summary, the Siracusa Principles recommend that limitations on human rights must:

- Respond to an urgent situation;
- Pursue a legitimate objective;
- Be proportionate to that objective;
- Be for a designated period;
- Be objectively considered; and
- Any limitations must be the least intrusive on the human right(s) in question (1A(11–12) and).

In 1994 the Red Cross developed a voluntary *Code of Conduct for The International Red Cross and Red Crescent Movement and NGOs in Disaster Relief* (ICRC, 1994). This Code also emphasises human rights. In general, these guidelines and codes emphasise the need to provide assistance in an impartial, neutral, humane and respectful manner and in a way that maximises the benefits to affected populations and minimises harms and risks.

Infectious diseases – One area in which there is binding international law is in response to disease outbreaks that have the capacity to constitute global public health threats, for example, the COVID-19 pandemic. The international health regulations (IHR) directs (WHO, 2005):

- nation states to report (with a specified level of detail) to the World Health Organization (WHO) all diseases (infectious or otherwise) that might constitute a public health threat of international concern; and
- nation states to develop their capacity to detect, assess, notify, report, and respond to public health emergencies.

It also grants the WHO the power to issue non-binding recommendations, to require nation states to provide additional information and for the WHO to share information without the consent of the nation state, amongst other things. The adequacy and effectiveness of the IHR have been called into question by the COVID pandemic. Some critics suggest it needs to be strengthened, while others that implementation, both by the WHO and nation states has been flawed. Nation states have been asked to present proposals for reform, in tandem with proposals for a global pandemic treaty, but any change is some way off (Lancet Global Health, 2022).

DOMESTIC LAW ARRANGEMENTS

The primary responsibility for managing the response to any disaster or emergency lies with the government of the affected state (here referring to 'state' as a nation state rather than sub-national states or provinces) (UN, 1981, 1991; Fidler et al., 2005). Nation states have options as to how they make their emergency management arrangements, for example, in Canada [*Emergency Management Act*, SC 2007 c 15; *Emergencies Act*, RSC 1985, c 22 (4th Supp)], New Zealand [*Civil Defence Emergency Act 2002* (NZ)], and the UK [*Civil Contingencies Act 2004* (UK)] emergency management is a significant matter for the national government. In Australia primary responsibility for managing the response to disasters is vested in the states. The national government's role is generally limited to providing financial support to affected states and individuals (*Social Security Act 1991* (Cth); Australian Government, 2017) and providing direct assistance at the request of the states (Australian Government, 2020). Following catastrophic bushfires over the 2019/2020 summer, the Commonwealth legislated to allow for the provision of direct disaster intervention in the context of national emergencies [*Defence Act 1903* (Cth) s 123AA; *National Emergency Declaration Act 2020* (Cth)]. The Commonwealth is also taking a more proactive role in coordinating the national response to and recovery from disasters (Australian Government, u.d). The US gives primary responsibility for emergency management to local governments, but management can be moved up to State and then the Federal government depending on the size and impact of the event [*Robert T. Stafford Disaster Relief and Emergency Assistance Act*, Public Law 93–288, as amended, 42 U.S.C. 5121 et seq].

Most jurisdictions have specific disaster (emergency) management legislation which identifies when a disaster can be declared and creates powers that can be exercised during a disaster. Many other items of legislation contain specific provisions that will apply in the event of a disaster and with few exceptions, other legislation will continue to apply even during a disaster. Domestic laws are essential to create appropriate organisations such as national emergency management offices, as well as local fire brigades and rescue services [*Fire and Rescue Services Act 2004* (UK); *Fire and Emergency New Zealand Act 2017* (NZ); *Fire Services Act* (RSBC, 1996) Chapter 144 (British Columbia, Canada); *Health and Safety Code, Division 12 Fires and Fire Protection* [13000–14960] (California, USA); *Fire and Rescue NSW Act 1989* (NSW)]. Laws also define who is responsible for formulating emergency plans and for giving agencies both the authority and the obligation to take part in disaster planning [*Emergencies Act*, RSC 1985, c 22 (4th Supp); *Civil Defence Emergency Act* 2002 (NZ); *Civil Contingencies Act 2004* (UK); Australian Government, 2020; *State Emergency and Rescue Management Act 1989* (NSW)]. Where there is an international obligation, for example, to facilitate the entry of relief personnel and to allow licensed health professionals to practice in the affected country, then it is up to states to ensure that their domestic laws give effect to those international obligations (ICRC, 2007). Domestic laws are required to set out the powers that may be employed to control an emergency (*Emergency Management Act*, SC 2007 c 15; Australian Government, 2020; Lee, 1984).

Public health emergencies are often, but not always, addressed in separate legislation focused on public health, recognising the different dynamics between public health emergencies and disasters more generally and the need for specialist expertise to respond to different forms of emergencies. [*Public Health (Control of Disease) Act 1984* (UK); *Public Health Act 2010* (NSW); *Biosecurity Act 2015* (Cth); *Public Health Service Act* 42 U.S.C. ch. 6A § 201 et seq., *Health Act 1956* (NZ); *Quarantine Act* (S.C. 2005, c. 20)]. The COVID-19 Pandemic demonstrated the need for law to allow governments to take steps to control public health threats and therefore *prevent* overwhelming medical emergencies.

Both emergency management laws and public health emergency laws grant additional powers to specified actors to protect the public, property and the environment during the duration of the emergency. These powers may include:

- entering private property;
- destroying private property;
- using or moving private property;
- requiring people to evacuate or quarantine in specified places;
- the creation and use of border controls, curfews, stay-at-home orders and/or exclusion zones; and
- requirements for the public to wear protective equipment, take protective measures or be vaccinated.

These measures impose limitations on the legal and human rights of individuals and could be abused by governments. Accordingly, to balance the need for such powers against the limitations imposed upon individual rights and interests, most emergency management and/or public health emergency legislation will contain checks and balances, including:

- clear criteria as to what constitutes a disaster or public health emergency which must be met before a disaster/public health emergency is declared;
- clarity as to who in what circumstances has the power to declare a disaster or public health emergency;
- time limitations on declarations that an event is a disaster or a public health emergency (although extensions are possible); geographical limitations within which emergency powers can be used (so can be national, state, province or territory-wide, regional or local depending on the emergency);
- emergency powers can only be exercised by designated individuals for the duration of the declared disaster/emergency;
- The exercise of those powers is subject to oversight and review by the courts and other administrative bodies.

Those who lawfully exercise these powers (i.e. apply the criteria and are the appropriately authorised persons) and do so in good faith are generally immune from civil liability as individuals. Those who exercise these powers outside of the circumstances permitted by law or in bad faith could face legal proceedings. But decisions of this type can also be subject to review. For example, in Papua New Guinea a government declaration of an emergency in the Southern Highlands Province was successfully challenged and the use of emergency legislative powers under that declaration was overturned by the court [*Southern Highlands Provincial Government v Somare, Chairman of the National Executive Council* [2007] PGSC 2; SC854]. Other challenges to the use of emergency public health powers (e.g., lockdowns, border closures), have been less successful [*Dolan and others v Secretary of State for Health and Social Care and others* [2020] EWCA Civ 1605; *Loielo v Giles* [2020] VSC 722; *Palmer v State of Western Australia* (No 4) [2020] FCA 1221]. The English Court of Appeal stated in Dolan [2020, 89]:

> on public health issues which require the evaluation of complex scientific evidence, the national court may and should be slow to interfere with a decision which a responsible decision-maker has reached after consultation with its expert advisers.

Thus, emergency managers need to have a broad understanding of the legislative environment in which they work.

CASE STUDY 9.1 – SARS IN SINGAPORE

The Political response to SARS in Singapore fostered a spirit of public collaboration and solidarity which contributed to control of the virus. Recognising early that containing SARS was the only way of restoring the confidence of tourists and trade partners, control and containment efforts were made a priority of the government at the highest level to regain economic recovery. Strong public partnerships were fostered between the government and the people largely due to the frank, open, complete and constant information which was being disseminated to the public (Deurenberg-Yap et al., 2005).

Singapore's high vigilance in initiating containment measures to control the outbreak of SARS meant the disease was only prevalent in the country for less than four months. Specific SARS ambulances transported patients to dedicated SARS hospitals which were closed to visitors. Frequent and regular temperature monitoring with every household being issued thermometers, early case identification, isolation of patients, contact tracing, and home quarantine of contacts were integral in controlling the outbreak. Movement of healthcare workers, patients and visitors within and between hospitals was restricted and the military in Singapore was deployed to assist with contact tracing and to enforce quarantines. Education of healthcare workers and audits of infection control practices were also implemented. Cross-border transmission was monitored with incoming travellers from SARS-affected areas completing health declarations and all outgoing travellers monitored for fever. The public was urged to restrict non-essential travel to SARS-affected regions, schools were closed and sporting activities suspended. Increased public education programs on good hygiene were implemented and information was made readily available to the public. There were mandatory biosafety precautions for laboratories testing for SARS virus culture and all laboratory workers were counselled on biosafety guidelines (Deurenberg-Yap et al, 2005).

When faced with an emergency or disaster, decisions must be made with both limited time and limited knowledge. In the post-incident review, it may be thought that the decision was not the best that could be made, or that it resulted in poor outcomes. Laws are required to ensure that a responder:

> … is not to be charged with negligence if … faced with a situation which requires immediate action of some sort and if, in the so-called 'agony of the moment', he [or she] makes an error of judgment and takes a step which wiser counsels and more careful thought would have suggested was unwise.
>
> [*Leishman v Thomas* (1958) 75 WN (NSW) 173, 175]

Judge made law

The common law tradition is a legacy of English colonial imperialism and is shared with other former English colonies including the US, Canada, and New Zealand. The essential feature of the common law is that judges who deliver detailed reasons when deciding cases that come before them develop the law. The earlier decision of a superior court such as a Court of Appeal or the national Supreme or High Court defines the law that other subsequent courts must follow.

In the area of disaster and emergency management, law common law courts have been sympathetic to the dynamic and information-poor environment in which decisions have been made (Eburn, 2013). Litigation against those who respond during a disaster to provide emergency assistance is rare and to date, has been unsuccessful [*Capital and Counties v Hampshire Council* [1997] QB 2004; *Electro Optic Systems Pty Ltd v NSW* [2014] ACTCA 45]. Further courts have shown great latitude to appointed decision-makers recognising that decisions have to be made with imperfect knowledge. Provided the decisions made are within the range of available options a court will not intervene even if others would argue that an alternative response would have been more effective or less restrictive [*Kassam & Henry v Hazzard & Ors* [2021] NSWSC 1320; *Larter v Hazzard* (No 2) [2021] NSWSC 1451; *Loielo v Giles* [2020] VSC 722; *Gerner v The State of Victoria* [2020] HCA 48; *Palmer v Western Australia* [2021] HCA 5; *Dolan and others v Secretary of State for Health and Social Care and others* [2020] EWCA Civ 1605].

Medical emergencies

Even though there has been no successful litigation against people stepping forward to provide emergency medical care (Graham et al., 2015) at an accident or in a disaster, there is an expressed fear that people will be subject to some legal liability for their actions, taken in good faith to assist others. Many states now have Good Samaritan laws (named after the biblical parable), to protect a person who steps forward to provide emergency medical care [*Social Action, Responsibility and Heroism Act 2015* (UK); *Good Samaritan Act*, RSBC 1996, c 172 (British Columbia, Canada); *Civil Code, Division 3 Obligations Part 3 Obligations Imposed by Law* [1714.2–1714.23] (California, USA); *Civil Liability Act 2002* (NSW) s 57)].

This shows the importance of law in emergency management. The presence of international and domestic laws should remind those involved in planning for and responding to emergencies that they do not operate in a legal vacuum. It is not, or should not be, the case that governments when faced with emergencies, whether pandemics or fires, must try to create law 'on the run' or govern outside the law (Fatovic, 2009). Rather legislation must be in place before the event to allow governments to exercise the extra-ordinary powers that are required to deal with the dynamic situation of any emergency.

People and organisations who are part of the disaster management process need to be aware of the relevant international and domestic laws that apply to facilitate disaster assistance. At the same time, they should have little concern that they will be sued or found liable for their honest attempts to deal with the situation that presents itself.

ETHICAL CHALLENGES

Disasters place unprecedented demands on health systems and expose emergency healthcare workers to a range of risks. Despite this challenge, legal guidelines and emergency service professional codes of ethics are largely silent on the issue of professional obligations during disaster. This provides little to no guidance on what is expected of healthcare workers or how they ought to approach their duty to treat in the face of risk.

Ethical challenges for individual health professionals

In 2022, the outbreak of COVID-19 is ongoing. The WHO estimated that between January 2020 and May 2021 approximately 115,000 health and care workers died from COVID-19 (WHO, 2021). Healthcare professionals had to choose between providing care and protecting themselves and their families and friends – crystalising (as had earlier pandemics) an ethical challenge and fundamentally changing our assumptions about duty and risk (McConnell, 2020; McDougall et al., 2021). This was particularly so with COVID-19 as its rapid global spread, large case numbers, and airborne nature saw widespread shortages in protective equipment necessary to offer some protection for health workers.

Should they work?

The professional obligation to face risks has been referred to as part of a larger duty to care (Annas, 1988; Daniels, 1988). Contemporary ethical standards offer some guidance on treating patients during emergency siuations, but they are largely silent on the issue of healthcare worker professional responsibility (Ruderman et al., 2006) and the ramifications of failing to fulfil this responsibility. Healthcare professionals are arguably not required to accept life-threatening risk and the burden of psychological stress associated with that risk whilst caring for patients, but there appears to be no uncontroversial way to establish a threshold at which risk acceptance becomes a duty (Iverson et al., 2008). Morally speaking, when does the right to protect oneself from serious risk outweigh the duty to care for patients in need?

The obligation to continue caring for patients in the face of personal risk has been a central tenet of medical professionalism in some places since 1847. In the American Medical Association's (AMA) first Code of Ethics (Zuger and Miles, 1987; Huber and Wynia, 2004), it was written that when pestilence prevails, it is the professionals *'duty to face the danger and to continue their labours for the alleviation of suffering, even at the jeopardy of their own lives'*. This statement helped formalise a sense of physician duty that was sustained until the 1950s and 1960s. When domestic threats of infectious diseases such as Smallpox and Polio dissipated, such heroic statements vanished from the AMA Code (Huber and Wynia, 2004). The AMA (2001) now states that

> …because of their commitment to care for the sick and injured, individual physicians have an obligation to provide urgent medical care during disasters. This ethical obligation holds even in the face of greater than usual risks to their own safety, health or life.

But it also states

> … the physician workforce is not an unlimited resource. Therefore, when providing care in a disaster with its inherent dangers, physicians also have an obligation to evaluate the risks of providing care to individual patients versus the need to be available to provide care in the future.
>
> [Opinion 8.3]

However, many Codes of ethics or conduct or guides to good practice remain silent on this issue. After the SARS epidemic some ethicists suggested that there was an argument for some duty to treat in the context of that pandemic. This was because appropriate safety measures could be and were taken, resulting in lower infection rates for health workers, at least after the initial outbreak (Emmanuel, 2003). These approaches imply a need to balance the risks to patients with the risks to health workers, with an eye to the sustainability of the system in the face of ongoing patient need. However, others argue that any duty must be mediated by consideration of the vulnerabilities of the health worker and/or their family members (McConnell, 2020; McDougall et al., 2021).

Healthcare workers hold similar values when it comes to professional responsibility and duty of care, and this duty is an integral part of what it means to be a health professional. Alongside professional integrity, duty of care is largely based on patient's rights, professional virtue, beneficence, and social utility. However, despite these various ethical reasons to uphold a duty of care in all circumstances, both historic and recent events have highlighted that not all healthcare workers will be willing and ready to respond during a disaster.

Ethical challenges for health systems

There are several ethical considerations for health systems during disasters or public health emergencies. In this section we focus on two challenges: ethical responsibilities for ensuring a safe place of work; and resource allocation in an environment of significant resource scarcity due to high demand.

Responsbilities to staff

The ethical issue of the safety of those who respond to disasters and public health emergencies is not new. Health workers are particularly vulnerable to the effects of infectious diseases due to increased exposure, with that risk reducing with the availability and use of appropriate protective equipment, including training about how to maximise safety, and well-designed facilities. Similarly, those who respond to disasters also require appropriate equipment, training, and other resources so that they can work in an environment that manages risks appropriately. Aside from the physical risks, it is also clear that disasters and public health emergencies place health workers under emotional and psychological pressure. But during an emergency or pandemic health workers' well-being is 'both intrinsically and instrumentally valuable' (McDougall et al., 2021, 320). McDougall et al. (2021) have suggested an ethical framework for healthcare organisations to assess risks and balance risks to patients and health workers.

Resource allocation

One ongoing issue with the management of disasters and public health emergencies is how to allocate medical services to patients, such as ventilators or ICU beds, when demand surges and overwhelms resources. For example, the Italian Society of Anaesthesia, Analgesia, Resuscitation, and Intensive Care issued guidance to clinicians, after reports that COVID patients in some over-whelmed Italian hospitals were denied access to ICU, ventilators, or oxygen due to the level of demand. The guidance aimed to address the risk of unfair choices that might arise from a first come first served model of allocation. The guidance suggested that age, comorbidities, and pre-existing functional status should be considered in making access-related decisions (ability to benefit). This was critiqued on the basis that the approach was ageist and discriminatory towards older patients (Craxì et al., 2020) and persons experiencing disabilities or chronic illness. Other proposed models of prioritisation have included greatest clinical acuity, prioritisation of populations with traditionally poorer health outcomes, prioritisation of health workers and essential workers, and, very controversially, prioritisation of the COVID vaccinated over the non-COVID vaccinated.

Health systems across the world have been re-examining or creating policies to determine the basis on which prioritisation for access to health services or evacuations should occur in disasters and public health emergencies (Craxì et al., 2020). The ethical implications of this type of prioritisation for fairness and equity are clear, as is the need for such policies to be developed with broad consultation, before the disaster or public health emergency.

CONCLUSION

This chapter has provided an introduction into key elements of the legal framework at the international and domestic levels, followed by an introduction to some of the most significant ethical issues for health professionals in disaster management and public health emergency contexts. It has demonstrated that law and ethics are an important aspect of disaster management and public health emergency practices both domestically and internationally and, as such, knowledge of both is an important part of professional practice.

ACTIVITIES AND READINGS

Activity:

1. Detail the legislative arrangements in a jurisdiction with which you are familiar.
2. What do you see are the weaknesses in this framework?

References

American Association for the International Commission of Jurists. *The Siracusa principles on the limitation and derogation provisions in the international covenant on civil and political rights* [Internet]. 1985. Available from: https://www.icj.org/wp-content/uploads/1984/07/Siracusa-principles-ICCPR-legal-submission-1985-eng.pdf

American Medical Association. *Physicians' responsibilities in disaster response & preparedness* [Internet]. 2001 [updated 2017; cited 2022]. Available from: https://policysearch.ama-assn.org/policy-finder/detail/opinion%208.3?uri=%2FAMADoc%2FEthics.xml-E-8.3.xml

Annas, G. Legal risks and responsibilities of physicians in the AIDS epidemic. *Hastings Centre Report*, 1988. **18**(2): p. 26–32.

Association of South East Asian Nations. *ASEAN agreement on disaster management and emergency response.* 2005 Jan 06; Vientiane, Laos.

Australian Government. *Comdisplan 2020: Australian government disaster response plan.* 2020, Canberra: Commonwealth of Australia.16p. Available at https://www.homeaffairs.gov.au/emer-gency/files/plan-disaster-response.pdf.

Australian Government. *Natural disaster relief and recovery arrangements determination 2017.* 2017, Canberra: Commonwealth of Australia. Available from https://www.disasterassist.gov.au/disaster-arrangements/natural-disaster-relief-and-recovery-arrangements.

Australian Government. *National recovery and resilience agency: About us (undated).* Available from https://recovery.gov.au/about-us

Biosecurity Act 2015 (Cth)

Capital and Counties v Hampshire Council [1997] QB 2004.

Civil Code, Division 3 Obligations Part 3 Obligations Imposed by Law [1714.2–1714.23] (California, United States of America).

Civil Contingencies Act 2004 (UK)

Civil Defence and Emergency Act 2002 (NZ)

Civil Liability Act 2002 (NSW) s 57.

Craxì, L., M. Vergano, J. Savulescu, and D. Wilkinson, Rationing in a pandemic: Lessons from Italy. *Asian Bioethics Review*, 2020. **12**(3): p. 325–330.

Daniels, N., Duty to treat or right to refuse? *Hastings Centre Report*, 1988. **21**(2): p. 36–46.

Deurenberg-Yap, M., L. L. Foo, Y. Y. Low, S. P. Chan, K. Vijaya, and M. Lee, The Singaporean response to the SARS outbreak: knowledge sufficiency versus public trust. *Health Promotion International*, 2005 **20**(4): p. 320–326.

Dolan and others v Secretary of State for Health and Social Care and others [2020] EWCA Civ 1605.

Eburn, M. *Emergency law.* 4th ed. 2013, Annandale: The Federation Press.

Electro Optic Systems Pty Ltd v NSW [2014] ACTCA 45.

Emergencies Act 1985 (CAN)

Emergency Management Act 2007 (CAN)

Emmanuel, E.J. Lessons of SARS. *Annals of Internal Medicine*, 2003. **139**(7): p. 589–591.

Fatovic, Clement. *Outside the law: Emergency and executive power.* 2009, Baltimore: The Johns Hopkins University Press.

Fidler, David P. Disaster relief and governance after the Indian Ocean Tsunami: What role for international law? *Melbourne Journal of International Law*, 2005. **6**(2): p. 458–473.

Fire and Rescue Services Act 2004 (UK)

Fire and Rescue NSW Act 1989 (NSW)

Fire Service Act 1975 (NZ)

Fire Services Act 1996 (CA)

Gerner v The State of Victoria [2020] HCA 48.

Good Samaritan Act 2002 (CAN) c 172

Graham, R., M.A. McCoy, and A.M. Schultz, *Strategies to improve cardiac arrest survival: A time to act.* 2015, Washington, DC: National Academies Press. 459p.

Health Act 1956 (NZ)

Health and Safety Code, Division 12 Fires and Fire Protection [13000–14960] (California, United States of America).

Huber, S.J., and M.K. Wynia, When pestilence prevails…physician responsibilities in epidemics. *The American Journal of Bioethics*, 2004. **4**(1): p. W5–W11.

Inter-Agency Steering Committee. *Operational guidelines on the protection of persons in situations of natural disasters*. 2011.

International Committee of the Red Cross. *Agreement of the organization of the international activities of the components of the International Red Cross and Red Crescent Movement – The Seville Agreement*. 1997 Nov 25–27; Sevilla, Spain.

International Federation of Red Cross and Red Crescent Societies and the International Committee of the Red Cross. *Code of conduct for the International Red Cross and Red Crescent Movement and NGOs in disaster relief*. 1994.

International Federation of Red Cross and Red Crescent Societies. *Law and legal issues in international disaster response: A desk study*. 2007, Geneva: IFRC. 216p.

Iverson, K.V., C.E. Helne, G.L. Larkin, J.C. Moskop, J. Baruch, and A.L. Aswegan, Fight or flight: The ethics of emergency physician disaster response. *Annals of Emergency Medicine*, 2008; **51**(4): p. 345–353.

Lancet Global Health. The future of the International Health Regulations. *Lancet Global Health*, 2022; **10**(7): p. e928.

Larter v Hazzard (No 2) [2021] NSWSC 1451.

Lee HP. Emergency Powers. Sydney: Law Book Company; 1984.

Leishman v Thomas (1958) 75 WN (NSW) 173, 175.

Loielo v Giles [2020] VSC 722.

Kassam & Henry v Hazzard & Ors [2021] NSWSC 1320.

McConnell, D. Balancing the duty to treat with the duty to family in the context of the COVID-19 pandemic. *Journal of Medical Ethics*, 2020. **46**: p. 360–363.

McDougall, R.J., L. Gillam, D. Ko, et al. Balancing health worker well-being and duty to care: An ethical approach to staff safety in COVID-19 and beyond. *Journal of Medical Ethics*, 2021. **47**: p. 318–323.

Palmer v Western Australia [2021] HCA 5.

Public Health Act 2010 (NSW)

Public Health (Control of Disease) Act 1984 (UK)

Public Health Service Act 42 U.S.C. ch. 6A § 201 et seq.,

Quarantine Act (S.C. 2005, c. 20)

Robert T. Stafford Disaster Relief and Emergency Assistance Act 2013 (US)

Ruderman, C., C.S. Tracy, C.M. Bensimon, et al. On pandemics and the duty to care: Whose duty? Who cares? *BMC Medical Ethics*, 2006. **7**(5): p. 1–6.

Southern Highlands Provincial Government v Somare, Chairman of the National Executive Council [2007] PGSC 2; SC854.

Social Action, Responsibility and Heroism Act 2015 (UK)

State Emergency and Rescue Management Act 1989 (NSW)

United Nations. *Convention on the Rights of Persons with Disabilities*. 2006.

United Nations. *Convention on the Safety of United Nations and Associated Personnel*. 1994.

United Nations. *General Assembly Resolution 36/225 Strengthening the Capacity of the United Nations System to Respond to Natural Disasters and Other Disaster Situations*. 36th session; 1981 Dec 17; New York, United States.

United Nations. *General Assembly Resolution 46/182 Strengthening of the coordination of humanitarian emergency assistance of the United Nations*. 78th Plenary Meeting; 1991 Dec 19; New York, United States.

United Nations. *General Assembly Resolution 57/150 Strengthening the effectiveness and coordination of international urban search and rescue assistance*. 57th session; 2003 Feb 27; New York, United States.

United Nations. *International Covenant on Civil and Political Rights*. 1966a.

United Nations. *International Covenant on Economic, Social and Cultural Rights*. 1966b

United Nations. *Sendai framework for disaster risk reduction 2015–2030*. Geneva: UN; 2015. 37p.

United Nations High Commissioner for Refugees. *The Guiding Principles on Internal Displacement*. 2004.

World Health Organization. *Health and care worker deaths during COVID-19*. 2021. Available from: https://www.who.int/news/item/20-10-2021-health-and-care-worker-deaths-during-covid-19

World Health Organization. *International Health Regulations*. 2005.

Zuger, A. and S.H. Miles. Physicians, AIDS, and occupational risk. Historic traditions and ethical obligations. *JAMA*, 1987. **258**: p. 1924–1928.

Part 3
Healthcare considerations

10

Health systems impacts and responses to disasters

Andrew Johnson, Gerry FitzGerald, Penelope Burns,
Stacey Pizzino, and Colin Myers

INTRODUCTION AND OBJECTIVES

Disasters pose significant challenges to the provision of health services in response and recovery. At the very time when health systems are required to surge to meet the growth in demand associated with a major event, they are subject to the devastating impact of the event. In the period following the disaster, sustaining and rebuilding health services are crucial to prompt management of disaster health effects presenting in the weeks and months after the disaster.

Disasters have direct and indirect impacts on the health system. Direct impacts include damage to health infrastructure, resources and supplies, including disruption and personal injury to personnel. Indirect impacts result from loss of support functions such as power, transport and supply chains, disruptions to school and childcare facilities and staffing, and longer-term relocation of medical personnel from the area.

Disasters adversely affect the health and wellbeing of people who will require disaster healthcare but also deprive people of access to their normal healthcare.

These considerations were well evidenced during COVID-19 when the system's ability to meet the surging demand for healthcare was further limited by the loss of key staff either from infection or isolation and disrupted supply chains. The closure of schools and childcare facilities aggravated staff availability. The risks associated with the pandemic dissuaded people from attending for both urgent and routine healthcare and disrupted screening and vaccination programs. This is likely to have adverse long-term population health impacts.

Health leaders need response and recovery plans that will guide responses in the context of the local environment. The plans for one region may be quite different from another and need to reflect not only the hazards and threats in their community, but the local capacity and resources available, and the local culture. A disaster will challenge healthcare providers to look for ways of coping with rapidly evolving changes over which they have little control while considering the need to sustain healthcare as an ongoing process during and after the event. Consideration of these matters in advance and, ensuring that everyone knows and understands their roles, will allow a more resilient response and better outcome.

DOI: 10.4324/9781032626604-13

The aim of this chapter is to explore the health system's role in disasters. On completion of this chapter, you should have the ability to:

1. Identify and discuss the impacts that disasters have on the health system.
2. Identify and evaluate strategies required to enable the health system to respond.
3. Critically evaluate strategies required to build health system resilience.

UNDERSTANDING HEALTH SYSTEMS

The WHO defines health as:

> "*a complete state of physical mental, and social wellbeing*", not merely the absence of disease [1, 2]

This broader view of health calls upon health systems to extend well beyond narrow perspectives of the treatment of the sick and injured and has relevance for the breadth of understanding of the impact of disasters. The WHO defines health systems as:

> A health system consists of all organizations, people and actions whose primary intent is to promote, restore or maintain health. [3]

Health systems include the 'continuum of health promotion, disease prevention, diagnosis, treatment, disease-management, rehabilitation and palliative care services, through the different levels and sites of care within the health system over the course of a lifetime' [4]. This comprehensive perspective is critical to understanding the roles played by health systems in the prevention and management of the adverse impacts of disasters. Healthcare prevention continues through the continuum of disaster management.

Routine population health services designed to prevent and control disease outbreaks and ensure healthy physical environments may also be conceptualised as disaster prevention and mitigation strategies.

Health systems vary across the globe reflecting the level of development, funding models, levels of access and resources available to service delivery. WHO supports countries in moving their health systems towards universal health coverage, through increased access to safe, high-quality, effective, people-centred and integrated services [4]. The extent and quality of health systems can determine the impact any event may have, and the capacity of the system to respond and minimise community impact.

Thus, disaster health management (DHM) and disaster risk reduction for health (DRR) is an *all of health, all of system activity*. Health system managers should (ideally) develop a holistic understanding of their respective health systems, the way each part functions and interacts during non-disaster periods, and how that changes to respond to disasters. This is not so as to focus on the clinical care of patients, but rather on the management and coordinating processes that are necessary to ensure patients are cared for efficiently and effectively.

To deal with these challenges, it is important for healthcare leaders and disaster managers to understand the way their system works. It is not a hierarchical, top-down system, but rather an organic, evolving, and ever-changing interconnected world that responds to leadership and not reliably to direction. Understanding these concepts builds resilience within the healthcare system, that is, the capacity to adjust and deal with threats and challenges and still achieve required outcomes.

This has significance for DHM, which should focus not only on the treatment of the sick and injured, but also on the promotion of resilience both of the individual and of the system. As both health systems and risk management move to a community-based approach, it is necessary to ensure that the community and all health stakeholders are involved. There has been a tendency to take a hospital-centric approach to DHM. However, COVID-19 has demonstrated the critical role played by community healthcare services. Both in the immediate response to a disaster but also importantly in the longer-term management of its health consequences.

During disasters the healthcare system will be stretched, and novel system-wide strategies will be required including maximising the whole of system response, enhanced use of telehealth and establishment of purposive facilities such as fever clinics, vaccination and testing centres, enhanced use of alternative infrastructure, as seen in mass entertainment centres, pop-up tents, shipping containers, parking lots, covered walkways, community buildings and churches, and local ovals.

Within this comprehensive concept of health systems there are particular aspects that play a leading role and are worthy of special consideration.

Population (public) health

The primary focus of population health is to protect the health of the population through the prevention of death, disease and disability in populations, and the promotion of health. Health protection has a critical role in DHM, particularly in the traditional fields of environmental health (water, sanitation, vector control, and shelter), communicable disease control and epidemic management. A broader role of public health is to reduce the overall level of risk to the community during the prevention and mitigation, preparedness, response, and recovery phases. This is particularly relevant in the post-disaster phase when normal public health protections may be damaged, increasing the risk of infectious and environmental hazards. It is also relevant in displaced populations where public health protections are absent and prompt provision of safe food and water, basic sanitation, and healthcare is required.

Population health activities to reduce risk in disasters include:

- Reducing the vulnerability of a community to environmental hazards through the control of dangerous goods, vector control, air quality, food safety, potable water, and effective sewerage management.
- Infectious disease surveillance and control systems including testing and contract tracing capability.
- Immunisation programs.
- Outreach medical/health services.
- Public information on potential health impacts, and personal and community measures to prevent disease.
- Promotion of healthy options to build individual resilience.
- Developing personal skills and strengthening community action.

Population health also contributes to system coordination and control [5] and to the preparedness for disasters, for example, the management of stockpiles of antiviral agents or personal protective equipment [6]. Population health services were stretched to the limit, or overwhelmed in some countries, during the COVID-19 pandemic screening for disease, determining case definitions, contact tracing, and establishing isolation and quarantine regulations. For this reason, a clear pathway to rapidly enhance recruitment to public health functions must be available within the health system

Emergency healthcare

Emergency Healthcare System (EHS) or Emergency Medical Systems (EMSs) has been defined as:

> A field of practice based on the knowledge and skills required for the prevention, diagnosis and management of acute and urgent aspects of illness and injury affecting patients of all age groups with a full spectrum of episodic undifferentiated physical and behavioural disorders; it further encompasses an understanding of the development of pre-hospital and in-hospital emergency medical systems and the skills necessary for this development. [7]

A well-developed EHS consists of the following components:

- Community-based primary care and first responder programs, including walk-in or urgent care centres.
- Pre-hospital care service (ambulance) with well-equipped vehicles, trained staff, and clear triage protocols.
- Healthcare facilities, including primary care and hospital Emergency Departments (EDs), with appropriate equipment and well-trained staff to provide triage and management of ill and injured patients.
- Interhospital transfer and retrieval services including aeromedical services
- Supportive critical care services such as surgical and intensive care services.

The EHS will be called upon to mount a rapid response to most major events and therefore system managers must have in place plans for scaling up response capacity to meet the sudden surge in demand and to sustain the capability over sometimes prolonged period.

MAINTAINING HEALTH SERVICES

To be able to maintain services and provide definitive care to the sick and injured during a disaster, Emergency Departments and receiving facilities must have plans to rapidly increase their capacity.

The capacity of the EHS to respond appropriately depends on its regular capability. A response in an urban centre may include paramedics and emergency medicine specialists while many rural communities may be served by small numbers of volunteers, co-responding personnel (i.e., Fire), along with rural nurses and general practitioners (GPs).

Some jurisdictions use hospital-based teams that deploy in a pre-hospital role [8]. This should be carefully planned for, so as not to place hospital staff in an unfamiliar role and environment, and also to not reduce the capacity at the receiving facility. Regardless of the role, any such teams must be prepared, appropriately trained, equipped, coordinated, and requested by the pre-hospital clinical lead. A special example of these teams is DMAT, which are multidisciplinary teams comprising task-specific mixtures of primary care, acute care, and public health capabilities. This is covered in detail in Chapter 17.

Coordination and communication structures need to be appropriate to the scope of the service. For example, it may be appropriate for a large hospital to have an incident management team and emergency operations centre (EOC), but coordination within a primary care facility may only be by radio or phone to a single person. A system-wide structure for communication between facilities and with disaster management agencies will be required. Different communication modes, including runners, radio, satellite and cell phone, email and data transmission may be useful in different environments. Systems such as bed management systems or emergency management systems all have appropriate roles and should be tested and exercised.

Whilst response pathways in a disaster should be as similar as possible to normal (just faster and with more capacity), some disasters may require significant reconfiguration of the emergency healthcare services. Professional services may need to be complemented by community-based organisations including primary care services and volunteer services. It is important to consider how such services will be engaged in the disaster response and how they are appropriately engaged in planning, training, and exercising. Initial responders will always be from the affected community and first aid competency and access to basic supplies should be encouraged.

> COMMUNICATION
> A system-wide structure for communicating between facilities and with disaster management agencies is needed. This requires different, and at times, innovative communication modes, including: runners, two-way radio, satellite and mobile phone, email and data transmission including inter/intranet and facsimile.

Following the London Bombings in 2005, survivors testified in the inquiry that they had to improvise first-aid supplies whilst clinical help arrived. Health agencies in London subsequently installed mass casualty first-aid kits, consisting of quantities of basic dressings and stretchers in underground and railway stations across London. The Coroner's report on the London bombings can be found at https://www.gov.uk/government/publications/coroners-inquests-into-the-london-bombings-of-7-july-2005-review-of-progress

---

FRAMEWORKS FOR HEALTH SYSTEM MANAGEMENT

All major disaster incidents require a multidisciplinary and coordinated mitigation and response and health management framework, that must necessarily fit within the broader community-wide systems and structures.

The 2011 World Health Assembly resolution 64.10 [9] provides a global mandate for DHM. This Resolution urges member states to 'Strengthen all-hazards health emergency and Disaster Risk Management (DRM) programmes'. This policy direction is reinforced by the Sendai Framework for Disaster Risk Reduction 2015–2030 [10] which sets four specific priorities for action, all of which have application to health agencies and health disaster managers. These are:

- Understanding disaster risk.
- Strengthening disaster risk governance to manage disaster risk.
- Investing in DRR for resilience.
- Enhancing disaster preparedness for effective response, and to build back better in recovery, rehabilitation, and reconstruction.

In response, many countries have developed national policy and legislation encompassing common elements of the Sendai DRM frameworks which provides a contemporary framework for health to develop resilience alongside other sectors.

These broader international directions are articulated by WHO at a regional level. For example, the WHO Western Pacific Region has six of the ten most vulnerable countries in the world according to the 2014 World Risk Report [11] (based on risk to natural hazards against exposure, susceptibility, coping capacity and adaptive capacity with a wide range of hazards including tropical cyclone, earthquake, tsunami, volcano, drought, and sea-level rise) impacting countries from a population of 1200 (Niue) to over 1.3Bn (China). Following consultation, a regional framework for health DRM was adopted in 2014 that identifies four key components as critical: development of governance, policy, planning and coordination; provision of information and knowledge management; capacity building for health and related services and resources; and support all-hazards DHM [4].

At the national level, health policy and legislative frameworks vary along with the roles and responsibilities of health agencies in disasters. In many instances health will be a support agency and national disaster management strategies will be implemented in accordance with the whole of community systems and structures. Health will be responsible for ensuring the ongoing delivery of health system functions during an emergency. It may also be the lead agency for human health emergencies such as heatwaves and pandemics. Disaster managers need to have consider how health will provide leadership and response coordination in these circumstances.

Jurisdictions may also have an established framework of contracts, services or standards for healthcare providers. Providers can be incentivised to participate in specific risk reduction activities, such as planning and participation in health DRM exercises. A business continuity management framework could be a contractual requirement. This is mutually beneficial in that the provider can remain in business whilst the affected community can continue to access health services.

At the local level, a mixture of private and public providers typically deliver health services. In any area, these may be coordinated by a sub-national entity such as a health district, or primary health network, or by a voluntary or corporate group. Understanding the relationship between different providers, especially around finite acute capacities such as operating theatres or ICU beds is critical. It is also important to ensure that community providers, including those funded through the social sector, are also considered. Providers such as aged care or disability providers can help reduce the impact on vulnerable people. Avoiding the evacuation or relocation of residents from a care facility through good preparedness will reduce the impact on all responding agencies. It is important to recognise that during a disaster, previously unknown vulnerable populations may emerge and the demand for some services, such as mental health and chronic disease management, may significantly increase.

System coordination and control

The legislative and policy frameworks will usually provide for the roles and responsibilities of health and other agencies in both routine emergencies and disasters. The development of plans for surge capacity, continued service delivery (business continuity) or leadership may be a mandatory requirement or may be directed and required by the policy framework. These plans need to describe the system of command, control, coordination, and communication that will be used (in an emergency or disaster) and enable local solutions to be developed that meet its intent. One solution is unlikely to work across all parts of a country. Typically, legislative and policy frameworks will include:

- A *legislative framework for disaster management*, national security, or civil defence. These typically outline Ministry or Department roles and responsibilities, often by hazard or consequence.
- Within the health system a range of *advisory committees or working groups*. During the pandemic there have been an extensive range of expert clinical groups collaborating internationally, providing advice on SARS-CoV-2 vaccinations and prioritisation groups, clinical management of COVID-19 patients, and following the 2019 Australian Black Summer bushfires, a national child trauma advisory group, all feeding back to key decision makers.
- The *roles and responsibilities* of various bodies which will be reflected at regional and local levels. Jurisdictions may have different approaches regarding the hazard and consequence management lead. For example, the response to Ebola in West Africa in 2014–2015 saw the overall response coordination allocated to central departments such as the Prime Minister, President, NDMA or Defence, however health remained responsible for managing the impact on the health system.
- The regulatory bodies including those responsible for *registration* of health professionals, regulation of pharmaceutical, consumables and devices and the protection of consumer interests. Consider the regulatory impediments to the use of foreign medical teams.
- The key *role of professional clinical associations and unions* in protecting their members' interest, safety and livelihood, being mindful that with early engagement these bodies can provide assistance in developing and supporting official policies and occupational health and safety. For example, during preparedness activity for Ebola virus disease, the professional bodies of several unaffected countries provided interpretation and dissemination of official advice, as well as identifying emerging issues to policy makers.
- The responsibility of associations and colleges for *training and the ongoing development* of health professionals. Many have working groups focussed on disaster medicine, or mass casualties. There is a role for colleges in providing stewardship and enhancing the capability of their professionals. They are often a key stakeholder in reaching health professionals and their population.

A considered approach to DHM throughout its continuum, demands a comprehensive understanding of key stakeholders in the jurisdiction, as these will be influential in setting policy direction and in sustaining major responses. Identification of these stakeholders and their roles and responsibilities is a critical component of planning and preparedness activities.

A considered approach to disaster health management demands a comprehensive understanding of key stakeholders, as these will be influential in setting policy direction and to sustain major responses.

THE IMPACT OF DISASTERS ON HEALTH SYSTEMS

Health systems are often affected by disasters. The range of ways in which impacts occur depends on many factors including the disaster hazard, the direct and indirect damage caused, the disruption to usual healthcare function, and the degree of mitigation from pre-disaster efforts in prevention and preparedness. Examples of direct and indirect impacts are explored below.

Direct impacts of disasters on health systems:
- Damage to critical infrastructure.
- Injury to staff.
- Loss of resources.
- Increased number of patients.

Direct impacts

Damage to critical infrastructure

In many disasters, the health system is in the disaster zone. On occasions, elements of the health system may in fact be the source of the disaster, for example, a hospital fire or terrorist attack. At other times, the health infrastructure may be damaged, for example, the destruction of hospital or community health centres in an earthquake. In the aftermath of Hurricane Katrina, makeshift hospitals were established in alternative venues such as airports and halls [12]. During the Brisbane floods health clinics were established in churches and halls. Damage to high technology services such as those providing ICU or renal dialysis can be particularly challenging to restore functionality. For example, clean water is vital to renal dialysis so contamination of water supplies may mean the transport of patients to a distant facility.

Injury to staff

One of the most challenging aspects of disasters for healthcare systems is the loss of its own people to the disaster. Not only does this have a direct impact on the capacity and capability of the service to respond, but it has a huge impact on the psychological wellbeing of the remaining staff. For example, early in the SARS epidemic in Hong Kong, key personnel, including the medical and nursing staff leading the response, fell ill with some staff dying. This can impact the willingness of staff to attend and continue to provide care. There may be an impact on both staff who were present and staff who *missed out* due to appropriate rostering practices. These concepts will be discussed in more detail in Chapter 12.

Loss of resources

As with loss of critical infrastructure, the supply caches of the health system may be impacted by the disaster or indeed they may be the source of the disaster. In a major centre, with greater redundancy, this may be less of an issue; however, in more remote population centres this can become a very significant issue. It is also impacted by 'just in time' delivery and stock holding policies. This may cause a failure of supply of medications and equipment for ongoing management of pre-existing conditions or for early treatment of conditions that could become life-threatening if not rapidly treated.

Increase in patient load

Indirect impacts of disasters on health systems:
• Decreased availability of staff due to loss of community infrastructure.
• Failure to resupply due to loss of supply lines.
• Loss of financial viability.

In a disaster, regardless of its nature, there is commonly a surge in demand. Each form of disaster brings with it, its own form of challenges, for example, a bomb blast or explosion will generate penetrating injuries, often multiple, and may be complicated by burns and smoke inhalation. A natural disaster such as a storm may give rise to blunt trauma, lacerations and, commonly, significant injury from clean-up efforts, for example, contaminated lacerations, falls from rooftops, and chain saw injuries [13]. As discussed in Chapter 11 disaster effects can continue for a prolonged period, with an increase in new physical and mental health conditions, and deterioration of chronic disease, in the months after an event.

Indirect impacts

Decreased availability of staff due to loss of community infrastructure

Health service managers rapidly discover how dependent they are on a complex interlinking of community resources when those resources are challenged. For example, in the lead up to a natural disaster such as a cyclone, *non-essential* services may be suspended. This can have a profound impact on health service staffing availability. For example, the closure of schools and childcare facilities can reduce the ability of parents to work. Similarly, disruption to public transport systems can affect the ability of staff to travel to work. Occasionally, the loss of staff may be the perverse consequence of the redistribution of local personnel. Foreign aid agencies arriving on disaster relief missions may take on local staff (both clinical and non-clinical staff such as drivers, interpreters etc.) to augment their response at the expense of local efforts. This represents a significant challenge to the delivery of both aid and normal services.

Failure of resupply due to loss of supply lines

Whilst destruction or contamination of stores and provisions can be seen as a direct impact, the capacity for resupply may be challenged. This is particularly the case for areas with poor transport infrastructure, or where transport mechanisms are disrupted. For example, after a tsunami there can be a near-total loss of supply lines, port infrastructure, airports, roads, and rail in the one event, whilst the health service infrastructure on high ground may be spared.

Loss of financial viability

Health systems are part of the economy, just like any other facet of society. They need money to run, to pay for staff, power, supplies and infrastructure. One of the early impacts of a disaster, or indeed the source of the disaster, can be financial crisis. For example, a private sector health service may be starved of revenue due to a collapse of the market for high-dividend elective surgery which may result in service failure. Similarly primary care services may lose income by the provision of free care to injured people. This can result in the closure of rural general practices leaving these disaster-affected communities with reduced healthcare services in the recovery phase.

Health system resilience

Each of the direct and indirect impacts described above is to a greater or lesser degree, predictable. This means they can be anticipated, planned for, and deliver more effective care despite those issues arising. This contributes to what is known as system resilience.

A resilient healthcare system is one that can anticipate and plan for the direct and indirect impacts of a disaster and still maintain an effective level of care despite these impacts.

In recent years, leading researchers in healthcare [14–17] have written about the concept of Resilient Health Care (RHC) outside of the context of disaster health. Their definition of RHC has evolved and resonates with the definition of resilience used in Chapter 1. An RHC system can adjust its functioning prior to, during, or following changes and disturbances, so that it can sustain required operations, under both expected and unexpected conditions [15]. The very qualities that make a health system robust and capable in normal times are the qualities required in the context of disaster.

Key elements of RHC are essential to reflect in disaster health, including healthcare as a complex adaptive system, safety-one and safety-two and work-as-imagined vs. work-as-done, further explained below [15].

Healthcare as a complex adaptive system (CAS)

Wiig and O'Hara [18] see resilience as *"a broad concept with a multi-sector and multi-level scope"*. *It involves multiple populations and organisations and is co-created as a "collective, dynamic responsibility"*.

Braithwaite et al. [14] challenged the orthodox *linear* thinking that prevails in healthcare. The dictum of *primum non nocere*, or *first do no harm* aims to eliminate unwanted outcomes, and to improve the efficiency of the healthcare system. It has led healthcare system leaders to adopt a *managerialism* approach to the delivery of healthcare, breaking care down into small, measurable and reproducible components which can then be standardised thus eliminating unwarranted variation. This has met with resistance from frontline workers who will often opine that standardised care cannot be achieved when the patient themselves is not standardised.

Suggesting an organic model of healthcare, Braithwaite et al. [14] describe a CAS that adjusts and evolves to meet the extant circumstances. A systematic review undertaken by Clay-Williams et al. [19] explored how organisational and cultural factors influence hospital-wide patient care interventions and the effects these interventions have on patients. The study examined organisational determinants including staff morale and organisational climate; organisational and patient safety culture; clinical and organisational leadership; education, training, promotion and awareness of interventions. Whilst the range of studies was limited, findings suggest there is potential to improve patient outcomes by changing organisational and/or cultural determinants. System-wide change can be most influenced by effective leadership, adequate funding and professional development, and career advancement opportunities [19].

According to Rouse [20], the CAS has a number of key features:

- Nonlinear and dynamic and not inherently reach fixed-equilibrium points; as a result, system behaviours may appear to be random or chaotic.
- Composed of independent agents whose behaviour is based on physical, psychological, or social rules rather than the demands of system dynamics.
- Goals and behaviours are likely to conflict because agents' needs or desires, reflected in their rules, are not homogeneous. In response to these conflicts or competitions, agents tend to adapt to each other's behaviours.
- Agents are intelligent. As they experiment and gain experience, agents learn and change their behaviours accordingly. Thus, overall system behaviour inherently changes over time.
- Adaptation and learning tend to result in self-organisation. Behaviour patterns emerge rather than being designed into the system. The nature of emergent behaviours may range from valuable innovations to unfortunate accidents.
- No single point(s) of control. System behaviours are often unpredictable and uncontrollable, and no one is *in-charge*. Consequently, the behaviours of complex adaptive systems can usually be more easily influenced than controlled.

The nonlinear, highly complex and *heterarchical* reality of the health system, means that it is not predisposed to work well when a hierarchical command and control disaster management approach is superimposed. One cannot command or force such systems to comply with behavioural and performance dictates using any conventional means. Agents in complex adaptive systems are sufficiently intelligent to game the system, find *work-arounds*, and creatively identify ways to serve their own or their patients' best interests. They will do so under both routine and non-routine challenges (such as disasters); for both positive and negative purposes.

The consequence is that the way work is actually delivered on the ground may bear little resemblance to the way that leaders and managers think it is being done. Hence, policies, procedures and plans, written by middle managers, may bear little resemblance to what is and can be done in the workplace.

For those who may lead in disaster health, this reinforces the need to ensure the engagement of the frontline workers in designing and implementing solutions to emergent problems. In health, unlike most industries, the smartest people are often at the frontline, and they understand the work they do better than anyone else. To be effective, the disaster health leader needs to lead and coordinate and not manage or direct, communicating outcomes desired, rather than methods and processes to get to those outcomes.

Safety one and safety two

Consider the work of Hollnagel, a systems engineer who recognised the intense scrutiny applied to rare failures within systems, rather than recognising and seeking to understand what goes right. Hollnagel et al. [21] describe the pursuit of eliminating variation and risk as *safety-one*, and the broader focus on understanding what happens to make things go right as *safety-two*. The implications of this for disaster health practitioners and indeed for much of the Health Quality and Safety infrastructure, are profound. Rather than focussing only on where things go wrong, and in taking a linear reductionist approach to understanding failure, analysis is often better to look at what goes well so this can be maximised when the system is stretched.

MANAGEMENT OF SURGE

One of the most predictable effects of a disaster is the surge in emergency health activity that it may produce. EHS worldwide, although very different in their structures, approaches and service delivery, share a common feature. They are overloaded in normal times, let alone in a disaster. This can lead to significant *brittleness* and vulnerability within the system.

Managing surge requires:
- Space.
- Staff.
- Stuff (supplies).
- Systems flow.

A key in the response to a surge is recognising that this is not just an issue for the EMS but rather the broader health system and the entire community. Community healthcare services often have considerable capacity to see large numbers of patients, particularly lower acuity, to keep EDs and other services less overwhelmed to manage the higher acuity patients.

This was seen post Hurricane Katrina when a group of general practitioners took responsibility for 3700 evacuees arriving in Texas, providing care to 45% over a fortnight. Commonest presentations were medications for chronic illnesses, and skin infections. The local ED saw 148 evacuees arriving separately with many not seriously ill.

(Edwards, 2007)

Mobilising community support can take the load off the over-stretched health system and allow it to function optimally. This can include: schools and childcare services working extra hours to look after the children of key staff; families or friends taking home patients not requiring acute care who are waiting for aged care placement; and other government agencies assisting with transporting stores. Health is a key priority for the community, and they will want to help, if given permission to do so and a role to play, and will contribute to building local community capacity and resilience.

The disaster health manager therefore is challenged to work within an already stretched system to achieve the required objectives, this is going to require changes; to priorities, to flows, and to the approach to care. In the reality of healthcare as a CAS, it is important to recognise the significant variation in context. Consider, for example, the variability between a regional and a metropolitan centre. Not only will the regional centre have fewer resources directly but will also lack access to other facilities that may characterise a metropolitan area.

Therefore, it is better to work on the basis of principles and concepts, rather than tightly defined rules and practices.

One such common approach applies to surge management. The well-drilled department will be able to *flip into disaster mode* without the need for external authority and will take a number of actions immediately. Disaster mode may require rapid expansion of capability that can be usefully considered under the categories of space, staff, stuff, and systems [22].

For example, the recent COVID 19 pandemic, challenged healthcare systems. However, the nature of challenge varied with stages of the pandemic. During the contain phase, enhanced community based social isolation measures restricted staff availability even though the demand for care was low. During significant outbreaks though, demand surged while availability of staff was also restricted by both active infections and enforced quarantine and isolation.

In contrast, a lull in healthcare presentations can also be seen when locals evacuate high-risk communities, or during the pandemic when patients stayed away from areas they saw as high risk. As noted above, for privately funded community healthcare services, this becomes a consideration for longer-term sustainability.

Space

Often the first warning of a major event may be the arrival of patients at health services or a report from the media on the waiting room television. Walk-in patients can arrive even before the first ambulances, and things can get very chaotic and very crowded very quickly. The leadership on the ground needs to have the delegated authority to initiate actions across the system. This will involve the creation of space to triage, assess and manage patients and to provide for definitive care. This is a whole of system issue, not just an EMS response, and can be based on the concept of *divert, decant, absorb and expand*. For example:

- Defer all non-emergency patients or divert to community-based services, particularly general practice.
- Decanting the acute health system by discharging everyone who is unlikely to come to harm or moving patients to outgoing care. Inpatient teams should conduct urgent discharge rounds. Consideration may be given to altering discharge criteria from

ready for discharge to *unlikely to come to harm if discharged*. The increased the load this may place on primary care doctors needs to be remembered.

- Absorbing additional patient numbers may require increased capacity within the available space regardless of normal capacity constraints. For example, most EDs have pre-prepared plans to rapidly expand their footprint by placing those with minimal injuries or illness into hospital outpatient areas in order to maintain the main area of the ED for complex and critical patients.
- Moving screening functions such as triage outside the ED may assist by improving patient flow to nearby clinical spaces that can be used for ambulant patients, e.g., outpatient clinic areas. These areas may also be used for *cohorting* of friends and relatives.
- Deferring all non-emergency surgery and ICU admissions and preserving critical internal infrastructure. For example, designating a number of theatres for trauma reception, same for ICU.
- Where patients are awaiting aged care placement and not requiring acute care, family may be called to take them home for the duration of the disaster or step-down facilities such as schools or hotels commissioned for this purpose.

Staff

Arguably augmentation of staff should come first, but in reality, the actions are required in parallel. Without staff, with the right skills, it is not possible to deal with a surge in attendances. The people who know best how to manage patients in a surge, are those who work in the emergency environment every day. They need to be preserved to do the things that only they can do and use others to undertake supportive tasks.

Things to consider include:

- Redeploying staff from other areas.
- *Buddying* extra staff with specialty staff to maximise staffing numbers and reduce disorientation for those staff working outside their usual area of expertise, or those staff recalled from retirement.
- Calling in staff whose specialised skills may be required, including the leadership team. This needs to be balanced with the requirement to maintain capacity over time and not *burning out* all human resources in the initial response.
- Cancellation of non-essential tasks such as training or projects.
- Consider utilising partly trained support personnel such as students.

Stuff (supplies)

This is a *catchall* expression to group all other resources required. Some elements are essential to cache and have at the ready; others can be sourced *just-in-time*. One essential to consider for caching is medical records. These are now usually accessible online in the form of electronic medical records. Early notification and mobilisation are essential for *just-in-time* resources.

Systems flow

Maintaining the flow of patients is essential to the normal business of EMSs. Patients should proceed in a single streamlined way from one point of care to the next. In any system, there are always bottlenecks, the rate-limiting component of care. Commonly these will be found in a resource-intensive, expensive component of care such as diagnostic imaging or operating theatre access. In maintaining flow in disasters, it is critical to ensure that patients only receive diagnostics that will inform or alter their care, and they should not be detained waiting for results unless that affects the direction of their care. This rationing of diagnostic imaging to improve overall patient flow is best accomplished by more senior medical staff.

In the COVID-19 pandemic, systems of flow were substantially affected by the need for strict observation of infection, prevention and control systems with spacing between patients, avoidance of time spent in smaller enclosed areas, and the need for access to PPE. Patients were streamed to infective and non-infective streams or were seen in outdoor tents, and in drive-through clinics particularly for diagnostic swabbing and vaccinations. The need to maintain infection control by separating COVID-19-infected patients from those who were not created high levels of additional work within all health services including Intensive Care Units, wards, operating theatres, and community healthcare services.

PREPARING THE HEALTH SYSTEM

Of course, usual healthcare need continues during disaster and not all is deferrable, e.g., birth of babies. Considering this in advance will assist in getting the best outcomes for the community. Critical to success, is the forward planning that allows staff and leaders (and the community) to assume familiar roles and use concepts, principles and practices that they understand well enough to be able to adapt them. Plans should not be rigid. Each disaster is unique. Health plans should delineate desired outcomes, and the principles and concepts needed to achieve the outcomes, allowing flexibility in application.

The preparation of the health system for disaster is a consequence of system-wide strategies built around the concepts of resilience healthcare systems. Greater success is likely to be achieved when disaster responses are familiar to all involved. Considering the relative rarity of disasters, this is best achieved by 'mainstreaming' DHM into routine activities.

Thus, disaster plans need to be developed that demonstrate an understanding of how the system operates in normal circumstances and how those operations can surge in response to both routine and rare events. The process and scope of planning are dealt with in Chapter 14.

Similarly, health system responses need to reflect a phased approach which recognises the confusion and uncertainty of initial responses. The phased approach is discussed in Part 4.

ISSUES WITH THE PROVISION OF HEALTHCARE IN DISASTERS

There are many significant issues specific to health planning and the provision of health services during disasters. The following are explored as examples only and not an indication of their importance or prevalence.

Clinical issues

- **Management of the deceased** is a critical factor, not only for the physical management of the bodies, but also for the recovery phase and achieving 'closure' for individuals and the community. Additional capacity for storage of the deceased may be necessary and access to similar facilities (e.g., anatomy teaching facilities) or refrigerated vans have been commonly utilised. Cultural and religious considerations as well as accurate disaster victim identification are critical to effective long-term management. Modern techniques using DNA sampling of victims, whilst time-consuming to process, may allow for body disposal by burial or cremation, whilst maintaining the opportunity for subsequent identification.

- In many catastrophic disasters, patients are identified as alive but requiring huge input for unlikely survival. It is always a challenging decision to take, but at times the dictum of 'greatest good for the greatest number' means that it may be considered unethical to expend extremely limited resources in likely **futile care**. Some health services address this through plans to identify and provide comfort care to those identified with 'non-survivable injuries' in an area separate to the rest of the emergency response. Treatment may be limited to oxygen therapy and pain control. As the disaster evolves, these patients may be reassessed and if their condition improves, reconsidered for definitive care.

- **Clinical standards** may need to vary from normal. Recently the concept of *Crisis Standards of Care* has been explored as a means of describing altered clinical standards [23]. Rapid progress of patients through operating theatres may be essential to avoid a critical bottleneck. Many of the presenting injuries may take several hours and enormous resources for definitive care. Initial stabilisation, haemostasis, and wound toilet followed by delayed definitive care can expedite care and reduce scarce resource utilisation in the early phase of the disaster. This may be characterised as damage control surgery and draws experience from a long history of military surgery. In General Practice this may mean limiting care to the immediate most urgent presentation with usual more comprehensive preventive care postponed until later visits.

- **Rationing** is a word commonly brought into discussions of disaster healthcare. The ethical challenges are real and confront the clinician in the front line who is charged with allocating scarce resources to people who may have competing needs. Such choices are invidious and are an extreme amplification of the daily dilemma faced by practitioners in many parts of the world. The process of rationing is generally achieved through triage and disaster triage is a significant issue in DHM.

- **Reduction in use of resources** is often achievable by rethinking our tolerance of *abnormal* clinical parameters. For example, only a few years ago, blood and blood products were used much more freely and given to patients with much better haemoglobin levels than now tolerated. Many products designed for medical use are labelled *single use only* when they can in fact, with appropriate care be reused multiple times with effective cleaning and sterilisation. Innovative clinicians and technicians will often be able to repurpose discarded items and should be encouraged to do so safely.

Human resource issues

In a disaster response augmentation of staff can be critical. On most occasions, domestic and international external relief will become available if required, but this can take some time to emerge. Some considerations in the early phases include:

- Disaster healthcare provision may place health care workers (HCWs) at personal risk, for example, the risk of nuclear contamination for HCWs working close to the exclusion zone during the Great East Japan Earthquake Tsunami, or the risk of personal infection and severe illness for HCWs during the current SARS-CoV-2 pandemic.

- Clinical governance and credentialing of clinical staff is an essential feature of health systems. Health services need to consider how they will verify the bona fides of volunteer clinicians. In the disaster context there is a need to ensure flexibility in response, and staff may be required at times to work outside their normal scope of practice.

- A key factor in staff making themselves available in a disaster is concern for the **safety and protection of their family**. An effective strategy used in many facilities in cyclone-prone areas of Australia is to allow staff to bring in their families during the event. They must be self-sufficient and depart the facilities as soon as it is safe to do so.

- Similarly **care of children** may be critical to maintaining staff availability during a response. This does not need to be complex and can offer meaningful and valuable duties to staff who are experts in dealing with children. It may be accommodated in areas of a hospital such as meeting rooms, office areas, or paediatric-friendly areas such as outpatient spaces designed for children. Allowing interaction between staff member parents and their children offers a huge psychological boost to both parties.

- For many staff and patients, **pets are considered family members**. People will risk their lives to save their pets. If an effective mechanism for providing pet care can be established for staff, it is likely that staff availability may well follow. As Cyclone Yasi approached Townsville in 2011, many staff smuggled pets into the campus, this was the only way they felt they could attend and meet their commitments.

- Reduced **access to work** is a significant issue in disasters. In fires, storms, earthquakes and other natural and indeed man-made disasters, simple issues such as road closures can mean the difference between having staff and not. Similarly, the suspension of public transportation may restrict access. Engagement with other agencies such as municipal councils, emergency response agencies and the military may assist in transport in these circumstances.

- Commonly there will be a flow of **volunteers** that can be both helpful and a hindrance. It is worth considering how their efforts may add value, freeing up skilled staff to do things that require their expertise. Building relationships with (organised) volunteer agencies, such as the Red Cross may help ensure volunteers are appropriately credentialed. The use of volunteers is limited in complex clinical environments which require specialist knowledge. However, systems such as buddying and the use of volunteers for support can be helpful. Volunteer clinicians are a common feature including those arriving as part of a disaster medical assistance team.

- In a disaster event, the nature of presentations will be significantly different to normal times, and the availability of resources may necessitate the use of different treatment modalities. Rather than continuing to try to provide the same care as normal, practitioners may need to adapt to what is available. Additionally **professional standards may need greater flexibility**. For example, an obstetrician and gynaecologist may be able to sufficiently skilled in basic surgical techniques such as laparotomy and haemostasis and may be able to assist experienced trauma surgeons.

Societal issues

- **Reconnecting families** and loved ones is a critical element of restoring community and social cohesion. In the confusion that often reigns in the aftermath of a disaster, where there are people missing, and friends and families will try to track them down. These people may congregate at health facilities and crowd control can become a real issue as well as communication with concerned relatives and friends. Setting up a dedicated facility for friends and families where they can be supported, register their interests and facilitate reunion can go a significant way to maintaining respect and order. In some countries police services will coordinate the compilation of patient identification from multiple sources and make that data available via dedicated phone lines for friends and relatives.

- It is worth remembering that many major incidents also require **forensic or criminal investigation and preservation of evidence**. The general principles of *bag, tag, seal, and secure* should ideally be followed, but liaison with local police services to determine what they require is advised.

- It is important to consider how the health service will **manage the media** during the event. Having a designated area for which is separate to and away from the relatives' area will help to control information that goes into the public domain and avoids unnecessary harassment of these families. The EOC needs to be aware of their need for up-to-date information and should provide regular and timely media briefings to meet these needs and avoid misinformation. Media engagement needs to be coordinated and consistent and therefore without seeking to restrain freedom of speech, it is more helpful if uncoordinated media engagement is avoided, particularly when it adds to confused messaging.

Health system issues

- Community providers can be a source of support and a source of demand. In many cases GPs and community-based providers will be available to provide care but may not be able to operate from their normal practice or may have issues with supplies and resources. However, GPs are used to being flexible and working with minimal resources. They are a critical resource for health services as they can provide care to people not requiring the specialised resources of a hospital and are responsible for long-term care of those affected by disaster. They are also the front line of services during pandemics. The health system must engage with the primary care sector to ensure they continue to function.

  The most appropriate location for GPs is in their usual practice, providing long-term continuity of chronic conditions and medications; preventative healthcare through surveillance and early management of disaster health effects, and vaccinations (COVID, tetanus, and influenza); and coordination of other healthcare provision across mental and physical health. If usual primary care patient healthcare and an expected three-fold increase in acute exacerbations of pre-existing conditions are not managed by GPs, EDs are more likely to be overloaded.

- Aged care is a significant component of modern health systems. Events that require evacuation of these facilities may put a great strain on an already overstretched acute health system. Prior planning with these facilities can avoid the use of hospitals as evacuation centres. For example, the Townsville Hospital in North Queensland has predetermined evacuation facilities including geriatrician supervision while other jurisdictions have worked closely with aged care facilities to develop their own evacuation and ongoing care options.

- In many cases, a hospital will be (literally) the 'beacon of light' in a ravaged community following a disaster. It will be amongst the first facilities restored to power, food supplies, and safety. Additional security, including engagement with police or military, may be required to preserve access to the health service to those who truly need it.

System leadership, direction, and communication

One of the most important issues for disaster health managers is to secure and maintain the engagement of staff critical to the response. Staff must be informed of what it is the facility is trying to achieve and what is required of them. They also want to know what authority they have to come up with solutions. Communication with staff in a crisis is even more challenging than normal, the pace is often frenetic, and the gossip trail can often better define people's understanding of what is occurring than is achieved through formal communication channels.

Staff communication should be timely, accurate, regular, targeted to the audience, and convey what is known, what is not known, what is expected, and what is being done. This communication must be carefully constructed and delivered; giving purpose and avoiding a sense of distress and panic. A calm recognised trusted senior authority figure should deliver the message. Depending on the size of the organisation this may be face to face or via telecommunications. In protracted disasters, an effective mechanism may be to use regular bulletins that include an up-to-date status report, and what has changed since the last reporting period (see Chapter 9).

Ensuring communication has been received and understood is critical to establish the effectiveness of that communication. Regular face-to-face visits by senior staff within organisations is an effective mechanism. For example, the Townsville Hospital used links to a website to establish if staff had sufficient information and understood their roles during cyclones. This enabled the incident management team to tailor further communications to address information needs. An interesting facet was that administrative staff opened email communications most quickly and were then asked to ensure that subsequent communications were then printed out, prominently displayed and put in front of the clinicians who most needed to be informed.

ACTIVITIES

Activity one

1. What do you see is the role of primary care (e.g., General Practices) in the continuum of health DRM?
2. If you were asked to coordinate the redevelopment of health services for a small island nation devastated by a cyclone – what components would you wish to include and what priority would you give to each?

Activity two

1. What are the phases of a disaster response in a health service?
2. You are the Emergency physician on duty in your busy department at 6 PM on a Friday evening. You are notified by the ambulance service that there has been an

accident involving a bus full of schoolchildren and a train. What are your immediate actions?

3. You get a further call after 30 minutes telling you that there are 15 dead, 10 critical including 5 major burns, and 10 with minor injuries. Are there any further considerations?

4. As Health Incident Controller, how will you communicate with your hospital staff?

Activity three

1. Think about your community and the types of disaster it is most likely to experience. Describe a disaster's potential effects on the health and wellbeing of the community.

2. Identify the potential public health consequences.

KEY READINGS

1. Hollnagel, E., J. Braithwaite, and R.L. Wears, *Resilient healthcare: The resilience of everyday clinical work*. 2nd ed. 2015, Farnham, Surrey: Ashgate.

References

1. World Health Organisation. *Preamble to the Constitution of the World Health Organisation. As adopted by the International Health Conference*. 1946, New York (NY).
2. World Health Organisation. *Constitution*. 2023 [March 11, 2023]; Available from: https://www.who.int/about/governance/constitution.
3. World Health Organisation. *Everybody's business: Strengthening health systems to improve health outcomes: WHO's framework for action*. 2007, Geneva (CH): World Health Organisation.
4. World Health Organisation, *Western Pacific Regional framework for action for disaster risk management for health*. 2015, Geneva (CH): World Health Organisation.
5. World Health Organisation, *Safe hospitals initiative: Comprehensive safe hospital framework*. 2015, Geneva (CH): World Health Organisation.
6. Leggat, P.A., Oseltamivir and its role in influenza prevention and treatment. *Annals of the ACTM*, 2011. **12**: p. 61–63.
7. International Federation of Emergency Medicine. *IFEM definition of emergency medicine*. 2008 [23 April 2016]; Available from: www.ifem.cc/about-us/.
8. Hirsch, M., et al., The medical response to multisite terrorist attacks in Paris. *The Lancet*, 2015. **386**(10012): p. 2535–2538.
9. World Health Organisation. *World Health Assembly Resolution 64.10: 'Strengthening national health emergency and disaster management capacities and resilience of health systems'*. 2011 [17 May 2016]; Available from: https://www.who.int/publications/i/item/10665-106547.
10. United Nations. *Sendai framework for disaster risk reduction 2015–2030*. 2015. Geneva: United Nations.
11. United Nations University, A.D.W., *World risk report 2014*. 2014, Berlin (DE), Bonn (DE): Alliance Development Works and United Nations University - Institute for Environment and Human Security.
12. Lister, S.A., *Hurricane Katrina: The public health and medical response*. 2005, Washington, DC: Library of Congress. Congressional Research Service.
13. Aitken, P., et al., Emergency department presentations following tropical cyclone Yasi. *PloS One*, 2015. **10**(6): p. e0131196.
14. Braithwaite, J., et al., Healthcare as a complex adaptive system, in *Resilient healthcare: The resilience of everyday clinical work*, E. Hollnagel, J. Braithwaite, and R.L. Wears, Editors. 2013, Surrey (UK): Ashgate.
15. Hollnagel, E., J. Braithwaite, and R.L. Wears, *Resilient health care: The resilience of everyday clinical work*. 1st ed. 2013, Surrey (UK): Ashgate.

16. Ellis, L.A., et al., Patterns of resilience: A scoping review and bibliometric analysis of resilient health care. *Safety Science*, 2019. **118**: p. 241–257.

17. Wears RL, S.K., Van Rite E., Patient safety: A brief history, in *Patient safety: Perspectives on evidence, information, and knowledge transfer*, L. Zipperer, Editor. 2014, Gower: Farnham, Surrey.

18. Wiig, S. and J.K. O'Hara, Resilient and responsive healthcare services and systems: Challenges and opportunities in a changing world. *BMC Health Services Research*, 2021. **21**(1): p. 1037.

19. Clay-Williams, R., et al., Do large-scale hospital-and system-wide interventions improve patient outcomes: A systematic review. *BMC Health Services Research*, 2014. **14**(1): p. 1–13.

20. Rouse, W.B., Health care as a complex adaptive system: Implications for design and management. *Bridge-Washington-National Academy of Engineering*, 2008. **38**(1): p. 17.

21. Hollnagel, E., J. Braithwaite, and R.L. Wears, *Resilient health care: The resilience of everyday clinical work*. 2nd ed. 2015, Surrey (UK): Ashgate.

22. Koenig, K.L., et al., Surging to the right standard of care. *Academic Emergency Medicine*, 2006. **13**(2): p. 195–198.

23. Gostin, L.O. and D. Hanfling, National preparedness for a catastrophic emergency: Crisis standards of care. *JAMA*, 2009. **302**(21): p. 2365–2366.

11

Physical health impacts of disasters

Penelope Burns, Colin Myers, Joris Yzermans,
and Michel Dückers

INTRODUCTION & OBJECTIVES

The World Health Organisation (WHO) defines health not merely as an absence of disease, but as a state of physical, mental and social well-being [1]. A potential omission of this definition is 'the ability to adapt and self-manage in the face of social, physical, and emotional challenges' [2]. Disasters are an extreme source of such challenges, and health risk exposure, with notable profound effects on human physical, mental and social health [3], as well as economic and environmental effects [4], and access to healthcare services.

Although we discuss the physical health consequences of disaster in this chapter and the mental health consequences in the next chapter, substantial evidence and knowledge clearly identify the need to consider a person's health holistically across physical and mental health and, as alluded to by WHO, the broader social determinants of health [1]. This is important as different aspects of health are interrelated, health vulnerabilities (or risk factors) fitting within one domain (e.g., mental, physical, functional of social) can be a predictor for health effects in another domain [3, 5].

Epidemiologic studies in disasters provide the distribution and determinants of health-related states in disaster populations, allowing clinicians to prepare for, and monitor, these presentations, as well as presenting opportunities for early identification and management to improve disaster health outcomes. Predictable patterns of illness, disease and injury effects can be shown over time, and identify more affected subgroups [6].

Under the realisation of this complex interplay of physical, mental, social and environmental factors, the aim of this chapter is to provide an overview of the impact of disaster on the physical health, to identify higher-risk groups and to consider disaster risk reduction (DRR) strategies to improve disaster health outcomes.

On completion of this chapter students should be able to:

1. Discuss the physical health effects associated with all hazard disasters.
2. Recognise the temporal nature of these physical health impacts.
3. Identify factors creating a higher risk of adverse health outcomes.

DOI: 10.4324/9781032626604-14

4. Identify higher risk groups and understand the rationale for their higher risk.
5. Consider DRR strategies that might improve physical health and well-being outcomes following an acute disaster incident.

PHYSICAL HEALTH IMPACTS OF DISASTERS

Chapter 21, Natural Disaster, details hazard-specific health effects such as increased fractures and crush injuries in earthquakes, increased drownings in floods and tsunamis, increased mortality rates during extremes of temperatures and increased suffocation in landslides and avalanches. However, *a substantial proportion and volume of disaster health effects are consistent across hazard types* [7]. Therefore this chapter discusses the health impacts associated with all hazard disasters.

The disaster literature demonstrates an association between many symptoms and clinical conditions with exposure to a disaster [7]. Researching this association immediately after disasters is challenging. Issues include the unpredictable nature of disasters requiring rapid development of ethical, relevant research protocols; access and safety in chaotic, dangerous environments; inclusion of vulnerable potentially traumatised populations; and potential impedance of rescue activities [8]. Cross-sectional and cohort studies in the latter half of the 20th century have provided a view of potential associations between health effects and disasters. Randomised controlled trials are ethically and practically difficult in the disaster environment. Over the last 20 years, increasing numbers of longer-term prospective cohort studies have provided stronger evidence of an increase in prevalence, incidence and association of many health conditions and symptoms following disasters, over immediate, intermediate and long-term periods, along with new incident conditions, and deterioration of pre-existing, chronic conditions. Case studies have contributed by describing new conditions such as tsunami lung and tsunami sinusitis.

For example, large prospective longitudinal cohort studies are ongoing following the 2001 World Trade Center (WTC) attacks involving the hijacking and crashing of two planes into the Twin Towers in New York City (NYC). The early death toll due to trauma and injury was 2,973.

> I heard a turbine smash into one of the buildings. I remember the sounds and the people jumping…Muzak was playing… People were jumping, and debris was flying. It was awful.
> Perez, licensed emergency medical technician and volunteer [9]

The people of NYC, survivors and rescuers, were televised layered with a thick grey dust that blanketed Ground Zero. The majority of long-term damage to physical health in these survivors is now attributed to this dust. Local residents, school children, rescuers, emergency services, volunteers and recovery workers were all exposed to this dust in the Lower Manhattan area for many months. Over 400,000 people are now thought to be at risk for long-term health effects including predominantly respiratory, but also cardiovascular, endocrine, gastrointestinal, psychological, ophthalmological and otic diseases. Twenty years later the effects of that exposure are still emerging from longitudinal scientific studies. Potential associations between disasters and diseases with a longer latency period such as cancer, peripheral neuropathy and autoimmune disease are beginning to emerge [10].

Longer-term studies have also affirmed the association between physical and mental health effects. For example, in a large prospective longitudinal study conducted two to six years after the WTC, researchers found that measures of dust cloud exposure, personal injury on 9/11 and post-traumatic stress disorder (PTSD) were all associated with an increase in heart disease almost three years after the attacks [11]. This was supported by Brackbill et al. who showed that comorbidity of physical injury and PTSD increased the likelihood of developing heart disease [12]. Broader life effects are also being studied examining the effect of income loss, or earlier retirement, in those with multiple 9/11-associated health effects.

Communicable, or infectious, health effects

In well-resourced countries, infectious outbreaks are uncommon following disasters, except where the primary disaster is infectious itself (e.g., the global SARS-CoV-2 (Severe Acute Respiratory Syndrome-associated Coronavirus 2) pandemic discussed in Chapter 24). Even with significant disruption to utilities, studies from Hurricane Katrina and Hurricane Sandy showed no significant increase in infectious disease outbreaks [13, 14].

However, in lower-resourced countries and in humanitarian disasters, infectious diseases are a major concern, predominantly due to increases or changes in locally endemic organisms including acute respiratory infections and gastroenteritis. Disruption of water and sanitation, displacement of populations, crowding in evacuation centres, poor pre-event health status and disruption of health services, may all impact on the risk of water, food or airborne infectious disease. In poorly vaccinated populations, vaccination programs for highly infectious and deadly diseases such as measles and tetanus, need to be urgently established.

Infectious disease tends to present a different time course to acute injury in disasters. Following the Great East Japan Earthquake Tsunami (GEJET) a significant increase in infectious disease hospitalisations occurred later, at two weeks, and was predominantly pneumonia due to usual community-acquired pathogens. Mortality attributed to pneumonia was significantly increased in the first 12 weeks peaking in the second week [15]. Half the cases of pneumonia were contracted whilst in evacuation centres [16].

Non-communicable, or non-infectious, health effects

The scientific literature reports disaster health effects on most body systems, including cardiac, respiratory, endocrine, dermatologic, musculoskeletal, gastrointestinal, ocular, otologic and neurological effects. This section aims to provide a broad overview of non-communicable health effects with discussion of new incident disease and symptoms, including Medically Unexplained Physical Symptoms (MUPS), and of chronic disease.

To fully realise the physical health impact of disasters it is crucial to understand the temporal nature of these effects. The physical health epidemiological disaster knowledge base is more nascent and possibly less rich than the mental health dimension [5]. That said, we are making progress in developing insights on the temporality of physical health impact [7], although we are not yet at the point where we can reliably plot the prevalence or risk for particular health problems over the course of weeks, months and years in detail.

Cardiac effects

An increase in the incidence of acute cardiac events such as hypertension, acute myocardial infarction (AMI), cardiomyopathy and non-cardiac chest pain (NCCP) following disasters is increasingly well-documented with early evidence of an influence on heart failure (HF) and ventricular tachyarrhythmia [17–20].

Hypertension was considered one of the greatest burdens to healthcare in the early stages of the GEJET and Hurricane Katrina. A high background prevalence of pre-existing hypertension in these populations was compounded by an increase in blood pressure (BP) in those with no history of hypertension (92%), and in those with pre-existing hypertension, both in those taking their usual medications (10%), and those not taking them [21].

A significant increase in AMIs was associated with the 2010 Christchurch earthquake, occurring during the first two weeks post-event [18]. The WTC attack was associated with a significant increase in cardiovascular admissions of lower Manhattan residents to NYC hospitals within the first five weeks. During the second week there was a 72.7% relative increase in cardiovascular admissions compared with 14.7% in the control area [22]. Post Hurricane Katrina an increased incidence of AMI was sustained at two years [23] and three years [24] with a three-fold increase observed over both periods [23, 24]. Linking back to mental health, an association has been reported between PTSD and vascular conditions following disasters [25].

Early evidence suggests that the time of day of an earthquake may affect cardiac presentations. Cardiac admissions following the Christchurch earthquakes increased significantly but showed very different presentations for each quake. Significant increases in AMI and NCCP presented following the first early morning quake; with significant stress cardiomyopathy presentations following the second midday quake [18].

Following Hurricane Katrina, longer-term change in the chronobiology of AMI was seen where onset of AMI increased significantly during nights and weekends, and decreased significantly during the more expected times of mornings and weekdays [26].

The contemporary evidence on the temporal nature of cardiovascular events following all hazards disasters can be summarised as immediate, covering the first days to weeks, intermediate, covering weeks to months, and longer term, covering one year to over a decade [7]. Immediate effects are particularly hypertension, AMI, cardiomyopathy, NCCP, cerebrovascular accidents (CVA) and arrythmias. Intermediate effects include exacerbations and deteriorations of chronic disease including hypertension, HF and CVA. Longer-term effects include AMI, CVA, HF and hypercholesterolemia [7]. This longitudinal effect suggests that targeted early preventative management for these conditions in those at higher risk should be worthwhile.

Respiratory effects

Extensive literature exists on the respiratory effects of disasters on adults and children, particularly in incidents with increased particulate matter such as the WTC attack in 2001, and increasingly from huge wildfires such as the 2019 Black Summer bushfires in Australia [27]. An estimated 417 excess deaths, and exacerbation of cardio-respiratory conditions, were attributed to the latter during 19 weeks of continuous fire activity resulting in extensive prolonged bushfire smoke along the eastern coast of Australia [27].

Following the WTC attacks, those most exposed to the dust cloud were most at risk [28, 29]. In the first days immediate health effects included new or worsening upper or lower respiratory symptoms, with almost a quarter experiencing gastroesophageal reflux [30, 31]. Over half the children who were residents, schooling or volunteering in the dust-affected area, reported symptoms post 9/11 including shortness of breath, cough, wheezing and sinus or throat irritation [32].

New conditions such as WTC cough, tsunami lung [33], tsunami sinusitis [33] and thunderstorm asthma are also being described and documented in the immediate disaster period.

Tsunami lung, due to submersion during a tsunami, may involve aspiration of oil, waste and soil in the water, resulting in a chemical-induced pneumonitis complicated by infection from organisms. Contaminated sludge has also been found in sinuses and stomachs. The majority of deaths following the GEJET were attributed to drowning in the tsunami [33].

Power outages contribute to effects on health including respiratory. In the first two weeks post-landfall of Hurricane Sandy in NYC in 2012 significant numbers of carbon dioxide exposures were reported, attributed to activities such as indoor grilling, inappropriate generator placement and residential fires [34]. Other effects seen included aggravation of existing respiratory disease [16]; respiratory infections [15, 16]; sinusitis and chest injuries.

From a temporal perspective, examples of deleterious effects of disasters on respiratory health can be found over ten years post-disaster [7]. An increased incidence of asthma and ongoing deterioration in pulmonary function with persistent lower respiratory symptoms (LRS) has been seen for over ten years following exposure to dust during the WTC attack [29, 35, 36]. The most prevalent physician-diagnosed respiratory conditions post-WTC attack were asthma, chronic bronchitis and chronic sinusitis [36].

Effects on diabetes

People with diabetes in particular, face increased risk in disasters due to reliance on regular medication, exercise, diet and routine for glycaemic control. The effect of the acute disaster, difficulty accessing medications and monitoring equipment, alterations to diet provided in evacuation centres, and increased exercise in the clean-up, can all affect glycaemic control.

From a temporal perspective, several key messages arise from the diabetic literature. Firstly an increase in new incident diabetes is seen in the immediate aftermath [37, 38], in the first years in evacuees [38], and over at decade later in those post-WTC attacks with PTSD [37]. Secondly, potential higher-risk groups have been identified including pregnant women exposed to traumatic experiences during disasters [39]; those with existing Insulin Dependent Diabetes Mellitus (IDDM) [40]; evacuees [38]; and those with mental health co-morbidity [37]. Thirdly the literature demonstrates a variable worsening control of pre-existing diabetes [40–43], both in the short term and the long term, emphasising the need to optimise post-disaster care to minimise this effect. Examples of effects on diabetes are described in the literature up to ten years after the disaster [7].

Dermatological effects

Skin effects are predominantly seen in the first days to months. Sunburn, inflammatory and traumatic skin conditions are frequent in residents and clean-up workers in the post-incident environment [44]. Less common effects may include severe fire or chemical burns, or traumatic wounds, and may be life-threatening. Other apparently less urgent dermatological conditions, such as more minor wounds, may become life-threatening due to infection if not treated promptly and may contribute considerable distress and morbidity.

Chronic diseases

Immediate management of acute injuries and environmental risks is the priority of current disaster management. However, continuity of care for chronic diseases has been identified as the major healthcare provision after disasters reflecting the substantial prevalence of pre-existing chronic disease in disaster-affected populations. In Australia, for example, a significant proportion of younger adults now have chronic conditions, with almost half of the population having at least one chronic condition.

Individuals with chronic conditions have greater healthcare needs [45]. Following the Northbridge earthquake in Los Angeles, a longitudinal cohort study examined burden of illness at one year pre-, and three months post-earthquake. A significant difference in post-earthquake healthcare needs was seen between those with zero, one or two+ chronic conditions for pain for ≥ two days, difficulty refilling prescriptions, severe stress of > two weeks, lack of necessary medical equipment and inability to access medical help [46].

Those with a chronic condition are also three times more likely to present with an acute presentation, either an exacerbation of their chronic condition or a separate acute condition that might also adversely affect their underlying chronic condition [45]. During the week following Hurricane Sandy there were statistically significant increases in emergency department presentations for chronic conditions including diabetes, AMI, hypertension, chronic bronchitis, kidney disease, dialysis dependence, prescription refills and drug dependence; usually for several conditions at the same time [42].

Miscellaneous symptoms

MUPS, or non-specific symptoms, are subjective symptoms with no objective pathological condition or external cause found to explain them. Post-disaster explanations for 'non-specific symptoms' can be ambiguous and disputable. Symptoms, most commonly fatigue and headache, but also dyspnoea, back pain, muscle pain, gastrointestinal symptoms, palpitations, dizziness and sleeping problems have all been described post-disaster. However pre-disaster studies are often not available for comparison and study methodologies vary widely, so it is difficult to draw conclusions. A review by Yzermans et al. suggested the prevalence of MUPS ranged from 3% to 78% with longitudinal studies demonstrating a waning of symptom prevalence with time [3].

The next section examines some of the subpopulations considered at high risk of poor health outcomes in disasters.

RISK AND PROTECTIVE FACTORS, AND VULNERABILITIES

It is essential to understand the degree of risk from exposure to a hazard, and the protective value of available personal and community resources. People, and communities, experiencing the same disaster can experience very different health outcomes. Based on the existing literature we can attempt to provide an overview of the factors that might affect this experience, categorising them in Table 11.1 by:

- time period prior, during and post disaster incident, and
- levels ranging from individual, community to society [47–50].

Table 11.1 Risk and protective factors

Pre-disaster
- Pre-existing population health and well-being.
  - Prevalence and incidence of illness and disease.
  - Social determinants of health, and lifestyle including health-risk factors.
  - Level of public and preventive health activities (including vaccination and population screening rates).
  - Demographics (higher risk at extremes of age).
- Local population resources – community connectedness and resources, culture, social support, physical and socioeconomic environment, health services.
- Pre-existing individual health and well-being.
  - Number and severity of existing (chronic) diseases and chronic illnesses
  - Social determinants of health
- Individual resources – strength and resilience, family, community/social support and connectedness, employment, economic/financial, gender/age.

During disaster
- Impact, duration, and characteristics of the particular disaster incident.
  - Malevolent events may have greater psychological impact.
- Size of effect on basic needs, including damage to infrastructure, shelter food, water, health services, local community.
- Duration of effect including evacuation and long-term displacement.
- Individual experience and loss during the disaster, including personal injury and experience of loss of loved ones including pets.

Post-disaster
- Sustainability of all levels of primary, secondary, and tertiary healthcare services.
- Duration of community disruption and evacuations.
- Resilience and connectedness of local community.
- Active surveillance and early management of adverse disaster health effects including changes to social determinants of health.
- Secondary events (e.g., floods may follow bushfires due to changes to soil and vegetation) and 'new' life events.
- Level of impact on personal and community economics and business viability.

While the additional impacts of factors such as war, famine and population displacement must be acknowledged they will be covered in detail in Chapter 22 – Complex Humanitarian Emergencies.

These temporal and societal effects are linked:

- an individual with multiple chronic conditions taking multiple medications pre-disaster will have more need for ongoing access to medication and healthcare during the disaster when it may not be available, and this may contribute to a greater risk of deterioration in their conditions post-disaster [7].
- a low-income country with, low level of private and public health expenditure, poor access to GPs and hospitals offers less opportunity to detect and treat physical (and mental) health problems than a high-income better-resourced country [51].

Vulnerabilities: specific high-risk groups

Characteristics of specific population groups can create higher risk in disasters but can also bring strengths and capabilities. In this section we discuss key populations with characteristics that place them at higher risk, however this is not a comprehensive list, and you may be able to identify other high-risk groups.

Babies, infants, children and adolescents are a high-risk group physically and psychologically, and account for 30–50% of all global disaster-related deaths [52]. Children are not small adults. Depending on their age, and stage of development, children are at risk due to differing anatomy, physiology, immunology, cognition and psychology. Childrens' vulnerabilities are compounded by the need for particular equipment, dosages, and approaches to treatment, and the need for paediatric disaster knowledge and skills. As with all high-risk groups, children's resilience can be augmented by recognising their strengths and facilitating their contribution to disaster preparedness, response and recovery activities.

Pregnant women are physiologically and physically higher risk in disasters due to their immunocompromise, increased risk of gestational diabetes, and restricted mobility. Mendez-Figueroa et al. [53] reported an increase in maternal and neonatal morbidity post Hurricane Harvey of 27% and 50% respectively. For those caring for young infants, disruption of breastfeeding, or of supply of appropriate infant formula if bottle feeding, are important issues in the chaotic disaster environment.

The **elderly** may have increased risk in disasters related variously to physical limitations, including sensory restrictions (reduced vision and hearing); reduced balance, physical strength and mobility; reduced immunocompetence; cognitive effects exacerbated by stress and evacuation;[54] all compounded by an increased prevalence of chronic diseases and multi-morbidity. This greater risk continues after the disaster. Following the GEJET, women over 84 years had the highest mortality risk over the first three months [55]. Following Hurricane Katrina and Sandy the elderly were at higher risk for morbidity in the first three months. Following Hurricane Sandy Restricted access to food and water significantly increased hospitalisation rates for dehydration in those over 65 years, and an increased prevalence of cardiovascular disease, respiratory disease, and injury was seen in the first 12 months [56].

The elderly may also have increased resilience due to previous experience and successful management of disaster exposures, or prior immunity to infectious agents. For example, during the 2009 H1N1 pandemic elderly populations were less vulnerable, with lower morbidity and mortality, due to presumed previous exposure to the similar

H1N1-like viruses. Compared with usual seasonal influenza outbreaks, where those over 65 years accounted for over 90% mortality, during H1N1 it was 13% [57]. However, during the 2019 SARS-CoV-2 pandemic, the elderly were, in fact, more vulnerable, due to their physiology and a lack of prior exposure and hence immunity.

DISASTER RISK REDUCTION

The essence of a disaster is that there is chaos, risk, uncertainty and a serious lack of resources, including professional healthcare service capacity; a problem that is exacerbated in poorly resourced low-income countries. Substantial opportunities exist for DRR of disaster health effects, in primary and secondary prevention. The *Sendai Framework 2015–2030* calls for timely integration of DRR, and resilience-building strategies, into policies, planning and programs at all levels of disaster management [58]. Knowledge of the epidemiology of the health effects of disasters and the time period post-disaster when these may occur creates an opportunity for DRR in disaster healthcare across all phases of PPRR, and across all levels of healthcare. Through ongoing surveillance, early diagnosis, early management and targeted review of chronic conditions, the potential to improve disaster health outcomes for individuals and populations exists. Knowledge of the risk of deterioration of social determinants of health suggests benefit in health promotion activities ranging from protective and preventive measures, screening to healthy lifestyle activities (including good diet, exercise, weight control, sleep and limited substance use) and establishing an operational and accessible stepped care healthcare system.

Many health-focused DRR activities, increasingly being realised as an indispensable aspect of emergency management, are similar or even identical to routine non-disaster healthcare delivery. For many potential physical health effects, affected individuals/populations, especially potentially vulnerable groups, might benefit from general practitioners or more specialised rehabilitation expertise that is not always available in disaster settings.

CONCLUSION

Knowledge of the epidemiological patterns of illness and disease following disasters can inform DRR activities at all levels of healthcare; activities that are similar to 'normal' evidence-based health practice across the stages of illness and disease. The growing knowledge base of disaster epidemiology provides opportunities for prevention, and health and well-being promotion, with the potential to improve disaster health outcomes for individuals and communities over the short, intermediate and longer-term periods post disaster incident.

ACTIVITY

Consider being asked to undertake a locum as a resident doctor in the days following a bushfire disaster in a small rural community, in either a local community general medical practice or in the local hospital emergency department. Considerable environmental smoke presence continues for the whole four months of your locum.

1. What medical conditions might you expect to see in the first weeks, and alternatively after four months?
2. How do the two roles – community general medicine and hospital emergency medicine – differ in their contributions to disaster healthcare management in a disaster?

KEY READINGS

Fonseca, V.A., H. Smith, N. Kuhadiya, S.M. Leger, C.L. Yau, K. Reynolds, et al. Impact of a natural disaster on diabetes: Exacerbation of disparities and long-term consequences. *Diabetes Care*. 2009. **32**(9): p. 1632–1638. [41]

Brackbill, R.M., J.M. Graber, and W.A. Robison, *Long-term health effects of the 9/11 disaster*. 2019, MDPI - Multidisciplinary Digital Publishing Institute. [10]

Dirkzwager, A.J., P.G. van der Velden, L. Grievink, and C.J. Yzermans, Disaster-related posttraumatic stress disorder and physical health. *Psychosomatic Medicine*. 2007. **69**(5): p. 435–440. [25]

Bonanno, G.A., C.R. Brewin, K. Kaniasty, A.M. Greca, Weighing the costs of disaster: Consequences, risks, and resilience in individuals, families, and communities. *Psychological Science in the Public Interest*, 2010. **11**(1): p. 1–49. [5]

References

1. World Health Organisation, *Constitution of the World Health Organization*, W.H. Organisation, Editor. 2005, Geneva, Switzerland: World Health Organisation.
2. Huber, M., et al., How should we define health? *BMJ*, 2011. **343**: p. d4163.
3. Yzermans, C., B. van den Berg, and A. Dirkzwager, Physical health problems after disasters, in *Mental Health and Disasters*, Y. Neria, S. Galea, and F. Norris, Editors. 2009, Melbourne: Cambridge University Press.
4. Beyer, J., et al., Environmental effects of the Deepwater Horizon oil spill: A review. *Marine Pollution Bulletin*, 2016. **110**(1): p. 28–51.
5. Bonanno, G.A., et al., Weighing the costs of disaster: Consequences, risks, and resilience in individuals, families, and communities. *Psychological Science in the Public Interest*, 2010. **11**(1): p. 1–49.
6. Greenough, P.G. and F. Burkle, Practical applications of disaster epidemiology, in *Disaster Medicine*, G. Ciottone, Editor. 2006, Philadelphia, PA: Mosby Elsevier. p. 327–332.
7. Burns, P., The role of general practitioners in disaster health management, in *Academic Department of General Practice*. 2022, Canberra, ACT: The Australian National University.
8. Hunt, M., et al., The challenge of timely, responsive and rigorous ethics review of disaster research: Views of research ethics committee members. *PLoS One*, 2016. **11**(6): p. e0157142.
9. Goodman, L., The Hurting Heroes of 9/11, in *Newsweek*. 2016, New York: Newsweek LLC. p. 24–33.
10. Brackbill, R.M., J.M. Graber, and W.A. Robison, *Long-term health effects of the 9/11 disaster*. 2019: MDPI - Multidisciplinary Digital Publishing Institute: Basel Switzerland.
11. Jordan, H.T., et al., Heart disease among adults exposed to the September 11, 2001 World Trade Center disaster: Results from the World Trade Center Health Registry. *Preventive Medicine*, 2011. **53**(6): p. 370–376.
12. Brackbill, R.M., et al., Chronic physical health consequences of being injured during the terrorist attacks on world trade center on September 11, 2001. *American Journal of Epidemiology*, 2014. **179**(9): p. 1076–1085.
13. Greene, S.K., et al., Assessment of reportable disease incidence after Hurricane Sandy, New York City, 2012. *Disaster Medicine and Public Health Preparedness*, 2013. **7**(5): p. 513–521.
14. Cavey, A.M., et al., Mississippi's infectious disease hotline: A surveillance and education model for future disasters. *Prehospital and Disaster Medicine*, 2009. **24**(1): p. 11–17.
15. Aoyagi, T., et al., Characteristics of infectious diseases in hospitalized patients during the early phase after the 2011 great East Japan earthquake: Pneumonia as a significant reason for hospital care. *Chest*, 2013. **143**(2): p. 349–356.
16. Ohkouchi, S., et al., Deterioration in regional health status after the acute phase of a great disaster: Respiratory physicians' experiences of the Great East Japan Earthquake. *Respiratory Investigation*, 2013. **51**(2): p. 50–55.
17. Zhang, X.Q., et al., Effect of the Wenchuan earthquake in China on hemodynamically unstable ventricular tachyarrhythmia in hospitalized patients. *American Journal of Cardiology*, 2009. **103**(7): p. 994–997.

18. Chan, C., et al., Acute myocardial infarction and stress cardiomyopathy following the Christchurch earthquakes. *PLoS One*, 2013. **8**(7): p. e68504.
19. Steptoe, A., The impact of natural disasters on myocardial infarction. *Heart*, 2009. **95**(24): p. 1972–1973.
20. Huang, K., et al., Prognostic implication of earthquake-related loss and depressive symptoms in patients with heart failure following the 2008 earthquake in Sichuan. *Clinical Cardiology*, 2011. **34**(12): p. 755–760.
21. Tanaka, R., M. Okawa, and Y. Ujike, Predictors of hypertension in survivors of the Great East Japan Earthquake, 2011: A cross-sectional study. *Prehospital and Disaster Medicine*, 2016. **31**(1): p. 17–26.
22. Lin, S., et al., Respiratory and cardiovascular hospitalizations after the World Trade Center Disaster. *Archives of Environmental & Occupational Health*, 2010. **65**(1): p. 12–20.
23. Gautam, S., et al., Effect of Hurricane Katrina on the incidence of acute coronary syndrome at a primary angioplasty center in New Orleans. *Disaster Medicine and Public Health Preparedness*, 2009. **3**(3): p. 144–150.
24. Jiao, Z., et al., Effect of Hurricane Katrina on incidence of acute myocardial infarction in New Orleans three years after the storm. *American Journal of Cardiology*, 2012. **109**(4): p. 502–505.
25. Dirkzwager, A.J., et al., Disaster-related posttraumatic stress disorder and physical health. *Psychosomatic Medicine*, 2007. **69**(5): p. 435–440.
26. Moscona, J.C., et al., The incidence, risk factors, and chronobiology of acute myocardial infarction ten years after Hurricane Katrina. *Disaster Medicine and Public Health Preparedness*, 2019. **13**(2): p. 217–222.
27. Borchers Arriagada, N., et al., Unprecedented smoke-related health burden associated with the 2019–20 bushfires in eastern Australia. *Medical Journal of Australia*, 2020. **213**(6): p. 282–283.
28. Cohen, H.W., et al., Long-term cardiovascular disease risk among firefighters after the World Trade Center Disaster. *JAMA Network Open*, 2019. **2**(9): p. e199775.
29. Mauer, M.P., K.R. Cummings, and R. Hoen, Long-term respiratory symptoms in World Trade Center responders. *Occupational Medicine* (Lond), 2010. **60**(2): p. 145–151.
30. de la Hoz, R.E., et al., Reflux symptoms and disorders and pulmonary disease in former World Trade Center rescue and recovery workers and volunteers. *Journal of Occupational and Environmental Medicine*, 2008. **50**(12): p. 1351–1354.
31. de la Hoz, R.E., et al., Occupational toxicant inhalation injury: The World Trade Center (WTC) experience. *International Archives of Occupational and Environmental Health*, 2008. **81**(4): p. 479–485.
32. Thomas, P.A., et al., Respiratory and other health effects reported in children exposed to the World Trade Center disaster of 11 September 2001. *Environmental Health Perspectives*, 2008. **116**(10): p. 1383–1390.
33. Hiruma, T., et al., Tsunami lung accompanied by multiple disorders. *American Journal of Respiratory and Critical Care Medicine*, 2013. **187**(1): p. 110–111.
34. Chen, B.C., et al., Carbon monoxide exposures in New York City following Hurricane Sandy in 2012. *Clinical Toxicology* (Philadelphia), 2013. **51**(9): p. 879–885.
35 Ekenga, C.C. and G. Friedman-Jimenez, Epidemiology of respiratory health outcomes among world trade center disaster workers: Review of the literature ten years after the September 11, 2001 terrorist attacks. *Disaster Medicine and Public Health Preparedness*, 2011. **5**(Suppl. 2): p. S189–S196.
36. Webber, M.P., et al., Physician-diagnosed respiratory conditions and mental health symptoms 7–9 years following the World Trade Center disaster. *American Journal of Industrial Medicine*, 2011. **54**(9): p. 661–671.
37. Miller-Archie, S.A., et al., Posttraumatic stress disorder and new-onset diabetes among adult survivors of the World Trade Center disaster. *Preventive Medicine*, 2014. **66**: p. 34–38.
38. Satoh, H., et al., Evacuation after the Fukushima Daiichi Nuclear Power Plant Accident Is a Cause of Diabetes: Results from the Fukushima Health Management Survey. *Journal of Diabetes Research*, 2015. **2015**: p. 627390.
39. Xiong, X., et al., Hurricane katrina experience and the risk of gestational diabetes mellitus. *American Journal of Epidemiology*, 2011. **173**: p. S40.
40. Ng, J.M., et al., The effect of extensive flooding in Hull on the glycaemic control of diabetes patients. *Diabetic Medicine*, 2010. **1**: p. 108.

41. Fonseca, V.A., et al., Impact of a natural disaster on diabetes: Exacerbation of disparities and long-term consequences. *Diabetes Care*, 2009. **32**(9): p. 1632–1638.

42. Lee, D.C., et al., Acute post-disaster medical needs of patients with diabetes: Emergency department use in New York City by diabetic adults after Hurricane Sandy. *BMJ Open Diabetes Res Care*, 2016. **4**(1): p. e000248.

43. Leppold, C., et al., Sociodemographic patterning of long-term diabetes mellitus control following Japan's 3.11 triple disaster: A retrospective cohort study. *BMJ Open*, 2016. **6**(7): p. e011455.

44. Rusiecki, J.A., et al., Disaster-related exposures and health effects among US Coast Guard responders to Hurricanes Katrina and Rita: A cross-sectional study. *Journal of Occupational and Environmental Medicine*, 2014. **56**(8): p. 820–833.

45. Hassan, S., et al., Management of chronic noncommunicable diseases after natural disasters in the Caribbean: A scoping review. *Health Affairs (Millwood)*, 2020. **39**(12): p. 2136–2143.

46. Der-Martirosian, C., et al., Pre-earthquake burden of illness and postearthquake health and preparedness in veterans. *Prehospital and Disaster Medicine* 2014. **29**(3): p. 223–229.

47. Joshi, S. and M. Cerda, Trajectories of health, resilience and illness, in *Textbook of Disaster Psychiatry*, R. Ursano, et al., Editors. 2017, Cambridge: Cambridge University Press.

48. Schultz, J., et al., Disaster ecology, in *Textbook of Disaster Psychiatry*, R. Ursano, et al., Editors. 2017, Cambridge (UK), New York (US), Victoria (AU); Delhi (IN), Singapore (SG): Cambridge University Press. p. 44–59.

49. Dückers, M.L.A., A multilayered psychosocial resilience framework and its implications for community-focused crisis management. *Journal of Contingencies and Crisis Management*, 2017. **25**(3): p. 182–187.

50. Lowe, D., K.L. Ebi, and B. Forsberg, Factors increasing vulnerability to health effects before, during and after floods. *International Journal of Environmental Research and Public Health*, 2013. **10**(12): p. 7015–7067.

51. Dückers, M.L., R.J. Ursano, and E. Vermetten, A global perspective on the mental health response to terrorism, in *Risk management of terrorism induced stress. Guidelines for the golden hours (who, what and when)*, E. Vermetten, et al., Editors. 2020, Brussels: North Atlantic Treaty Organisation. p. 10–17.

52. Ronan, K. and B. Towers, Child-centred disaster risk reduction project: July 2014, in *Bushfire and natural hazards CRC annual report 2014*, B.A.N.H. CRC, Editor. 2015, Bushfire and Natural Hazards CRC

53. Mendez-Figueroa, H., et al., Peripartum outcomes before and after hurricane harvey. *Obstetrics & Gynecology*, 2019. **134**(5): p. 1005–1016.

54. Dosa, D., et al., To evacuate or shelter in place: Implications of universal hurricane evacuation policies on nursing home residents. *Journal of the American Medical Directors Association*, 2012. **13**(2): p. 190.e1–e7.

55. Morita, T., et al., Excess mortality due to indirect health effects of the 2011 triple disaster in Fukushima, Japan: A retrospective observational study. *Journal of Epidemiology and Community Health*, 2017. **71**(10): p. 974–980.

56. Swerdel, J.N., et al., Rates of Hospitalization for Dehydration Following Hurricane Sandy in New Jersey. *Disaster Medicine and Public Health Preparedness*, 2016. **10**(2): p. 188–192.

57. Verma, N., et al., Influenza virus H1N1pdm09 infections in the young and old: Evidence of greater antibody diversity and affinity for the hemagglutinin globular head domain (HA1 Domain) in the elderly than in young adults and children. *Journal of Virology*, 2012. **86**(10): p. 5515–5522.

58. United Nations International Strategy for Disaster Reduction, *The Sendai framework for disaster risk reduction 2015–2030*, U. Nations, Editor. 2015, United Nations.

12

Psychosocial impacts of disasters

Jane Shakespeare-Finch and Paul Scully

INTRODUCTION AND OBJECTIVES

Disasters can have a significant impact on mental health, which can be aggravated by poor forward planning, inadequate management of the recovery phase, and a lack of responsive and coordinated mental health aimed to support individuals, communities, and frontline personnel [1]. In recent times these disasters have included the COVID-19 pandemic. People respond to traumatic events in different ways yet psychosocial research in this area has predominantly focussed on the detrimental impacts of exposure. For example, a meta-analysis of the health impacts of natural disasters revealed increased levels of anxiety, depression, and post-traumatic stress disorder (PTSD) [2], as well as physical symptoms of disease. Although PTSD is the most documented outcome following trauma, it is a minority of people that will sustain a serious mental illness [3], and the majority of these will respond, recover, and return to pre-event functioning [4].

Traumatic experiences can also provide a catalyst for significant positive changes termed *post-traumatic growth* [5]. Most people recover from traumatic events in very sound ways psychologically. Post-event reactions/behaviours which may be different from the way in which the individual behaves in *normal* circumstances are not necessarily a symptom of psychopathology. Rather, responses such as intrusive thoughts, avoidance, numbing, and hyperarousal are likely to be normal reactions in the short term to events that are extraordinary.

Significant preparation and appropriate response planning and support should be available to mitigate the potentially negative impacts on the mental health of all members of the affected community [6, 7]. This chapter outlines the potential impacts that disasters can have on mental health and wellbeing. It also identifies ways in which individuals, organisations, healthcare workers, and others in positions of responsibility relating to disasters, can aim to prevent and to manage the adverse psychosocial impacts of experiencing trauma and promote mental health and wellbeing. On completion of this chapter, you should:

1. Understand the impact of disasters on mental health and wellbeing.
2. Understand factors that influence mental health and wellbeing in disasters.
3. Be able to identify strategies likely to prevent and manage adverse mental health consequences.

RISKS TO MENTAL HEALTH IN DISASTERS

Beyond the physical harm that may be inflicted upon victims and survivors of disasters, there is also potential harm to mental health. Stressors may include exposure to the evolving hazard and threat of injury or death, to family, friends or pets, loss of property and possessions, or loss of work and income. An understanding of potential psychological injury following disasters is essential. Such injuries are serious and may be made worse if appropriate steps are not taken. While most people do not suffer a diagnosable psychological disorder following a traumatic experience [4], recovery and return to pre-event mental health functioning can take a long period of time for people. For example, Dai and colleagues [8] conducted a study of people who had been diagnosed with PTSD following floods and were then followed up 13–14 years later. While most people had recovered from PTSD, nearly 16% of participants had not.

POST TRAUMATIC GROWTH

A minority of people sustain psychological injury from exposure to a disaster, but most people are resilient or experience post traumatic growth.

The impact of disasters on individuals may cause a range of reactions which can be described as *normal* for the circumstances. These include shock, denial or disbelief, as well as irritability, anxiety, mood swings, guilt, shame or self-blame. Such reactions should not be minimised or ignored, but nor should they be immediately *characterised* as a psychological disorder. People affected by disasters may have feelings of hopelessness or confusion and can have difficulty concentrating, a tendency to withdraw, a sense of disconnection, or a feeling of numbness. In the short term, these may simply be normal reactions to a situation that is far from normal. The stress of disasters may also have impacts on the emotional and behavioural aspects of a person's life, interrupting and/or changing relationships, and limiting the ability to function at work, at home, or in normal social interactions.

For some people these reactions do not easily dissipate, and for a minority, symptoms of distress may increase over time. Left unchecked, a diagnosable disorder such as acute stress disorder (ASD), PTSD, or depression may become evident alone or in combination for example, with anxiety and/or depression.

PTSD

REACTING TO TRAUMA

Reacting to trauma is a normal response to a situation that is far from normal.

Broadly speaking, symptoms of PTSD cluster into three areas: intrusive thoughts and images, avoidance, and hyperarousal. The following symptoms are detailed thoroughly in the DSM-V.

Intrusive thoughts or re-experiencing the traumatic event is often regarded as the hallmark feature of PTSD. Re-experiencing symptoms may be unwanted images that pop into a person's head; flashbacks to the traumatic aspects of the experience. People can become upset or distressed when reminded of what happened and have intense physical reactions like sweating, and a rapid heart rate. Unwanted images and thoughts may be present in dreams or when awake.

Avoidance and numbing symptoms are common in people suffering from PTSD. Avoidance is characterised by deliberate attempts to keep memories of the traumatic event out of mind; this can result in a person going to extreme lengths to avoid people, places and activities that trigger distressing memories. Numbing symptoms are reflected through a loss of interest that formerly brought enjoyment as well as detachment or estrangement from others and restricted emotional responses (e.g., to experience joy or love). Intentional avoidance is not to be confused with unintentional avoidance. Sometimes, choosing to remove yourself from situations you predict will be distressing is an adaptive strategy for coping (discussed later in this chapter).

Hyperarousal symptoms are experienced by the individual as though the *Fear System* has been recalibrated to a higher idling level. When people are experiencing increased arousal they may be easily startled, have poor concentration and memory, have increased irritability or anger, and experience sleep difficulties. Essentially, the person is in a state whereby they are constantly alert to signs of danger; they are in a state of high arousal and therefore, a state of hypervigilance. This is a fundamental activity of the brain whose role is to keep us from danger. In people with PTSD, this survival response does not dissipate as it does with people who do not have PTSD. In other words, trauma can alter the structure and functions of the brain [9]. This does not mean the effects cannot be easily overcome as discussed later in this chapter.

According to the Diagnostic and Statistics Manual – 5th edition, PTSD is a severe and enduring condition that may be diagnosed if symptoms remain and are sufficiently severe for more than 30 days [10]. PTSD is specified as acute when the duration of symptoms is less than three months and chronic if the duration of the symptoms is three months or more.

ASD

According to the DSM-V [10], ASD shares the above symptoms of PTSD however the duration of the symptoms is shorter. ASD also has an emphasis on dissociation. The symptoms in this instance last for between three days and one month [p. 279]. Symptoms differ to the reactions to trauma in severity and in levels of distress, impacting negatively on the way a person is functioning in occupational or personal contexts. Initially, ASD as a diagnosis was developed in order to identify people who were at a high risk of developing PTSD. However research demonstrates little evidence to support this proposition [11]. Bryant [11] argues that the majority of people who develop PTSD are not initially diagnosed with ASD.

Depression

Depression can also be a significant after a disaster, especially when the individual has suffered losses. It is worth noting that the incidence of depression following disaster can be very high. For example, Marthoenis and colleagues [12] found a prevalence rate of 58.3% in adolescents following an earthquake and Mamun and colleagues [13] revealed 64.9% of their participants had depression following a cyclone and associated flooding. It should be noted that acute depression following a disaster can follow a distinct course that is independent of PTSD.

Although some depression is likely in the aftermath of a disaster, a picture of severe depression, accompanied by hopelessness, unremitting despair and a loss of belief in any worthwhile future indicates a severe response [14].

Bereavement reactions and complications

Sometimes a disaster will have a double impact on individuals, for example, from the direct impact of the event as well as the death of a loved one. In these circumstances the individual must deal with the personal impact with perhaps loss of property, possession, income and the fear associated with the experience, as well as the pain of bereavement. The memories and post-incident complications will compound this bereavement. Traumatic bereavements include those that encompass the additional element of sudden, perhaps horrific, shocking encounters with death and trauma, with the death of a loved one. Descriptions of traumatic bereavements stand in stark contrast to the experiences of a quiet death in the home, without mutilation, bodily distortion, shock, threat, horror and helplessness. Bereaved and traumatised people may experience similar symptoms in terms of intrusive recollections, persistent thoughts and images, avoidance reactions and high levels of arousal. However, despite significant overlap, there are substantial differences in these two types of experiences [15]. The primary message here is that the concepts of ASD and PTSD, and that of traumatic bereavement are independent entities and care must be taken to ensure that they are dealt with appropriately, supportively, and where necessary clinically.

Compassion fatigue

Compassion fatigue is a term that denotes the emotional residue or strain of exposure from working with those suffering from the consequences of traumatic events [16]. In the context of disasters, people at risk of experiencing compassion fatigue include those who listen to stories of trauma and loss in the aftermath of the crisis and those who respond to the crisis. Emergency service workers such as paramedics, police, and fire crews may be witnesses to the suffering of others in addition to risking their own lives to respond to victims of disasters. Compassion fatigue can be conceptualised as comprising two factors: secondary traumatic stress (STS) and burnout [17]. STS has all of the symptoms of PTSD. Although in these cases, STS is caused by bearing witness to the trauma of others rather than being the direct victim. Burnout, the second concept that comprises compassion fatigue, refers to the emotional exhaustion, depersonalisation, and reduced sense of personal accomplishment that can occur for some people as a result of aspects of their work context. Burnout as a result of trauma exposure shares features with STS, such as feelings of depression, anxiety or helplessness, but onset tends to be gradual rather than sudden [16]. Burnout results from a cumulative build-up of excessive workplace stress (e.g., exposure to trauma, shift work, time pressure) or the emotional demands of working with

RESILIENCE

Being resilient or experiencing growth does not deny ongoing distress for some people.

clients. There is usually an immediate outpouring of concern following any disaster. However, the repetitive nature of disasters and the prolonged time of the recovery phase can lead to compassion fatigue. People who respond to the community in crisis and those who conduct the recovery efforts (e.g., body retrieval teams) are at added risk of compassion fatigue.

RESILIENCE AND GROWTH

Although many of the above reactions seem negative, it must be emphasised that people also show a number of positive responses in the aftermath of a disaster and other potentially traumatic events. These include resilience and coping, altruism, helping save or comfort others, relief and elation at surviving disaster and a sense of excitement [14]. The struggle that a disaster survivor may experience in to coming-to-terms with life following trauma, or a response worker may experience in coming to the aid of victims, can provide a catalyst for positive changes. Such changes include a greater sense of self-worth and personal strength, changes in a person's philosophy about life, and enhanced relationships with others [5]. What is important to remember is that people who are resilient and people who experience growth are not immune to the negative impact of disasters.

Resilience

The term *psychological resilience* is used to describe abilities or protective factors that enable an individual to maintain a stable equilibrium in situations of adversity or trauma, following only a brief interruption to functioning. Researchers [4] have provided convincing evidence that resilience is the most common outcome following such experiences. Despite literature indicating resilience is not equal to the absence of psychopathology, past research has typically assessed resilience by exactly that; the absence of negative mental health outcomes. It is only recently that **resilience has begun to be investigated by measuring its presence rather than the absence of pathology such as PTSD and depression** [18].

DISTRESS & GROWTH
Even people who experience significant distress can also grow and develop from those same distressing experiences.

Post-traumatic growth

Post-traumatic growth (PTG) is a term coined by Tedeschi and Calhoun [19] that refers to positive changes a person may perceive to have occurred following the struggle they engage in to coming-to-terms with life following a traumatic experience such as a disaster. PTG represents a movement beyond pre-event levels of adaptation. In other words, unlike resilience which indicates a person returns to their pre-event levels of functioning, PTG represents transformative positive changes such as an increased appreciation of life, a greater sense of personal strength, changes in philosophy, or in relationships [5]. Theoretically PTG rests on the assumption that the disaster or other traumatic experience is severe enough to metaphorically create a psychological earthquake that disrupts a person's view of the world and themselves within that world. For example, an individual's way of seeing the world prior to trauma may be that good things happen to good people, that life is mainly predictable. Experiencing a disaster and losses, can fundamentally shatter a person's view of the world and create a sense that the world is not safe, that unpredictable and seemingly *unfair* things happen to good people. This shattering of previously held views provides an opportunity for a person to re-examine their life. PTG is not an automatic bi-product of these disrupted beliefs, but is an outcome for some people as a result of the work they engage in to develop a new life narrative with the traumatic or highly challenging experience included. In recent research PTG and resilience have been identified using epigenetic research methods [20]. In other words, PTG and resilience can be seen through epigenetic expression in addition to PTSD.

PREVENTING AND MANAGING MENTAL HEALTH RISK

There are ways in which the risk associated with exposure to disasters can be reduced at both individual and community levels. From an individual perspective, coping resources and strategies are important in minimising psychological injury. At a community level, response to the disaster by relevant authorities can have a significant impact on the likelihood of a community being resilient. Powerful predictors of individual wellbeing include social support; factors that influence the wellbeing of emergency responders such as workplace connectedness and peer support; and variables that influence community mental health such as timely responses to the event itself, insurance claims, and open lines of communication.

Social support

Social support refers to the levels of care, love, comfort, esteem, and help received from and given to others. The perception that support is available if required may be as protective as actually receiving that support, but giving support has also been shown to be beneficial to mental health [21]. Social support systems may include family and colleagues as well as religious or other community affiliations. For example, religion has been positively linked to cognitive coping processes and to finding meaning in loss [5]. Although disasters introduce stressors that challenge the wellbeing of individuals and communities, they also provide an environmental context where functional social support may be extensively given and received. Receiving high levels of instrumental and emotional social support during and immediately after a natural disaster may improve perceptions of social wellbeing. For example, Kaniasty [22] found that the positive experience of social support in the first two months following a flood in Poland led to moderate increases in psychological wellbeing. Receiving adequate social support after a natural disaster provides needed material assistance, but also helps individuals to reframe their social experience, seeing others as dependable and kind [22]. In the study mentioned earlier [8], although nearly 16% of participants still had PTSD 13–14 years following their experiences of flooding, social support was found to be a significant predictor for those who had recovered.

Workplace connectedness

Workplace connectedness refers to the extent to which an employee feels valued and respected by the organisation they work for, their supervisors and colleagues. Connectivity or a sense of belonging to an organisation has been found to be related to reduced reports of anxiety and depression symptoms [23]. Within a group of Australian volunteer firefighters Tuckey and Hayward [24] found that feeling supported and connected to other volunteer fire-fighters was a protective factor against burnout and post-traumatic stress. Examining post-trauma responses in professional firefighters, Armstrong et al. [25] found the sense of connection or workplace belongingness was a significant predictor of PTG. A recent study of mental health in paramedics, organisational belongingness was the strongest predictor of professional quality of life, distress, and resilience [26].

Peer support

Peer support programs have emerged as standard practice for supporting staff in many high-risk organisations, that is, organisations which routinely expose their personnel to potentially traumatic events such as emergency services and the military [27]. With respect to emergency service staff, Shakespeare-Finch et al. [28] point out that good social support in the work setting can be enhanced by well-trained, skilled and respected Peer Support Officers who are available to assist and support personnel following traumatic incidents in the work context. This concept is related to connectedness but is more specific in its focus and is especially applicable in the aftermath of disasters.

Community wellbeing

The Australian Emergency Management Institute (AEMI) [29], and other similar organisations around the world, provide guidelines for effective management of the recovery phase of disasters in order to promote mental health. These principles may be summarised as follows:

- *Effective communication* – Often people can deal with bad news, but no news or lies are much more distressing. A key to reducing anxiety levels is to provide as much information as possible and ensuring communication is truthful, frank and open, even if those responsible may not have all the answers.
- The provision of *practical support* builds sense of community and tells people they are not alone. This may be in the form of assistance with clean up, rebuilding, taking children to school, or cooking a meal. However, it is important that the person being helped has a sense of agency that the help they are receiving is what they want.
- Providing *emotional support* is important to sustaining people during difficult periods of their lives such as after a disaster.
- *Validating the emotions* being experienced may help people restore a sense of normalcy even when nothing is normal. Providing reassurance that the processes of grief are normal and not evidence of psychopathology may help people to contain the extent of anxiety being experienced.
- *Identifying coping strategies and resources* will help people reduce anxiety and restore functionality. These strategies may include behavioural, emotional, and physical ones.
- Providing *information on, and access to resources* available to help, both physically and emotionally will help reduce anxiety levels.

CONCLUSION

Throughout this Chapter, two primary and important elements have been identified. Firstly, a small number of individuals who are impacted by a disaster or significant critical event may sustain a diagnosable psychiatric disorder. However, the vast majority will cope and indeed perform well in the face of adversity. Importantly, many within this *majority* will actually develop an enhanced sense of resilience and coping as a result of their experience with the event, and as a result of the way in which they have helped others, or have been helped by others. In adversity, people adapt in remarkable ways. Full recovery is not always likely to occur immediately, but evidence supports the view that with appropriate support and care, the majority of people do respond well. Some people, more than the prevalence of PTSD, will go on to experience PTG; most will be resilient or recover from their difficulties.

Given the significant body of available material informing our understanding of mental health, the second element relates to the compelling need for post-disaster mental healthcare and response to be clearly understood and focused. Further, appropriate steps need to be taken to ensure education and supportive intervention through raising awareness and continuing to conduct research that provides an evidence base for responses, be they proactive or reactive. Pro-active mental health education and support strategies to minimise, and where possible to prevent adverse reactions may be adopted (e.g., in workplaces, community groups and school settings). This is particularly important in disaster management planning contexts and emergency service and response settings.

ACTIVITIES

1. Consider a disaster with which you are familiar. What are the factors that may have impacted on the mental health consequences and how could those consequences be mitigated?
2. If you were asked to set up a mental health support services for a community, what would be its key elements?

References

1. Crompton, D., et al., Responding to disasters: More than economic and infrastructure interventions. *Insights on the Depression and Anxiety*, 2018. **2**(1): p. 14–28.
2. Ahern, M., et al., Global health impacts of floods: Epidemiologic evidence. *Epidemiologic Reviews*, 2005. **27**(1): p. 36–46.
3. Sayed, S., B.M. Iacoviello, and D.S. Charney, Risk factors for the development of psychopathology following trauma. *Current Psychiatry Reports*, 2015. **17**: p. 1–7.
4. Galatzer-Levy, I.R., S.H. Huang, and G.A. Bonanno, Trajectories of resilience and dysfunction following potential trauma: A review and statistical evaluation. *Clinical Psychology Review*, 2018. **63**: p. 41–55.
5. Tedeschi, R.G., et al., *Posttraumatic growth: Theory, research, and applications*. 2018, New York: Routledge.
6. Anderson, G.S., et al., Peer support and crisis-focused psychological interventions designed to mitigate post-traumatic stress injuries among public safety and frontline healthcare personnel: A systematic review. *International Journal of Environmental Research and Public Health*, 2020. **17**(20): p. 7645.
7. Opie, E., et al., The usefulness of pre-employment and pre-deployment psychological screening for disaster relief workers: A systematic review. *BMC Psychiatry*, 2020. **20**(1): p. 1–13.
8. Dai, W., et al., Association between social support and recovery from post-traumatic stress disorder after flood: A 13–14 year follow-up study in Hunan, China. *BMC Public Health*, 2016. **16**(1): p. 1–9.
9. Mucci, C. and A. Scalabrini, Traumatic effects beyond diagnosis: The impact of dissociation on the mind–body–brain system. *Psychoanalytic Psychology*, 2021. **38**(4): p. 279.
10. American Psychiatric Association, *Diagnostic and Statistical Manual of Mental Disorder*. 2013, Washington DC: AMA.
11. Bryant, R.A., Acute stress disorder. *Psychiatry*, 2006. **5**(7): p. 238–239.
12. Marthoenis, M., et al., Prevalence, comorbidity and predictors of post-traumatic stress disorder, depression, and anxiety in adolescents following an earthquake. *Asian Journal of Psychiatry*, 2019. **43**: p. 154–159.
13. Mamun, M.A., et al., Prevalence of depression among Bangladeshi village women subsequent to a natural disaster: A pilot study. *Psychiatry Research*, 2019. **276**: p. 124–128.
14. Raphael, B., *National Health and Medical Research Council. Disaster Management*. 1993, Canberra (AU): Australian Government Publishing Service.
15. Raphael, B. and N. Martinek, Assessing traumatic bereavement and posttraumatic stress disorder. in *Assessing Psychological Trauma and PTSD*, J.P. Wilson and T.M. Keane, Editors. 1997, New York: Guildford Press.
16. Figley, C.R., Compassion fatigue: As secondary traumatic stress disorder. An overview, in *Compassion Fatigue: Coping With Secondary Traumatic Stress Disorder In Those Who Treat The Traumatized*, C.R. Figley, Editor. 1995, Hoboken (NJ): Taylor and Francis.
17. Stamm, B., *The Concise ProQOL Manual*. ProQOL.org: Pocatello.
18. Shakespeare-Finch, J. and E. Daley, Workplace belongingness, distress, and resilience in emergency service workers. *Psychological Trauma: Theory, Research, Practice, and Policy*, 2017. **9**(1): p. 32.
19. Tedeschi, R.G. and L.G. Calhoun, *Trauma & transformation: Growing in the aftermath of suffering*. 1995, Thousand Oaks, CA: Sage. https://doi.org/10.4135/9781483326931

20. Miller, O., et al., DNA Methylation of NR3C1 and FKBP5 predicts posttraumatic stress disorder, posttraumatic growth and resilience. *Psychological Trauma: Research, Theory Practice & Policy*, 2020. **12**(7): p. 750–755. https://doi.org/10.1037/tra0000574.

21. Shakespeare-Finch, J. and P.L. Obst, The development of the 2-way social support scale: A measure of giving and receiving emotional and instrumental support. *Journal of Personality Assessment*, 2011. **93**(5): p. 483–490.

22. Kaniasty, K., Predicting social psychological well-being following trauma: The role of postdisaster social support. *Psychological Trauma: Theory, Research, Practice, and Policy*, 2012. **4**(1): p. 22.

23. Cockshaw, W.D., I.M. Shochet, and P.L. Obst, General belongingness, workplace belongingness, and depressive symptoms. *Journal of Community & Applied Social Psychology*, 2013. **23**(3): p. 240–251.

24. Tuckey, M.R. and R. Hayward, Global and occupation-specific emotional resources as buffers against the emotional demands of fire-fighting. *Applied Psychology*, 2011. **60**(1): p. 1–23.

25. Armstrong, D., J. Shakespeare-Finch, and I. Shochet, Predicting post-traumatic growth and post-traumatic stress in firefighters. *Australian Journal of Psychology*, 2014. **66**(1): p. 38–46.

26. Shakespeare-Finch, J., et al. Caring for emergency service personnel: Does what we do work, in *2014 Australian and New Zealand disaster and emergency management conference: Book of proceedings-Peer reviewed*, 2014. Surfers Paradise: Association of sustainability in Business Inc. p. 1–20.

27. Levenson Jr, R.L. and L.A. Dwyer, Peer support in law enforcement: Past, present, and future. *International Journal of Emergency Mental Health*, 2003. **5**(3): p. 147–152.

28. Shakespeare-Finch, J. and P. Scully, *Ways in which paramedics cope with, and respond to, natural large-scale disasters*. 2008. Hauppauge, NY: Nova Science Publishers, Inc. p. 89–100.

29. Australian Emergency Management Institute, Community recovery: Handbook 2, in *Australian emergency management handbook series*. 2011, Canberra (AU): Commonwealth of Australia.

Part 4
Getting ready

13
Prevention and mitigation

Gerry FitzGerald, Benjamin Ryan, Richard Franklin, and Stacey Pizzino

INTRODUCTION AND OBJECTIVES

Chapters 1 and 2 outlined the evolution of thinking about disasters and the shift from a principal focus on response to a more comprehensive all-hazards approach throughout the pre-event, event, and post-event continuum. The evidence of the value of this approach is unquestioned and highlighted at the macro community level when damage is minimised in well-structured communities, while the same event can be catastrophic in less well-developed societies. Building resilient community infrastructure and resilient communities is the best protection that may be offered to a community against the ravages of disasters. The by-product of this investment is improved living standards more generally which is more impactful on people's lives, as disasters are generally rare.

Therefore, much public policy has the effect of preventing or mitigating disasters. However, these policies are not recognisable as disaster prevention. Rather they are directed towards broader community development goals.

The aim of this chapter is to outline the concepts and strategies underpinning disaster prevention and mitigation. On completion of this chapter, you should be able to:

1. Identify and critically analyse the concepts and principles of disaster prevention and mitigation.
2. Identify and critically evaluate the range of strategies used to build resilience and reduce vulnerability.
3. Evaluate public policy options regarding their disaster mitigation impact.

PREVENTION AND MITIGATION: BUILDING RESILIENCE

Prevention implies the hazard may be controlled and the event prevented or at least reduced in frequency or severity. Prevention strategies may be diverse, comprehensive, and integrated with broader policy initiatives. For example, the accepted social niceties of not spitting in public or covering your mouth when sneezing may be alternatively viewed as pandemic prevention. Seismic planning and engineering can improve city infrastructure while helping ensure critical functions continue during and after an earthquake.

DOI: 10.4324/9781032626604-17

Land-use restrictions can limit the settlement of high-risk zones and maintain amenity. Building better roads to speed the flow of traffic implies greater safety and reduced risk of major accidents. Safer security systems may reduce the ability of terrorists to cause disruption. Finally, dams built for water supply may aid with flood mitigation.

However, prevention may be not possible, too costly, or not achievable because of the influence of other factors. Where disasters cannot be prevented, it is often possible to take actions that reduce or **mitigate** the impact of hazards on individuals and on the community and its socioeconomic fabric. Earthquakes may not be preventable. Building the ultimate safe road may exceed the community's economic capacity. Major structural or functional changes to society may be fiercely opposed by sectional interests. Consider the resistance to reducing carbon emissions resulting from fears of the impact such initiatives may have on the economy and quality of life. At times, communities and individuals are determined to accept the risk to achieve broad social and community goals although this acceptance may be unstated.

Any distinction between prevention and mitigation strategies may be artificial as the same dam may prevent some floods and reduce the impact of others. Hence it is customary to group prevention and mitigation strategies together.

Prevention and mitigation strategies also intersect with the concept of infrastructure protection which describes the range of strategies required to protect critical community infrastructure. Such strategies can include security, surveillance, and rapid response. This is discussed in detail in Chapter 15. Community lifelines are an essential component of disaster mitigation ensuring reduced impact on the community. For example, resilient design and construction of transport infrastructure will ensure continued supply and the capacity for evacuation of communities. Additionally, safe houses or evacuation centres may be required to provide protection in the event of a disaster.

Prevention and mitigation strategies include those taken by the individual, the organisation, or the community and by various levels of government. These strategies can also be taken during or after a disaster or hazardous event to prevent secondary consequences, such as measures to prevent the contamination of water. It may be directed at both individual and community infrastructure and behaviours.

- Strategies may be directed at the **individual** by encouraging reduction in risk taking behaviours, or by requiring personal protections such as vaccinations.
- Alternatively, **community**-focussed strategies may include initiatives that reduce or avoid hazards or reduce exposure to hazards. For example, land use planning to prevent building on a floodplain reduces hazards and reduces the risk of exposure. Communities and governments initiate and then sustain planning and preparedness activities.

Prevention and mitigation strategies may be also viewed as structural and non-structural.

- **Structural** measures are those directed towards the design and engineering of structures. These include building dams, diverting water flows, levees and seawalls, windbreaks, freeways with flexible joints to reduce the impact of earthquakes.
- **Non-structural** measures include policy and guidelines which guide not only the design and construction of physical elements but also the design and performance of non-physical elements such as standard operating procedures, governance structures, or response arrangements.

A combination of structural and non-structural measures is required for a comprehensive approach. Structures alone are not sufficient. Physical barriers can create a false sense of security, for example, the tsunami barriers in Japan or the levees in New Orleans. Often the community believes the construction of defences is an absolute protection when really at best it can reduce the frequency or severity of impact.

However, the resilience of a community is the product of a complex interplay of individual, organisational and community actions. van den Brink et al. [1] describe the *adaptive capacity wheel* in which an array of strategies fit within six fundamental domains that they describe as leadership, governance, resources, variety, learning, and autonomous change. Disaster managers and community leaders require an understanding of this complexity but at the same time need to take action to encourage or direct those strategies over which they have control.

Categorisation of prevention and mitigation strategies may assist with understanding their range and scope. Day et al. [2] categorised mitigation strategies firstly into those that are permanent, responsive to hazard alerts or anticipatory of risk. Secondly, they provided a means of evaluating strategies on the basis of those that may be 'brittle' (sustainable to a level of impact then fail) or those that are 'flexible' (continue to sustain to some extent regardless of the level of impact).

Understanding prevention strategies may also borrow from Haddon's Matrix used in injury prevention research which describes the inter-relationship between the host, agent/vehicle, physical environment, and social environment throughout the pre-event, event, and post-event cycle. Prevention and mitigation strategies are diverse and permeate through the host, agent, physical, and social environment perspective of Haddon's Matrix.

Strategies directed at the **host** are those aimed at human behaviour to reduce the likelihood of behaviours that may cause disasters. At its most strategic level, this may focus on the collective use of energy which fosters greater consumption of the earth's resources and greater production of CO_2 which in turn impacts on climate change. More directly, these strategies may focus on risk-taking behaviours or on deliberate actions designed to cause terror. They may also focus on preventing the vulnerability of individuals through physical protections (e.g., safety helmets) or through personal resilience (e.g., immunisations).

The strategies aimed at human behavioural modification may be broadly categorised as restrictive, educational, or informational. Societies will act to eliminate behaviours placing the community at risk through legal enforcement actions. They may also seek to inform individuals of the consequences of their actions or to educate them to enhance awareness and understanding. The scope of these strategies is well beyond this text's capacity to detail.

Strategies directed at the **agent** are generally those aimed at reducing the presence or risk posed by hazards. For example, containing chemicals and ensuring safety in their accessibility, handling and application may reduce the likelihood of chemical events. Safety systems built into transportation systems will reduce the likelihood of major collision.

Strategies focussed on the **environment** are directed towards ensuring the physical infrastructure that supports communities is resilient. Such strategies include building standards and land-use planning. Fire risks can be minimised by vegetation planning and fuel load reduction through controlled burning or vegetation clearing. Similarly, firebreaks, levees and evacuation pathways, and centres can help protect people from the impact of disasters and thus mitigate their effects.

Strategies focussed on the **social environment** are directed towards building community resilience to either prevent or mitigate the impact disasters have on society. Such strategies may focus on both the hard (physical) and soft (systems) infrastructure and target building connectedness and support.

Prevention and mitigation measures may occur at all levels of society and at the strategic as well as the operational and tactical levels. On a national level, governments might implement large-scale mitigation measures. They may also be taken at the international level. If achieving domestic cooperation to reduce risk is difficult, gaining international cooperation is extremely challenging. Mitigation measures may also be internally conflicting. For example, the light wooden style of houses traditional in Japan is less dangerous in earthquakes but not resistant to tsunamis.

Tactical initiatives are those that can be taken on impact to mitigate the effects. For example, following an earthquake or cyclone authorities may shut down electricity grids to prevent fires, turn off gas supplies or build emergency shelters. Individuals may ensure protective mechanisms are in place such as incorporating sprinkler systems to protect houses in fire-prone areas or having a generator available to ensure water pressures can be maintained.

Preventive or mitigation strategies can take different forms to deal with different hazards specific to the local community. For example, Miami Beach's approach to strengthening street flood mitigation is locally led with public works undertaken complemented by matching of funds up to $20,000 for private property owners who are preventing flood damage. Tropical areas may also impose cyclone resistance standards that are less valuable in temperate areas. Prevention and mitigation strategies also need to be efficient in the competing demands for resources for other legitimate and worthwhile requirements. They also need to be sustainable.

Organisations both public and private, service delivery agencies and productive industries need to build their own resilience. Disasters may be low-probability, high-consequence events, therefore organisational resilience is necessary to ensure the continued functioning required to sustain communities. An Australian government paper on organisational resilience [3] emphasised that resilience is an *outcome*, not a *process* and is related to the ability of organisations to maintain effective Business as Usual (BAU) the capacity to change and adapt and the ability to shape the environment.

Broadly, more resilient societies are often those with stronger economies. They can build stronger and more costly systems and put in place the necessary organisational or governance arrangements. More resilient societies are those that are more interconnected with strong social support systems such as family, religious, and social connections. Building societal systems helps build resilience and thus mitigate the impact of disasters.

DRIVING CHANGE

The old medical adage that *an ounce of prevention is worth a pound of cure* equally applies to disaster management. Prevention and mitigation not only reduce the human impact, but have also been repeatedly shown to reduce the economic costs of response and recovery. However, there are practical and political constraints to these simple cost-benefit analyses. For example, while insurance companies may be most adversely affected by events, they are generally not in the position to pay for mitigation or protective works, as these are not the purpose for which people pay their premiums.

There are several theories that seek to help understand the basis of prevention and mitigation action including Protection Motivation Theory, Person Relative to Event Theory, Protective Action Decision Model, Social Cogitative Preparation Model, and Theory of Planned Behaviour. Analysis of these competing theories is beyond the scope of this text, but it is sufficient to note that they emphasise the need to both convince players of the need for change but to provide them with the skills and means to do so [4].

Equally comprehensive approaches to managing risk such as the Risk Governance Council framework require inclusive interdisciplinary, transdisciplinary adaptable and problem-orientated approaches [5].

The policy drivers of mitigation and prevention particularly in democracies are often indirect and difficult to link to direct action. While government may be able to direct initiatives they fund, they are generally not in a position to direct the actions of private individuals and organisations. Evidence suggests that people are prepared to spend more on prevention and mitigation and that financial incentives directed towards the individual may deliver benefit in excess of the costs to the public purse [6]. It should be noted that the majority of critical community infrastructure is held by the private sector. Prevention and mitigation measures may need to be encouraged by governments or communities through strategies that are more indirect. These may be broadly grouped into five categories.

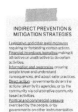

1. *Legislative and other legal measures* that require or forbid certain actions. These may range from direct legislative imposition of certain actions to the creation of standards forming benchmarks against which common-law judgements may be made. Examples may include land-use planning legislation, construction standards, and road safety activities.
2. *Financial incentives* either through taxation or price mechanisms make it financially attractive to take certain measures, or on the contrary impose financial penalties such as higher insurance premiums or direct fines for actions that are not appropriate.
3. *Information and awareness* programs that ensure people know and understand the consequences allowing for necessary protective actions to be taken.
4. *Direct action* where governments may determine the actions taken by agencies it directly controls, or by the community through collaborative community-based activities.
5. *Political and commercial pressure* may be exercised on governments (by the people) or by governments on other instrumentalities. This may involve the media and may include commercial pressure when governments take action against companies that devalue the safety of workers.

The difficulties confronting the implementation of prevention and mitigation strategies are the multiplicity of agencies involved in those strategies and the conflicting and confounding imperatives. For example, the finance department may be pushing for increased efficiency to improve productivity, while injury prevention advocates (and unions) may speak to safer production. The employment department may wish to lower occupational health and safety (OH&S) injuries whilst consumers are begging for lower costs.

The challenge of modern societies is to determine how mitigation strategies may fit within the complex and competing priorities and influences. How does a community exact the prevention and mitigation strategies and where is the authority for, and the sustainability of such decisions?

LAND MANAGEMENT
PRACTICES

Greater prosperity, the loss of historical knowledge through the passage-of-time, and a false or misguided belief that modern systems will prevent any ill-effects of a disaster have caused many communities to adopt high risk land management practices.

For example, people in floodable areas have previously built their houses on stilts to allow water to circulate relatively harmlessly under the house without damaging content. Greater prosperity, the loss of historical knowledge through the passage of time and the false or inappropriate belief that modern systems will prevent any ill effect, has allowed subsequent property owners to build-in under the house to expand the useable family space. However, this makes the property more vulnerable to the impact of flooding.

How can vulnerability be addressed in the light of competing demands and a reluctant community? Gaining coordinated approaches to disaster prevention and mitigation against conflicting interests is difficult not only within government, but across the entirety of society. Communities are likely to be tolerant of measures that address their own risk, but less so of measures to reduce the risk to others. How can individual interests be balanced against the greater good? The NIMBY (not in my back yard) perspective limits the creation of mitigation initiatives that disadvantage anyone. Societies often demand greater protection as long as someone else pays for it and it does not interfere with an individual's sense of comfort.

Comprehensive multimodal approaches are necessary as no single strategy is likely to be successful. Using floods as an example, vulnerability can be addressed through land-use planning, housing design and operational strategies such as alerts and evacuation. Furthermore, collective strategies to minimise the hazard may include:

1. Storage of excess rainwater in dams or flood protection ponds.
2. Channelling of water away from vulnerable areas using diversion channels or levees. Such channels need to be maintained to ensure they remain free of obstruction.
3. Water flow management ensuring absorptive land is maintained.

Contemporary management approaches emphasise the value of entrepreneurship and innovation in all stages of the disaster management cycle [7]. Consider a comprehensive strategic approach to drought management. This may include water conservation as well as soil conservation and management to prevent erosion through crop or plant selection. Understanding complexity and innovative approaches to management are the key to making a difference.

VULNERABILITY

The concept of vulnerability is often seen as the counterpane of resilience. This includes the social, physical, environmental, and economic factors, which increase the susceptibility of an individual, asset, or community to disaster or impacts of a hazard. However, the definition of vulnerability is unclear. Indeed, it could be posited that vulnerability like disasters is a relative term. Even the best swimmers may be vulnerable to the tsunami while some severely disabled individuals are heavily reliant on support at all times and thus highly susceptible to any changes in that equilibrium. There is clearly a range of vulnerability that balances the capability of the individual, organisation, or community against the extent and nature of the challenge confronting it.

Quantifying vulnerability within this notion of relativity is challenging. Weichselgartner [8] defines a process of analysis of the hazard, exposure, preparedness, and prevention response which leads to an overall view of vulnerability.

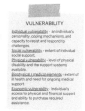

The vulnerability of people may be considered as comprising several interconnected components or perspectives.

- *Individual* vulnerability relates to the personality and coping mechanisms of the person and their capacity to resist and respond to challenges.
- *Social vulnerability* refers to the extent of social support the individual may have.
- *Physical vulnerability* concerns the level of physical disability and the system and structural supports available.
- *Biophysical/medical elements* concern the extent of ill health and the need for ongoing medical support. For example, a person with renal failure is highly vulnerability to the loss of transportation denying access to the dialysis machine or to the loss of power preventing the machines from operating.
- *Economic vulnerability* refers to the individual access to physical and financial support and the ability to purchase assistance when required.

Social and economic vulnerability is aggravated by the increasing complexity of modern society where the interconnectivity of human social systems becomes more vulnerable to the failure of component pieces. For example, modern western societies are particularly vulnerable to power failure on which relies much of our social system functionality from telling the time to communication and mobility. An individual in a wheelchair may be reasonably mobile in highly developed western societies until the power fails and they cannot use the elevator.

MAINSTREAMING MITIGATION AND PREVENTION

Often discussion of prevention and mitigation, implies these strategies occur in isolation of other public policy or social development. However, non-routine and rare events can never be the basis of social and economic development. After the 2011 Japanese earthquake and tsunami, people asked why they built those *fishing villages* in a tsunami-prone area. The nearness to the fish obviously outweighed any risks known or unknown of tsunamis. This concept of greater good must necessarily be taken into consideration in social and economic decisions. Most public policy decisions, as with most individual and organisational decisions, balance the risks of adversity against the potential benefits. Mines are built in dangerous and isolated places because that is where the minerals are. Human populations inhabit the alluvial (floodable) land because that is where the rich soil to support food production is.

Consideration of the cost-effectiveness of mitigation measures in their broadest sense must also be considered by balancing the economic and social perspectives.

- **Economic considerations**: Building high-level concrete houses to withstand the annual floods is optimal if the community can afford them.
- **Social consideration**: Some people enjoy the riverside aspects and are prepared to accept the risk of flooding. The danger inherent in this principle is that people will claim to accept the individual risk initially but loudly demand support and compensation when the inevitable disaster occurs.

CASE STUDY 13.1 – HOBART: TASMAN BRIDGE DISASTER, 9.27 PM SUNDAY, 5 JANUARY 1975

Bulk Iron Ore carrier 'the Lake Illawarra' travelling up the *Derwent River* collided with several pylons of the *Tasman Bridge*. Two piers of the bridge collapsed along with 127 metres of bridge decking. Four cars careered into the Derwent River killing all five occupants. Seven crewmen from the 'Lake Illawarra' were also killed. The disaster severed the main link between Hobart and its eastern suburbs with a population of approximately 40,000. This disaster is notable for the social impacts resulting from the loss of such an important road artery, as most of the city's hospitals, schools, businesses, and government officers were located on the western shore. A temporary one-lane bridge was constructed within the year, however, it was 34 months before the Tasman Bridge was reopened. The disaster did hasten the development of commercial and public facilities in the eastern suburbs

Except in the most high-risk areas, there is rarely a role for standalone approaches to mitigation but rather there is a constant need to take disaster mitigation and prevention into consideration in all public policy initiatives. This mainstreaming of disaster mitigation and prevention is more likely to ensure consideration is given, and that this consideration is encompassed in the broader perspective of the potential risks, costs, and benefits of community development.

Land-use planning is a classic example. As new development occurs, disaster impacts should be part of the contextual analysis. This mainstreaming of mitigation helps with a balanced consideration. The consideration of investment in a strong high-level bridge should consider not only the longevity and productive capacity of the bridge, but also its role in maintaining communication and access to vulnerable communities.

ACTIVITIES AND KEY READINGS

1. Produce a table which summarises strategies that may prevent or mitigate the impact of bushfires on a rural community. In doing so consider using the framework of host, agent, environment, and society but also the structural and non-structural measures.
2. Identify the legal, economic, physical, and social strategies that may help mitigate the effect of a tsunami on a coastal region.
3. Consider the cost and benefits of imposing lower speed limits on a highway.

References

1. van den Brink, M., et al., Climate-proof planning for flood-prone areas: Assessing the adaptive capacity of planning institutions in the Netherlands. *Regional Environmental Change*, 2014. **14**: p. 981–995.
2. Day, S. and C. Fearnley, A classification of mitigation strategies for natural hazards: Implications for the understanding of interactions between mitigation strategies. *Natural Hazards*, 2015. **79**: p. 1219–1238.
3. Ernst & Young and Australian Government, *Organisational Resilience: The relationship with risk related corporate strategies.* 2013, Canberra (AU): Commonwealth of Australia. p. 28.

4. Muzenda-Mudavanhu, C., A review of children's participation in disaster risk reduction: Opinion paper. *Jàmbá: Journal of Disaster Risk Studies*, 2016. **8**(1): p. 1–6.

5. Schweizer, P.-J. and O. Renn, Governance of systemic risks for disaster prevention and mitigation. *Disaster Prevention and Management: An International Journal*, 2019. **28**(6): p. 862–874. doi:10.1108/dpm-09-2019-0282

6. Donahue, A.K., Risky business: Willingness to pay for disaster preparedness. *Public Budgeting & Finance*, 2014. **34**(4): p. 100–119.

7. Sawalha, I.H., A contemporary perspective on the disaster management cycle. *Foresight*, 2020. **22**(4): p. 469–482.

8. Weichselgartner, J., Disaster mitigation: The concept of vulnerability revisited. *Disaster Prevention and Management: An International Journal*, 2001. **10**(2):p. 85–95. doi:10.1108/09653560110388609

14
Planning

Rosemary Hegner[1]

INTRODUCTION AND OBJECTIVES

The effective management of disasters begins well in advance of any event. Getting ready includes preventing and mitigating the risks to which the community is exposed, but it also involves organising the resources required including the people and their capability. Indeed, in the absence of frequent events, the only thing we can evaluate is how prepared the community is. Preparedness involves a range of strategies that in general aim to get ready for response and recovery. Key to preparation is the process of planning which provides the means by which other aspects of preparedness may be addressed.

Disaster planning should not occur in isolation of normal business planning. Modern organisations and communities have exposure to a range of risks including those associated with major incidents. Disaster planning should be part of the normal preparedness of organisations and communities to confront not only the routine risks associated with normal operations, but also the major non-routine risks that challenge the whole community.

The process of planning provides key stakeholders and participants with the means by which the context is identified and evaluated, relationships are formed, issues are identified and addressed and awareness is created. The process of planning is educational for all involved and by itself helps build awareness and capability.

The aim of this chapter is to address the issue of disaster planning for health and to outline the principles and practice of planning. On completion of this chapter, you should be able to:

1. Identify and critically discuss the value and importance of planning.
2. Identify the principles of disaster planning and its context.
3. Describe the process of planning and the activities required to achieve effective planning.

DOI: 10.4324/9781032626604-18

DISASTER PLANNING IN THE HEALTH CONTEXT

Good disaster management is about effectively coordinating and directing resources to achieve the *greatest good for the greatest number* when normal systems and processes are stretched to, or even beyond capacity.

Planning is the process of designing and documenting how an organisation or facility will respond to and manage a disaster to achieve the desired health outcomes. For many health services, a disaster response will be very complex and involve a diverse group from differing functional areas of health. This coordinated and joint approach must start in the planning process by identifying and engaging all those who will add value to and sustain an effective response and recovery during a critical period.

GOOD DISASTER MANAGEMENT
The ability to effectively coordinate and direct resources to achieve 'the greatest good for the greatest number' when normal systems and processes are stretched to or beyond capacity.

Engagement of the wider health system during business as usual presents its own challenges, as most health services work at, or close to capacity most of the time. This leaves little time to dedicate to planning and even fewer resources to dedicate to regular exercising of those plans. Ironically, the healthcare culture of continuing to serve and care no matter the circumstance can almost become an obstacle to effective planning. The argument *why should we plan, we always cope?* can almost be made, when a focused and dedicated workforce constantly adapts and overcomes in the face of adversity.

With changing demographics, cultures and climate and the heightened expectations amongst communities in the effectiveness of response to disasters, failing to plan can ultimately put at greatest risk well-intentioned health workforces who have limited time to meet and plan. So, it is never truer than in the health context that *failing to plan is planning to fail*, both for our people and our communities.

PLANNING PRINCIPLES

There are many and varied definitions of planning, but most will probably agree that it can be described as *an analytical and consultative process to help organisations or governments manage the risks presented from both common and extraordinary hazards.*

No amount of disaster planning, education and exercising will compensate for the confusion created from the departure from normal business or professional practice in the face of adversity.

Modern health services are under considerable stress, struggling to cope with the increasing demand for services within significant resource constraints. Health services can also be quite fragmented organisations with conflicting priorities, which means that planning activities, which are counter to or create challenges for normal business, will struggle to gain traction. This is one reason why consulting early with key stakeholders is a key principle in achieving the level of engagement critical to successful disaster planning. Equally important, however, is embedding normal business at the heart of our response to disasters. No amount of disaster planning, education and exercise will compensate for the confusion created by the departure from normal business or professional practice, in the face of adversity. Normal business may need to be augmented or supplemented of course, but familiarity in the planning of disaster systems and arrangements will enable health services to manage the surge in demand which accompanies any disaster.

Disasters present unique challenges to health services but can also present great planning opportunities. Disasters of course place systems under enormous stress, imposing extraordinary demands on staff and services. However, they can also present opportunities to step outside of normal boundaries and conventions, forging new relationships and arrangements borne of necessity. These opportunities must be anticipated in the planning process though, particularly if the principle that disaster planning must be rooted in *normal business* is to be applied. For example, where limitations in human, financial or technical resources are known, planners can anticipate the options that would normally be *off the table* such as accessing private health services or the capacity to modify staffing ratios. Disaster health plans will therefore strive to achieve a balance between those processes which are well-practiced and understood while providing permission for services to go beyond the normal.

PLANNING CONTEXT

Fundamental to the planning process is establishing and communicating the context within which the planning occurs, and the plan will operate. Central in establishing this context for health services is authority and governance.

The authority for the proposed plan will be relative to its strategic, tactical or operational application, but regardless, there must always be appropriate oversight and governance to ensure the efficacy of process, and accountability for development and delivery. At a jurisdictional level this may be informed by legislation outlining statutory obligations to plan, which in turn may inform government, department, health service or business unit planning. The mandate may not be legislated but may relate to organisational aims and objectives or public health priorities.

Wherever the mandate originates, it is essential to identify the authority to plan, the governance body with oversight, and the group or individuals responsible for the delivery of the plans. These aren't just considerations for the start of the planning process either. Throughout the journey the governance body will need to be consulted to approve finance and resources, stakeholder groups, endorsement of draft content and approval of finished plans. They will also have a crucial role in bringing the planning process full circle by:

- Setting review periods and exercising or training programs.
- Ensuring lessons identified during exercise or activation are incorporated into the plan.
- Inform the revision and update of the plan.

Therefore, identifying the appropriate governance body to provide oversight and direction is a critical early consideration.

Additionally, it is critical to understand the cultural, social, organisational and operational context within which the planning occurs. Establishing and understanding the planning context will therefore help clarify the ultimate objective and required output of the planning process. It may even change the initial perception of the plan's purpose and intent. The finished product must address the issues required without overreaching, must have oversight from the accountable body and, most importantly, must add value and understanding to those required to implement it.

THE PLANNING PROCESS

Whilst arguably this is a rather bleak assessment of the finished product, undeniably the planning process is an enormously beneficial and educative process in itself. By stepping through the planning process, planners and stakeholders will almost certainly build their organisational awareness, renew the links and relationships within their organisations, and have a better understanding of its capabilities, vulnerabilities and limitations. It may also be the case that where the disaster plan is perceived to be of little use, this could well be because the context was unclear, the process had failed to establish appropriate governance or scope, hadn't engaged the right stakeholders, or had been ambiguous in its aims and objectives.

Before progressing further in the planning process though, the first step is to *plan the plan!* Having obtained authority to plan, a project plan must be established with agreed deliverables, i.e., the plan's constituent parts. This chapter will not address the principles of project management, but a rudimentary understanding and application of these principles will not only be important in achieving a successful outcome to the project, i.e., delivering the plan in the agreed time frame and budget, but will also inform the planning process and deliver a better-finished product. There are number of key stages in the planning process:

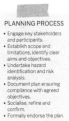

PLANNING PROCESS
* Engage key stakeholders and participants.
* Establish scope and limitations, identify clear aims and objectives.
* Undertake hazard identification and risk analysis.
* Document plan ensuring compliance with agreed objectives.
* Socialise, refine and confirm.
* Formally endorse the plan.

1. Engage key stakeholders and participants

    Most health services whether local, regional or jurisdictional in size, are complex organisations with many internal and external relationships and dependencies. Attempting to plan without first understanding the organisation and the stakeholders who will either be essential to the process, or who will be impacted by the application or activation of the plan, can at best result in ineffective plans, and at worst, create division and barriers which can delay or derail the planning process. Obtaining authority to plan through an appropriate governance body can help with this process, but the planner can't assume that this is so. Time spent in mapping out stakeholders and participants and those who will benefit or be affected by activating the plan will help to draw out all those who should be engaged or contribute to its development.

2. Establish scope and limitations – identifying clear aims and objectives

    Having identified key stakeholders and participants, the next question is how (or how much) they and their service or business should be incorporated into the planning process. Limitations in scope can be related to resources
    * Are there enough people to do this?
    * Can this be done in time?
    * Is this strategy affordable?
    * Is there the authority to do this?

    Whatever the limitations are, they need to be understood. This will save time and effort in developing an unworkable plan. As an example, a national disaster plan may include contingencies which will be activated at a national level, but which rely entirely on resources that are controlled by multiple jurisdictions. If the jurisdictions and/or their resources aren't well prepared or resourced, the national plan is unreliable.

    Logistical, financial, human resource or political issues may limit or deny the inclusion of key elements in the plan. If this is the case, the level of risk this presents to the plan and its success will need to be considered early in the planning process.

    Critically, the scoping process must identify the aim and objectives for your plan. Confusion between these two concepts is common with many and varying definitions. Simply put though the aim of the plan is a broad statement of the plan's purpose or intent, i.e., *the aim of this plan is to outline the health services strategy and arrangements for responding to, managing, and recovering from a natural disaster.* The objectives thereafter provide a detailed explanation of how to achieve that aim, i.e., a list of objectives for the above aim might include

a. To maintain an effective command and control structure with clear communication, notification and escalation processes for identifying and responding to disasters.

b. To establish effective incident response procedures to ensure the organisation is aware of and can respond to a disaster, including details of all departments and services involved in the response and their relationship to incident command.

c. To outline a recovery strategy to help the organisation recover from the impacts of the disaster, return to normal functioning, identify lessons and opportunities from the disaster and build capability through reviewing and updating the disaster plan.

Plans should be sustainable. Details should be avoided as they rapidly age the plan. Rather mechanisms need to be identified by which those details can be acquired in the event of an emergency. For example, phone numbers or individual names can change daily and should not be included in the plan. However, the plan may identify a source of this information and mechanisms developed whereby that source is maintained, up to date and accessible. A common example might be to reference the hospital's electronic telephone directory which is regularly maintained and updated by the telephony team.

3. Undertake hazard identification and risk analysis

Emergency risk assessments including hazard identification are well documented in international and national standards. Understanding hazards is an important element in health emergencies and clarity regarding the hazard(s) in the context of planning for emergencies affecting health services is essential. For example, a *Hospital Emergency Plan* is likely to be a very broad plan encompassing many hazards including fire (both internal and external to the facility), bomb threats, medical emergencies etc.

In the context of health disaster management, the hazard or source of potential harm is of less significance. The key consideration becomes the impact of the disaster on health services and their functionality, and the additional demands placed on the facility. Put simply, at the very time health services need to respond to the enhanced health service demands from an affected community, its ability to do so may be limited by adverse impacts of the event on the health facility and the people and other resources required. This was particularly evident during COVID-19 when health services' capability was reduced by staff absenteeism caused by illness or exposure. Earthquakes may damage or destroy the health facilities at the very time they need to care for those injured in the event. Maintaining health service functionality in the event of business disruption from whatever cause is often documented within business continuity plans, which are addressed in Chapter 6.

However, the aim generally is to not have different plans but rather one consolidated plan that addresses the core principles of response and establishes the systems and structures required to maintain services regardless of the cause of the disruption. This principle is termed the 'all hazards response'.

4. Document the plan's compliance with the agreed objectives then socialise, refine and confirm

Returning to the examples of objectives for a disaster plan above, the next step is to expand the detail of each objective and the processes and arrangements needed to help achieve them and make the plan work. For example, the first objective above '*To maintain an effective command and control structure with clear communication, notification, and escalation processes for identifying and responding to disasters*' can be broken down as follows:

a. Command and control structure.
b. Incident notification pathways – internal and external.
c. Escalation processes.
d. Incident management teams.

This process then informs the list of contents for the plan with the objectives being broken down into their constituent parts and detail on how to achieve them.

Documenting and circulating the plan also requires careful consideration. It is less common now that plans are printed. Electronic documentation has advantages in terms of rapid circulation and availability but poses challenges for version control and validation. The structure of the plan must allow for amendments.

5. Formal endorsement of the plan

As each objective is addressed in the planning process the key stakeholders will be able to provide agreement on content and informal endorsement of each element. Formal endorsement must be completed before the plan can be released and become a functional part of business practice. The governance body identified whilst establishing the context for the plan will have agreed upon the appropriate administrative endorsement process and this must now be undertaken.

Version control for disaster plans is extremely important. Identifying a source of truth for a health service or organisation is critical in ensuring those who activate the plan will be working with up-to-date and relevant documents and processes. This can also be part of the endorsement process and by making this the business of the governance body or committee rather than a bespoke group established solely for the planning process. The plan will benefit from well-understood administrative procedures and oversight.

PLANNING FRAMEWORKS

The purpose of a planning framework is not only to establish a hierarchy of plans but to ensure an understanding of the relevance of each plan and its relationship to the planning framework as a whole. National, jurisdictional, regional and local plans can often be developed in relative isolation and with little reference to the subordinate or superior arrangements and systems. Without good linkage between the vertical levels, a national plan for example may include objectives only achievable with resources controlled at the jurisdictional level. Equally, regional plans and services supporting local/hospital arrangements will fail if the horizontal interdependencies and relationships aren't understood. Efforts can often be wasted or duplicated without first establishing the planning framework and where consolidated arrangements can be developed and shared.

PLANNING

Effort can often be wasted or duplicated without first establishing the planning framework and where consolidated arrangements can be developed and shared.

Visual representation of planning frameworks can be a powerful tool in clarifying these vertical and horizontal relationships as in the example in Figure 14.1 below.

The example in Figure 14.1, the national health disaster plan at the strategic level can only function if the constituent jurisdictions understand their responsibilities in the national context. Equally they must be consulted in its development, if their capability and capacity are to be understood and integrated effectively.

Thereafter the jurisdictions' health disaster plan must outline in tactical terms how they will respond to the activation of national arrangements and to a jurisdictional event. The jurisdictions must consult with their regional health services so the regions can develop sub-plans/guidance to inform the whole-of-jurisdiction approach.

Finally, hospitals will then be able to plan their operational approach including supporting the regional and jurisdictional response, but importantly these operational plans will be consistent, and informed by the work done at the jurisdictional and regional level. For example, workforce health plans can be developed by the jurisdiction to ensure consistent application of Personal Protective Equipment (PPE) across all regions and then operationalised by hospital service units and staff.

If communicated clearly and consistently this approach ensures effort is not duplicated in policy development at the hospital and operational level, where attention and time can then be focused on the formulation of specific hospital clinical and administrative arrangements and plans.

In this way, understanding the interrelationships in the planning framework and knowing that these relationships work both ways, not only in a strictly top-down hierarchical sense, will ensure effort is expended in a more efficient and productive way.

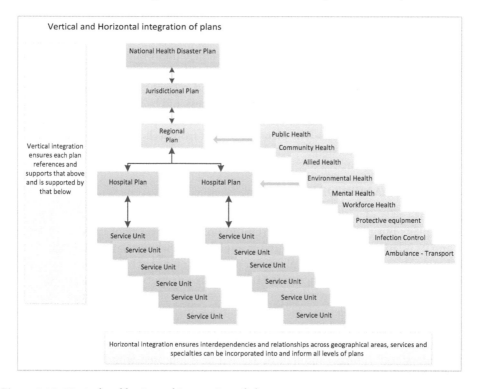

Figure 14.1 Vertical and horizontal integration of plans

STRUCTURE AND CONTENT OF PLANS

There is no magic formula or rigid structure for what should be in a plan. The aim and objectives of the plan though are a good place to start in understanding whether what is written (*the contents*) and how they are laid out (*the structure*) effectively achieve the objectives in a logical and workable order and thereby, hopefully, achieve the aim of providing a framework for operational staff to provide optimal care in a disaster.

It can be difficult sometimes to know from the outset whether all the key elements of the plan have actually been captured in the contents list and it's tempting (because they're usually located at the front of the document) to write the perceived contents list first, then flesh them out in the body of the plan. This can be successful if a clear and comprehensive picture of what is to be achieved and how already exists, but it's not necessarily a hard and fast rule. A perfectly reasonable approach would be to set out the administrative elements of the plan, already outlined when establishing the context, then apply some basic structure around which to frame the operational elements of the plan, for example:

- Authority and governance.
- Scope.
- Risk assessment/Hazard identification.
- Aims and objectives.
- Information/background.
- Method – operational guidance on how you will complete the objectives and achieve the aim.
- Glossary of terms.

Then just start writing! Almost certainly when stakeholders are engaged, discussions progress, and the plan takes shape, new information will come to light about the perceived scope and limitations. The plan may take more than one turn or new direction, but that is normal. The value in this kind of dynamic writing process is that it will confirm or change the understanding of the original intent and thereby result in a more accurate and robust final product.

TRANSLATING PLANS INTO ACTION

1. Embed, socialise and educate

    Confirming or dispelling the perception that plans are nothing, but planning is everything happens at this stage. Adding a plan or policy to an organisation's library, a shared drive, or a document repository, doesn't add value where it's needed. This only validates the common perception that *I can put this on the shelf with the others!*

    The planning process itself can be educative for those who undertake it or participate in it, but now it must be determined who are the education and socialisation audience. Many health services and large organisations will have communications departments to help with this and raise awareness of the disaster plan and its development. Whilst the audience may vary, and many will have an interest, the plan's aim and objectives will determine the people who really need to know about it and who must be reached. The focus ought to be on those who will need to use it, have a role in it, or who will rely upon it during a crisis. Expecting the organisation to passively adopt and embrace a plan which isn't well communicated to the right audience, will fulfil the prophesy of *planning to fail!*

2. Establish the exercise, validation, and review cycle

Belief that there's no value in plans is only true of the paper and plastic gathering dust on a shelf. The true value of a plan can only be measured in its application and validation and whether it lives in the minds of those who one day may have to use it. Therefore, a crucial component of the plan, which must be included in the endorsement process, is the exercise, validation, and review schedule.

Exercising can take many forms, field, functional, tabletop, discussion etc. and will be addressed in another section of this text. All have value and potentially any or all can be included in the exercising and evaluation cycle of the plan. But scale and complexity can often result in long gaps between exercises as they require planning time and release of resources. Smaller compartmentalised exercises focusing on key elements or sections of the plan (e.g., command and control, notification and escalation, ED clinical response etc.), can then be considered together to validate the plan as a whole and can be much easier to achieve.

This brings us full circle, back to the context and governance body. In establishing the authority to plan, the frequency of exercise, validation and review must be considered. This must be documented, mandated and regulated by the appropriate body or committee.

The exercising process must also be managed and communicated carefully. Often executives, senior clinicians and administrators will be required to participate in disaster exercises as they have a role in the disaster plan. But this is frequently by virtue of their position in the organisation, rather than any particular knowledge or experience in disaster response. This can result in avoidance and delays in the exercising cycle, perhaps not through indifference or neglect, but because nobody wants to fail, or to be seen to struggle, and this must be anticipated in planning and communicating exercises. Adherence to the principle of embedding normal business into the heart of our plan ought to reassure those who have a part to play, because all that is being asked of them is to do what they do every day, only with slightly different structures, resources or guidelines to help manage the crisis. Hopefully then the key players will understand that this is an opportunity to exercise the plan, and for the organisation to learn together, in a safe learning environment. It should not be regarded as a test of performance and knowledge but rather a test of the plan. In this way plans can be properly exercised and validated to determine where and how they need to be revised and improved.

It's also natural for the planner to feel protective of their plan; after all it's the product of much hard work. But as has already been stated, the real value of the plan is when it lives in the minds of those who one day may have to use it, not in the words on the paper. Validating the plan and identifying areas for improvement and refinement during an exercise, can only serve to better prepare organisations and their people for the day they'll need to use it for real.

The plan is just that, a plan, not a hard and fast, inflexible program which must be adhered to at all costs. Organisations will have the best chance of operationalising their plan and effectively responding to and recovering from a disaster if they

- Engage with the right people.
- Understand how and when the plan is intended to be used.

- Make it reflect what the people who'll need to use it do every day.
- Exercise the plan regularly.

ACTIVITY

1. Identify the key stakeholders from a community with which you are familiar and consider how their disparate interests may influence the development of a community plan.
2. What criteria would you use to ensure your planning process is effective?

KEY READINGS

Kahan. J. 2015 Future of FEMA – preparedness or politics? *Homeland Security & Emergency Management*, 2015. **12**(1): 1–21

United Nations. (2015, April). Sendaiframework for disaster risk reduction 2015–2030. Paper presented at the Third United Nations World Conference on Disaster Risk Reduction, Sendai, Japan. Retrieved from: http://www.wcdrr.org/uploads/Sendai_Framework_for_Disaster_Risk_Reduction_2015-2030.pdf

Note

1. With acknowledgement to Christie Duce and Deon Canyon, and previous author Mark Cannadine.

15

Preparedness

Benjamin Ryan[1]

INTRODUCTION AND OBJECTIVES

While planning is the critical component of preparedness and often a means of focussing discussion around readiness, there are strategies required to ensure the community and the health system are ready to respond to disasters. Preparedness involves a range of strategies and activities aimed at ensuring a community is resilient and able to respond rapidly to disasters. For example, a casual visitor to drought-affected areas of central Australia may be puzzled to find boats stored at the local authority, yet this is an essential component of the preparedness arrangements built around the identified community risks.

Preparedness considers the design, development and maintenance of systems and structures before, during and after a disaster. This may be complemented by the processes of surveillance, prepositioned personnel and resources and having equipment available to enable flexibility, responsiveness and adaptability. Another key aspect is preparing people, building their resilience and pre-arming them with skills and knowledge to respond appropriately. Additionally, it incorporates identification, training and availability of help through both paid and volunteer organisations and individuals.

The aim of this chapter is to explore the requirements for preparedness. On completion of this chapter, you should be able to:

1. Identify what constitutes resilience of individuals, communities and organisations.
2. Understand how to strengthen and maintain resilience.
3. Identify the strategies required to be ready.
4. Discuss the concept of critical infrastructure protection.

PUBLIC HEALTH SYSTEM

For public health system preparedness there is a need for sound analysis of disaster risks and good linkages with early warning systems. This includes considering the prospect of multiple hazards, contingency planning, stockpiling of equipment and supplies, the development of arrangements for coordination, evacuation and public information and associated training and field exercises [1]. These activities must be integrated with

DOI: 10.4324/9781032626604-19

PREPAREDNESS CYCLE

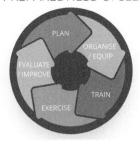

Figure 15.1 Preparedness cycle [2]

legal, financial and institutional capacities across the preparedness cycle, which includes planning, organising, training, exercising and evaluation (Figure 15.1).

Understanding the context of the disaster community and public health system is important for the recovery process. There needs to be an appreciation of the risks faced by communities along with an understanding of the existing strengths and capacity, including past experiences. For example, is there a hospital in a flood zone and how many times has flooding occurred? Also, if there were mitigation strategies in place did they work or is improvement needed.

A tool for understanding the context is the Public Health System Scorecard (Health Scorecard) addendum. This was developed after application of the Disaster Resilience Scorecard for Cities revealed a need for a deep dive into the health sector. The Health Scorecard was developed with input from a group of multisectoral experts, including the United Nations Office for Disaster Risk Reduction (UNDRR) and the World Health Organisation [3]. The Health Scorecard has been used by local and national governments to identify priorities and develop action plans for strengthening resilience. It is freely downloadable and provides a systematic process for emergency managers to better understand the context and priority areas for action.

INFRASTRUCTURE PROTECTION

In the past, key infrastructure items were physically independent but with the growing complexity of modern societies and advances in technology have made the interconnections automated and often invisible. UNDRR defines critical infrastructure as:

> "The physical structures, facilities, networks and other assets which provide services that are essential to the social and economic functioning of a community or society".

The infrastructure dependencies can take various forms (Table 15.1). For example, cybersecurity is now considered a key aspect for infrastructure protection. While technological advances have made systems more efficient it also increases vulnerability.

Over 90% of Australia's critical infrastructure is owned privately [5] and across OECD countries over 80% of people are employed in the private sector [6]. Thus, it is difficult for the government to directly influence its protection but rather attempts to achieve this strategically through partnerships and support arrangements with the private sector. The goal is to enable critical infrastructure owners to understand responsibilities and support mechanisms for securing their assets, apply risk management techniques, conduct regular

Table 15.1 Dependencies [4]

Class	Description	Example
Physical	Operations rely on other infrastructure and supply chains to provide services and/or commodities as an input.	A water facility relies on chemicals and electricity produced by external providers.
Cyber	Operations rely on information and data produced or managed by others.	A fuel terminal relies on IT and communication systems to operate accounting and billing systems to distribute fuel.
Geographic	Operations of multiple systems are collocated and susceptible to similar hazards or a single disruption.	Gas, electric, and water lines sharing a right of way can all be disrupted simultaneously.
Logical	Operations rely on other systems due to economic, policy, or human factors.	Travel restrictions enacted in one state may impact cross-state transportation of goods causing supply chain issues or new regulations on the chemical sector may impact the operations of sectors that use chemicals, such as water and food & agriculture.

reviews and develop and test business continuity plans. This has been recognised at a global level when ARISE was started by UNDRR in 2015 to support the private sector to become a key partner in reducing disaster risk. This group has over 400 members and 29 networks across the world [7].

Critical infrastructure protection describes the range of strategies required to protect critical community infrastructure, including public health. Such strategies can include security, surveillance, workforce availability, transport systems and rapid response. Particular components of society and its infrastructure are essential to the development of resilience and to the sustainability of the community throughout the response and recovery phases. For example, a computer virus that damages the IT system of a bank may have massive consequences throughout the economy as payrolls a frozen.

As a result, many countries have initiated special programs aimed at identifying the critical infrastructure and ensuring there are systems in place to build their resilience and to protect them from malicious or natural assault. For example, in the US the Presidential Policy Directive 21 (PPD-21) of 2013 set up a national program of "Critical Infrastructure Security and Resilience" and this was built on previous directives from 1998. The "European Programme for Critical Infrastructure Protection" is a framework used to identify and improve critical infrastructure.

Critical infrastructure sectors may include the following sectors:

- Banking and finance
- Transportation
- Power and energy

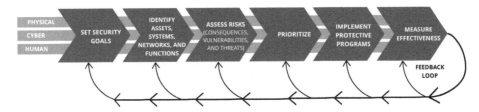

Figure 15.2 Critical infrastructure risk management framework [8]

- Information and communications
- Government agencies, particularly social services and law enforcement
- Healthcare and public health
- Water supplies, including storage
- Wastewater systems
- Agriculture and food supplies
- National monuments and icons.

Critical infrastructure, particularly iconic structures, is increasingly vulnerable to both natural failures (human error, weather, and seismic events) and to external attacks including cyber-attacks. Critical infrastructure protection does require organised approaches and these need to integrate government, private and not-for-profit sectors.

The United States Cybersecurity and Infrastructure Security Agency has developed a framework to identify, analyse, and allocate resources to prepare for threats [8]. The six-step process outlined in Figure 15.2 includes a feedback loop of prioritising vulnerability efforts, addressing physical factors and handling operational aspects that can increase the susceptibility of infrastructure to a disaster. This risk-based preparedness approach can provide a basis for mitigating the consequences of a disaster or other crisis proactively or as they occur.

The response and recovery phases of critical infrastructure protection interlink with business continuity planning particularly for service-orientated industries. For example, the maintenance of health services requires not only the protection of the physical asset but also the protection of the management system and the people required to maintain services. Business continuity requires an advanced understanding of the organisation's objectives and resources. The public sector must balance the drive to maximise return for taxpayers' funds, with the need to have a certain level of capacity in the event of a disaster.

Ultimately, the process of critical infrastructure protection is an interactive process throughout the cycle of getting ready, responding, and recovering. It is not possible to defend every critical asset in every location. Responsibilities need also to be delegated to individual asset owners and their operators.

SURVEILLANCE

Surveillance is an important component of preparedness as it sets up systems and structures that monitor risks within the community and identify when the risk is heightened. Traditionally the term surveillance has been used in the security services to monitor community threats and in the public health domain to monitor the outbreak of diseases.

However, the term surveillance does have a broader plain English meaning encompassing all the activities involved in the monitoring of risks and impacts.

Surveillance also occurs throughout the disaster management cycle. It involves proactive risk surveillance as would occur in any community and is informed not only by the history of what has occurred previously but also by the monitoring of events around the world. It also involves monitoring the impact of disasters and seeking to identify the potential adverse consequences including those that may emerge after the event. For example, it involves systems to monitor the possibility of infectious disease outbreaks and to identify the long-term health consequences including mental health consequences.

Australia has established the Trusted Information Sharing Network which provides access to surveillance information for a range of key community infrastructure operators. There is also a range of other surveillance tools available and freely accessible, which allow the sharing of information. These include the Pacific Disaster Center's DiasterAWARE° and Centre for Research on the Epidemiology of Disasters.

There is considerable experience in surveillance around infectious diseases. Compulsory reporting of certain diseases allows monitoring of the trends and patterns and supports early recognition and intervention. The formal reporting systems however tend to be slow, and attempts have been made to develop more timely surveillance through monitoring of emergency health service data or crowd-sourcing. For example, *Outbreaks Near Me*[2] uses public data to map outbreaks for COVID-19 and flu. This was developed by Boston Children's Hospital, Harvard Medical School, and volunteers from across the technology industry. This citizen-led approach (non-government) to outbreak monitoring is increasing and this has been applied to other public health issues such as air quality and will likely continue to evolve.

PREPARING THE PEOPLE

Building individual disaster management capability is a critical component of disaster preparedness. Most large organisations have recognised the risks of internal disasters and have in place individuals responsible for policy advice, planning, training and coordination. Thus, large hospitals or local governments or private sector industries will have one or more emergency management specialists whose responsibility is to facilitate training of key personnel, advising on policy, leading planning activities and ensuring systems are in place to ensure coordination in the event of a disaster.

Broader capability development is based on the training of other individuals whose normal responsibilities may extend to disaster management. This may include individuals whose normal role will be useful in a disaster (e.g., paramedics) along with individuals whose normal role may not be essential but who may be called upon to play a critical support role in a disaster. Thus, in health services, for example, part of the breadth of training of clinicians may include the extension of their clinical role to practice in resource-constrained environment both during major events and in rural or international environments. Equally others may need to be trained to take up roles in a coordination centre. The challenge for major organisations is to meet these development needs within the constraints of a challenging economic environment.

We address the educational needs in more detail in Chapter 28, but it is worth considering how any organisation or community would ensure sufficient personnel are trained to take up roles in a disaster. Community engagement, as discussed in more detail in Chapter

8, will engage with all sectors of society about disaster risks and can help inform and allow communication to an audience that may not be accessible to government officials. Depending on the community this could include leaders from schools, sporting clubs or faith-based organisations. This can be complemented by exercises to test preparedness arrangements and contribute to the educational needs of the individual, organisation, and community.

PREPARING THE RESOURCES

Equipment required in disaster may need to be prepositioned. Such equipment needs to be evaluated for its appropriateness in a disaster and positioned either on a standing arrangement or during a time of heightened risk. For example, in the event of an impending cyclone, flood boats or helicopters may be repositioned closer to the impact site. The goal is to ensure resources are ready to respond but at the same time may be safe from damage.

Consumables will be necessary to ensure business continuity and responsiveness. Often consumables and equipment will be **stockpiled** so that they are ready and protected. The nature, location and protection of such stockpiles is a necessary component of the planning process. In medical terms, the first line of defence is the "*imbedded stockpile*" which is the consumables and equipment currently located within health services. For example, the masks and drugs are in every health centre and hospital as well as in storage facilities and distribution centres. This stockpile is the essential component of the first response and needs to be identified and protected so that it can facilitate the response phase.

Preparedness focuses on preparing equipment and procedures for use when a disaster occurs. Preparedness measures can take many forms including the construction of shelters, implementation of an emergency communication system, installation of warning devices, creation of backup life-line services (e.g., power, water, sewage), and rehearsing evacuation plans. Planning for all different types of events and all magnitudes is of utmost importance, so that when a disaster does occur responders know exactly what their assignments are.

For evacuation, a disaster supplies kit may be prepared and for sheltering purposes a stockpile of supplies may be created. The preparation of a survival kit such as a "72-hour kit" is often advocated by authorities. These kits may include food, medicine, flashlights, candles, and money. Also, putting valuable items in safe area is also recommended.

PREPARING COUNTERMEASURES

There are a range of countermeasures that need to be considered during preparedness. This will depend on the type of disaster, crisis, and the context. From a hospital perspective, the World Health Organisation has developed a "*Rapid hospital readiness checklist*", to identify gaps and major areas that require investment and action [9]. For a disease outbreak, examples of countermeasures could include:

- Quarantine and containment
- Infection control
- Surveillance and contact tracing
- Social separation
- International boundaries, duties & foreign nationals.

The **state should meet standards** relating to surveillance and contact tracing. The state should demonstrate an important need to know, take decisions openly, consult with the relevant communities and use data only for legitimate purposes. Surveillance without names is far less effective but, in some countries, may be required. Depending on the novel nature of the outbreak, physicians and hospitals may have a moral obligation to report cases to ensure the most effective public health interventions. In this instance, the benefits and burdens of privacy invasions are equitably distributed. In many countries these obligations may be enforced by law.

Isolation is the separation, for the period of communicability, of known infected persons. Isolation takes place under conditions to prevent or limit the spread of infection. Quarantine is the restriction of activities of healthy persons who have been exposed to a communicable disease to prevent disease transmission during the incubation period if infection should occur.

Public health officials usually have police powers to enforce public health regulations. However, they generally prefer voluntary measures and only resort to mandatory measures as a last resort. Voluntary measures promote better cooperation and improved results of contact tracing. Mandatory enforcement will usually come at a higher cost, divert resources, cause confrontation, and undermine public cooperation.

Support should be offered quickly to those who are directly affected and vulnerable. This will facilitate a smoother transition into the recovery process. Information on impacts will be limited at first, meaning that it will be difficult to assist the diverse needs of the community. In addition, needs will evolve and change rapidly as the recovery phase unfolds. The key is to initiate quick actions to address immediate needs.

Conflicting knowledge values and priorities in a community will usually create tensions. Emergencies create a stressful environment where grief and blame also affect those involved. The achievement of recovery is therefore a long and challenging journey. The journey will be assisted by the acknowledgement of community knowledge and values, especially where these contrast with the assumptions of the outside community.

We need to protect the needs and interests of those who are identified as sick or exposed. This may require consultation with the representatives of the communities most at risk to ensure mental and physical welfare in the short and long-term.

Finally, a preparedness plan establishes arrangements in advance to enable timely, effective, and appropriate responses to specific potential hazardous events or emerging disaster situation [1]. Ultimately, the actions need to be focussed on enabling a seamless transition from response to recovery.

ACTIVITIES

1. Identify three critical infrastructures in your community.
2. Describe in broad terms how you would ensure that critical infrastructures are identified and protected.
3. What strategies would you consider essential in preparing an organisation/community for disaster response?
4. How would you develop an educational strategy for an organisation/community with which you are familiar so that it would be better placed to respond to a disaster?

KEY READINGS

Schlegelmilch, J., M. Stripling, T. Chandler, S. Marx, & P.B. Gu, Establishing a foundation for performance measurement for local public health preparedness. *Disaster Medicine and Public Health Preparedness*, 2022. **16**(3), 1208–1214.

World Health Organisation Rapid hospital readiness checklist https://www.who.int/publications/i/item/WHO-2019-nCoV-hospital-readiness-checklist-2020.1

Disaster Resilience Scorecard for Cities - Public Health System Resilience Addendum https://mcr2030.undrr.org/public-health-system-resilience-scorecard

Notes

1. With acknowledgement to previous authors Julian Meagher and Rosemary Steinhardt
2. https://outbreaksnearme.org

References

1. UNDRR. *Preparedness*. 2022; Available from: https://www.undrr.org/terminology/preparedness.
2. FEMA. *Developing and maintaining emergency operations plans*. 2010; Available from: https://www.ready.gov/sites/default/files/2019-06/comprehensive_preparedness_guide_developing_and_maintaining_emergency_operations_plans.pdf.
3. UNDRR. *Disaster resilience scorecard for cities - public health system resilience addendum*. 2020; Available from: https://mcr2030.undrr.org/public-health-system-resilience-scorecard.
4. Cybersecurity & Infrastructure Security Agency. *What are dependencies*. n.d.; Available from: https://www.cisa.gov/what-are-dependencies.
5. Feakin, T. *Building critical infrastructure resilience in the Asia–Pacific*. 2015; Available from: https://www.aspistrategist.org.au/building-critical-infrastructure-resilience-in-the-asia%C2%AD-pacific/.
6. OECD. *Government at a glance 2021*. 2021; Available from: https://doi.org/10.1787/1c258f55-en.
7. UNDRR. *About ARISE*. 2022; Available from: https://www.ariseglobalnetwork.org/explore/about.
8. Cybersecurity & Infrastructure Security Agency, *A guide to critical infrastructure security and resilience*. 2019: Cybersecurity and Infrastructure Security Agency.
9. World Health Organisation. *Rapid hospital readiness checklist: Interim Guidance*. 2020; Available from: https://www.who.int/publications/i/item/WHO-2019-nCoV-hospital-readiness-checklist-2020.1.

Part 5
Incident management and response

16

Principles of incident management

Gerry Fitzgerald, Jonathan Abrahams, and Stacey Pizzino

INTRODUCTION & OBJECTIVES

Incident management is a generic term that applies to the management of any potential and actual event. Effective incident management can help contain events and prevent them from becoming more complicated. Conversely, ineffective incident management can contribute to the escalation of the event and consequential effects that could have been avoided. In effect, disorganised management may cost lives and other assets. A comprehensive, predetermined and systematic approach based on core principles, organisational structures and agreed and tested procedures form the basis of incident management systems (IMSs) which are necessary to reduce confusion and manage events effectively. Organisation of the response, prevention of primary and secondary consequences, effective preparedness and transitioning to recovery are also key considerations in IMSs.

On a day-to-day basis, much of the focus of emergency response agencies is on the management of incidents that are relatively limited in scope and time. The systems and structures that underpin effective incident management are thus familiar to these agencies. The same principles used to manage a transport crash or localised disease outbreak can be used to support scaling up of arrangements to manage more complex events that cover a wide geographic area or are more prolonged disasters such as cyclones, earthquakes, epidemics or conflicts.

The management of response to disasters with multiple locations/loci should rely on incident management principles and practices to surge the response capability to meet the demands of an event.

Additionally, efficient and effective management depends on careful and detailed assessments of the event and its immediate and consequential effects/impact. The initial assessment must be carried out by an experienced, appropriately qualified practitioner and promptly relayed to all other agencies, including hospitals and trauma centres who will be involved in the management of the event.

Training and exercise scenarios often assume that full knowledge of the extent and effects/impact of the event will be immediately available. The reality is that information will be incomplete due to the complexity, confusion and chaos that may accompany the event. Bystanders and the media can be critical of this initial confusion. In reality, the full

DOI: 10.4324/9781032626604-21

extent of the impact of events such as a cyclone or epidemic/pandemic may not be known for months.

The aim of this chapter is to explore standardised approaches to incident management including the assessment and evaluation of an incident, and the core principles, systems and organisational structures that underpin the initial response. Chapter 17 will focus on the management of the scene and the role of emergency responders.

On completion of this chapter, you should:

1. Have an in-depth understanding of the factors influencing the type and scale of disasters, including the nature and magnitude of their impacts.
2. Be able to take a structured approach to incident assessment and reporting which will help define and initiate an appropriate response.
3. Have an in-depth understanding of the core principles of incident management and their application to disaster management.
4. Have an in-depth understanding of the importance of timely incident assessment and evaluation.

INCIDENT ASSESSMENT AND EVALUATION

Assessment and evaluation of the incident must consider the physical and social context within which the event occurs and the nature and scale of the event.

When responding in a known environment, the context will be familiar to those tasked with the initial assessment and should derive from the pre-planning and preparatory actions. However, when the response is in an unknown environment/community, responders may not immediately understand the context, therefore its identification is a critical part of the initial assessment. In these circumstances, responders should undertake the necessary preparations to "enter the community". This must include pre-deployment briefing information that allows them to understand the country or community context and dynamics and a detailed understanding of the event and its immediate impact. Responders will need to understand their role in incident management.

Understanding the community and its characteristics

- Early engagement with the local government or relevant Consulate, Foreign/Home Affairs to identify the local **policy and legislative environment** including common-law and other subsidiary regulations. It is also critical to identify the policy direction of the community as articulated by public statements as well as the standards expected.
- Identify the **planning environment** and the hierarchy of plans that are in place. This includes local and national plans, as well as international plans and protocols for international or cross-border assistance (see Chapter 14 – Planning).
- Understanding the **organisational environment** requires a knowledge of the systems and structures established by the community and country to plan and prepare for disasters and to support response. These include the consultative and coordination arrangements and the roles and responsibilities, resources and capabilities of the various organisations both formal and informal, i.e., community groups and volunteer organisations.
- Disasters are a social phenomenon and a critical aspect of the context evaluation is to understand the **nature and structure of the society** impacted by the disaster by identifying:

- What is the level of social cohesion and how well does the community work together?
- How stable is the community, will they accept instruction and direction from community leaders and/or outsiders?
- How does both formal and informal communication occur?
- What are the predominant attitudes and beliefs informed by culture and faith and how will these influence the behaviour and receptiveness of people to assistance and take personal or community actions?
- What is the level of security in the community?
- What are the other potential hazardous events, risks and priorities in the community, for example civil unrest, water supply, nutrition, poverty, employment, that may affect the response?
- Disaster management requires an understanding of the **political environment.** Many would say that a disaster is not the time to consider politics. However, local, national and even global politics are key to governance, leadership, trust, and confidence and to the management of the event. There are always political considerations, not necessarily party politics, but rather the access to decision-makers, resources and services, the interplay of powerful people and groups, religious and cultural beliefs and the clash of ideas and inequities.
  - Who are the key stakeholders and what interests do they have?
  - What authority will they exert?
  - How can they support the IMSs and the respective response and recovery strategies?

The key influencers are not necessarily those with formal authority, they could be religious or community leaders. Some seek political advancement through a high-profile role in the disaster response while others may lose political support because of their absence or poor handling of the leadership role. Policies and procedures need to be effectively administered to prevent actors seeking to derive personal benefit from donations or from diverting resources away from assessed priorities. On the other hand, adversaries and antagonists can become allies and assets in times of disaster.

The **physical environment** before the event and because of the event should be identified. Event-related and other risks (including disease) for the responders and affected communities along with current weather/forecasts and security.

CAN ADVERSARIES BE ALLIES IN TIMES OF NATURAL DISASTER?

Following the 1995 Sakhalin Island earthquake, Russia denied Japanese rescuers entry to the impacted region. It was thought the Russian Government was concerned Japan would use its access to take control of the island.

Both Humanitarian Needs Overviews and Humanitarian Response Plans are based on different forms of analysis of context, needs and resources that ultimately serve to determine priorities for actions at national or sub-national levels. They often begin with summaries of the "crisis context" which may include histories, trends and forecasts with reference to:

- Political, socio-cultural, demographic and economic profiles
- Security environment
- Infrastructure and technology
- Environmental profiles

It is also critical to understand the **operational environment** and the capability of the disaster-affected community. This includes:

- The organisations involved and their capacity.
- The available human resources including their number, skills and capability.
- The scope and range of local consumables including clinical (drugs and Personal Protective Equipment, PPE), fuel, food and water, power and supply chains.
- Facilities may be disrupted by the event, buildings, or access (roads) damaged and destroyed. Understanding what is available, what can be restored to functional use and what is required to achieve this is an important first step in the assessment.
- The available equipment necessary for recovery and equipment that can be restored to functionality. This may include highly specialised equipment (e.g., hospital ventilators) or equipment necessary for restoring functionality (e.g., generators).
- Finally, information sources are a critical component of the operational evaluation.

CASE STUDY 16.1 – YEMEN

The 2021 Humanitarian Response Plan for Yemen describes a range of factors related to the sources of the conflict, the vulnerabilities and assets of the population and the effect that these factors have on the provision of assistance. The analyses highlighted the devastating impact of years of conflict on health, economy, infrastructure, displacement, food insecurity and many other aspects of society. The analysis made reference to:

- Intensification of the conflict at the beginning of 2021.
- Difficulties in achieving a political settlement.
- High levels of internal displacement.
- Shrinkage of the national economy including people living below the poverty line and loss of revenue.
- Food insecurity, looming famine and record rates of malnutrition.
- Devastation on public services and infrastructure including water and sanitation services, road access and telecommunications.
- Impact of flash flooding following abnormally intense cyclone activity.
- Outbreaks of cholera, dengue, diphtheria, malaria, vaccine-derived poliovirus and COVID-19.
- The impact of COVID-19 on health and other services.
- Continued reversal of development gains in the poorest country in the Middle East.

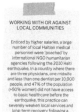

WORKING WITH OR AGAINST LOCAL COMMUNITIES

Enticed by higher salaries, a large number of local Haitian medical personnel were 'poached' by international NGO humanitarian agencies following the 2010 Haiti earthquake. In a country where there are three physicians, one midwife and less than one dentist per 10,000 people, and 47% of the population (>50% women) did not have access to basic healthcare before the earthquake, this practice can severely weaken local services and long-term recovery following a major disaster.

Any external assistance should be provided on the premise there are local capabilities that are providing the initial response and any external assistance will need to support this response. Failure to recognise the local resources is damaging to the speed and effectiveness of the response and to community recovery. The use of local resources not only ensures they are, and remain relevant to the local community, but also aids with health, social and economic recovery.

Understanding the incident

It must be emphasised that there will be limitations on the initial assessment. The full extent of the impact will not be known, often for years afterwards. This standardised approach can be adjusted to any incident including disease outbreaks. It is important initially to identify with the available resources across all agencies and all sectors what is known, but also to identify the limits of knowledge.

There are important principles behind this analysis and the reporting of the information including:

- **Objectivity** to ensure any information is restricted to what is known and does not speculate about things that are not known and recognises the unknowns for which information needs to be collected, analysed and interpreted.
- **Data informed** to ensure that where reasonable, deductions can be sustained.
- **Respectful** to the privacy and rights of individuals including their religious and cultural beliefs and to the performance of other responders.
- **Brevity** which helps with rapid communication leading to timely action.
- **Relevant and focussed** on what is needed to be known by those to whom the communication extends.

Initial evaluation/assessment of the incident needs to take a structured, systematic approach. The exact structure may be locally determined and may vary with each event. A structured approach may include the following elements:

- The nature of the incident; what caused it and its extent.
- The location and physical extent of the incident.
- Hazards/risks – known and potential.
- What are the access issues?
- The number of people directly affected in the incident (if known) and the population at risk of being affected.
- What has been the impact of the incident on the community, the services, the people and the society and the businesses and the economy?
- How severe are the illnesses or injuries caused?
- What resources are available to deal with the incident across multiple agencies and sectors of society and what are the evident gaps?
- What are the current levels of activity of responding agencies?
- Are there any safety or security concerns for those responding?

The outcome of the initial assessment is to determine what is required to be done and how that should be achieved. Objectives must be fashioned for each strategy along with issues of concern and the risks of the chosen strategies. Objectives will be reviewed daily and amended as necessary as more information becomes known about the event.

FOCUS ON HEALTH EVALUATION
Healthcare sector evaluation in a disaster focuses on identifying the number of people affected, type and severity of injuries, and the location of people who may require medical aid; including those who may be in need of public healthcare.

CASE STUDY 16.2 THE COVID-19 – PANDEMIC

The evolution of COVID-19 shows how information from many sources were put together to present an ever-increasing picture of all aspects of the disease and risk management including identifying and describing the pathogen, modes of transmission, measures to prevent spread, and abilities to provide diagnosis, vaccination and treatment. Several key milestones were passed, reflecting the dynamic nature of the virus, devastating global health and other effects, the adaptation of governance and scientific research mechanisms and the development, testing and use of capabilities aimed at managing the disease, its consequences and an equitable distribution of resources. Actions taken by WHO's response to COVID-19 for the period from 31 December 2020 to 10 April 2021, including the rapid activation of its Incident Management Support Team on 1 January 2021 are described in the Listings of WHO's response to COVID-19.

Who should do the assessment?

It is important that the evaluators with high levels of expertise, experience and training in the required process are used to assess an incident. Many countries now maintain capabilities for the assessment of damages, impacts and needs which are largely determined by the domestic risk profiles, requirements and resources.

At international level

The United Nations Disaster Assessment and Coordination (UNDAC) teams can deploy quickly at the request of the disaster-affected country, working cooperatively alongside the local authorities who are usually the national disaster management organisation or their equivalent. Similarly larger international aid agencies including NGOs will also maintain a disaster assessment capability [1].

Formalised approaches are used to undertake a rapid initial assessment in accordance with the UNDAC format and under the leadership of the United Nations. It provides information about the needs, possible strategies and resource requirements and aims to identify:

- The impact/effects and consequences that a disaster has on a society and its infrastructure, and the ability of that society to cope.
- The sectors of the population most in need of assistance.
- The level of response by the affected country, its internal capacity to cope with the situation and the level of response from the international community.
- The most urgent relief needs and potential methods of organising them most effectively.
- Coordination mechanisms.
- Significant political, cultural and logistical constraints.

The UNDAC system is designed to support national governments, with assessment and coordination during the first phase of a sudden-onset emergency. The UNDAC system comprises four components:

- Staff: Experienced emergency managers made available for UNDAC missions by their respective governments or organisations.
- Methodology: Pre-defined methods for establishing coordination structures and for organising and facilitating assessments and information management.
- Procedures: Proven systems to mobilise and deploy aUNDAC team.
- Equipment: Personal and mission equipment for UNDAC teams to be self-sufficient while on deployment [1].

The United Nations has also developed a formalised approach to needs assessment via the Post-Disaster Needs Assessment. This is an internationally accepted methodology for determining the physical damage, economic losses, and costs of recovery after disasters. The Damage and Loss Assessment that informs the needs assessment is quantitative in nature and is used to value damages and subsequent economic losses. It provides a standardised tool for the valuation of disaster damage.

Increasingly, information, communications and other technology are used to aid assessment. Satellite imagery has been shown to be an efficient and useful resource for informing damage assessments for decision-makers [2]. Drones are being used to make detailed analyses [3], and crowd-sourced information is increasingly used with analysis of both images and text to inform and support activities such as epidemic intelligence and community-based disease surveillance via mobile phones.

Reporting

There are personal, positional and professional responsibilities not only to report on what has occurred but also to evaluate the effectiveness of that response. Reporting helps with incident management at all levels and informs future planning and preparedness. Such reports may be broadly categorised into progress report and post-hoc evaluations (final reports).

- **Progress reports** (also known as situation reports or SITREPS) provide an assessment of what is currently known about the event, its impact and the response activities. There is no agreed formula about such reports except within particular agencies.
- **Final reports** are compiled after the event and seek to address the nature and scope of the event and the lessons to be learnt from the disaster.

Reports will rely on the availability of reliable information. Therefore, an efficient data management system that facilitates reliable data collection, analysis, interpretation, communication and storage will be required. Information management is a key function in an IMS and the role is usually managed by specialists whose primary role is to provide accurate, timely and useful information to those responsible for manag-

Disaster reports provide an opportunity to learn lessons from the response and identify any changes needed in planning and preparedness and how the response and recovery can be improved upon. Disaster reports must never be used to apportion blame.

ing the response. Variable data causes confusion and a loss of community and political confidence. Inefficient systems of data management will impose on the direction, priorities and effectiveness of operational responses and impose additional burden on both responders and victims.

INCIDENT MANAGEMENT SYSTEMS

The aim of IMSs is to provide organised and systematic approaches to the management of an incident. Originating from military command systems, these systems are frequently adopted by emergency services (Police, Fire and Ambulance) and other organisations that respond to emergencies (e.g., health authorities and hospitals) to organise day-to-day operations but can be scaled up during a major event. They can be applied to any emergency/disaster situation and provide a common/consistent standardised, flexible and economical approach at all levels of the system.

While national systems vary in detail, they usually share core functions including

- shared situational awareness,
- flexibility,
- management by objectives,
- unity of command,
- functional modular management and
- span of control.

They also share a modular approach to management in which functions are grouped by common purpose into core areas.

Examples of some IMS used in many countries are outlined in Table 16.1. Figure 16.1 shows, as an example, the structure an IMS could take during a major disaster.

The core functions of the local IMS used in countries or localities are locally defined but in broad terms:

1. **Planning** responds to the initial assessment of the incident and its consequences for the community, environment and business operations. The planning cell will use the intelligence acquired to plan for different scenarios and planning horizons.
2. **Operations** address the immediate issues and coordinate the day-to-day response activities.
3. **Logistics** manage legal and financial matters, human and material resources including rostering, accommodation, telecommunications, transport and supplies.
4. **Public Information (communication)** is responsible for identifying stakeholders, managing, and monitoring the media, development and issuing of key messages and official warnings, media conferences, site tours and any official visits.
5. **Investigation** is responsible for seeking specific information related to the cause and nature of the event.
6. **Intelligence** is responsible for gathering, analysing and modelling information about the current situation and making forecasts about future requirements. The importance of obtaining local knowledge should not be underestimated. Long-term locals particularly can provide a wealth of knowledge about their local area and community. Additional functional areas may include legal, finance, welfare etc.

The key advantages of IMS are that they clearly identify those with authority and delegate authority where appropriate. They ensure relationships between individuals and

Table 16.1 Examples of IMS

Name	Country of origin
National Incident Management System (NIMS)	United States
Australian Inter-Service Incident Management System (AIIMS)	Australia
Coordinated Incident Management System (CIMS)	New Zealand
Joint Emergency Services Interoperability Programme (JESIP)	United Kingdom

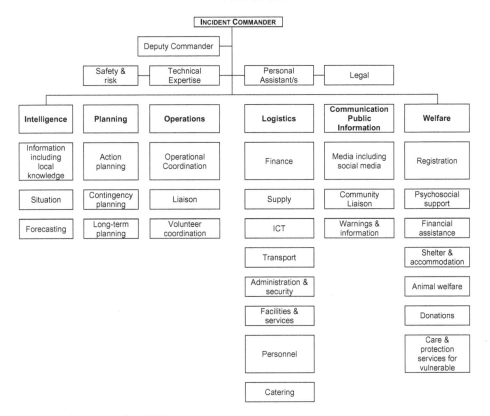

Figure 16.1 Structure of an IMS

organisations, provide a disciplined and structured approach to management which reduces uncertainty.

However, there are limitations. Organisations that are not emergency services or regularly involved in emergency response are often not familiar with these approaches. Public health organisations have their own approaches to the management of incidents. These have the potential to conflict with those familiar to emergency services and vice versa. Increasingly public health organisations are applying IMSs with adjustments to take account of the emphasis on technical and clinical management of the health aspects of the incident. Incidents without scenes are more challenging and do not readily fit into the highly structured IMS. Other forms of IMSs may be useful throughout the continuum of disaster management and suit strategic and tactical levels of management for events with increased complexity due to scale, impact, timeframe and other factors.

An alternate view of IMSs is to consider the level of management. For example, in the United Kingdom this is described as the "Gold Silver Bronze" levels but more commonly known as Strategic, Tactical and Operational. Figure 16.2 below summarises the focus of these three levels.

However, while structured approaches are important, the critical success factor is having a skilled leadership team that is well-connected and familiar with each other.

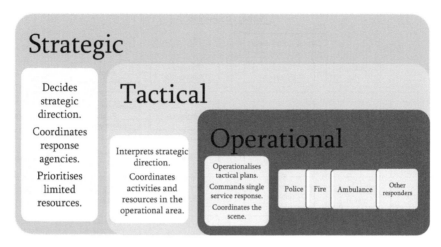

Figure 16.2 Strategic, tactical, and operational levels of response

INCIDENT MANAGEMENT STRUCTURES

Throughout the duration of a major incident, there will be a need to establish, or scale-up centres at which the incident may be coordinated and controlled. These will have various titles depending on the jurisdiction, for example Major Incident Rooms, Disaster Coordination Centre, Emergency Operations Centre. Emergency Coordination Centre etc. An incident may have several coordination centres depending on the size, scale and complexity of the disaster, the level of response required and the jurisdictional boundaries. There will be a coordination centre in the field, at the local hospital, health services and health department.

Countries with well-developed systems will have pre-determined coordination centres which are fully equipped and can be scaled up as needed. However, while a pre-designated facility will be the preferred option, a coordination centre may be a community hall or even a virtual location or house. It is important however that the centre has the necessary equipment, facilities and appropriately trained and skilled staff with the authority to commit resources and make decisions on behalf of their respective agency. In events in which public health is involved, Public Health Emergency Operations Centres (PHEOC) will be established at various levels including within the WHO. The PHEOC is a physical location for the coordination of information and resources to support incident management activities. Timely implementation of PHEOCs provides a mechanism for ensuring leadership, effective decision-making and resource utilisation.

IMPEDIMENTS TO EFFECTIVE IMSS

The increasing interconnectedness of modern societal support systems challenges those responsible for incident management, particularly during complex disasters. Furthermore, the people involved in disaster management bring a range of human factors that can affect system performance. Figure 16.3 outlines the human factors that influence multi-agency incident management.

The performance of the incident management team can be seen as a complex interplay between the human and technical aspects of the IMS, the nature of the event and the

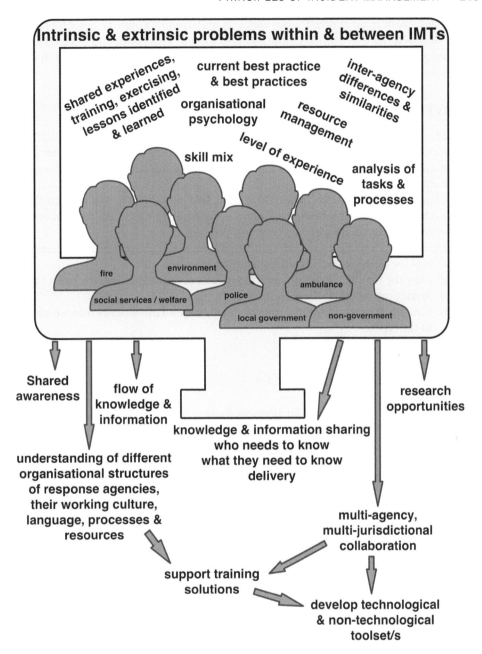

Figure 16.3 Human elements in multi-agency incident management

resilience of the team. It can be evaluated against a framework of recovery time, resource status and interactions [4]. Increased coherence in the IMS operations requires analysis of each component, and implementation of effective strategies to ensure there is a resilient connection between each component [5].

Novel conceptualisations of the challenge are required. Nowell and Steelman [6] explored the challenges of complex disasters in the US and identified novel concepts of *hybrid governance* and *network governance* as underpinning approaches. Hybrid governance they described as unified command systems and area command systems and networking governance builds on existing strategies by including joint information centres, agency liaison and multiagency coordinating groups.

ACTIVITIES

1. Identify a recent event in a community with which you are familiar. Draft a preliminary report on the event which describes the context and environment and the nature and impact of the event and identifies how the environment influenced the nature and extent of the impact.
2. Identify a national, sub-national or local IMS with which you are familiar and undertake an analysis of its strengths and weaknesses and make recommendations in regard to its utility for a recent major incident.
3. Examine the reports of recent inquiries or Royal Commissions into disasters. Discuss at the strategic, tactical and operational levels:
   a. How the rapidly changing event, the structure of the IMS and the role of the lead agency impacted on the response?
   b. Can you identify additional improvements beyond those of the recommendations of the reports?

KEY READINGS AND RESOURCES

1. FEMA National Incident Management System accessible at https://www.fema.gov/emergency-managers/nims
2. Power, N. Extreme teams: Toward a greater understanding of multiagency teamwork during major emergencies and disasters. *American Psychologist*, 2018. **73**(4): p. 478–490. doi: 10.1037/amp0000248. PMID: 29792462.
3. House, A., N. Power, and L. Alison, A systematic review of the potential hurdles of interoperability to the emergency services in major incidents: Recommendations for solutions and alternatives. *Cognition, Technology & Work*, 2014. **16**(3): p. 319–335.
4. Jensen, J., and W.L. Waugh, Jr. The United States' experience with the incident command system: What we think we know and what we need to know more about. *Journal of Contingencies and Crisis Management*, 2014. **22**(1): p. 5–17.
5. McAleavy, T., Perceiving the effects of scale on command and control: A conceptual metaphor approach. *Journal of Emergency Management*, 2020. **18**(2): p. 91–104. doi: 10.5055/jem.2020.0453. PMID: 32181865.
6. Hardy, K., and L.K. Comfort, Dynamic decision processes in complex, high-risk operations: The Yarnell Hill Fire. *Safety Science*, 2015. **71**: p. 39–47
7. Jensen, J. and S. Thompson, The Incident Command System: A literature review. *Disasters*, 2015. **40**(1): p. 158–182.
8. Rimstad, R. and G.S. Braut, Literature review on medical incident command. *Prehospital and Disaster Medicine*, 2015. **30**(2): p. 205–215.

References

1. United Nations Office for the Coordination of Humanitarian Affairs. *UN Disaster Assessment and Coordination (UNDAC)*. n.d.; Available from: https://www.unocha.org/our-work/coordination/un-disaster-assessment-and-coordination-undac.
2. Liou, Y.-A., S.K. Kar, and L. Chang, Use of high-resolution FORMOSAT-2 satellite images for post-earthquake disaster assessment: A study following the 12 May 2008 Wenchuan Earthquake. *International Journal of Remote Sensing*, 2010. **31**(13): p. 3355–3368.
3. Griffin, G.F., The use of unmanned aerial vehicles for disaster management. *Geomatica*, 2014. **68**(4): p. 265–281.
4. Son, C., et al., Modeling an incident management team as a joint cognitive system. *Journal of Loss Prevention in the Process Industries*, 2018. **56**: p. 231–241.
5. Hardy, K. and L.K. Comfort, Dynamic decision processes in complex, high-risk operations: The Yarnell Hill Fire, June 30, 2013. *Safety Science*, 2015. **71**: p. 39–47.
6. Nowell, B. and T. Steelman, Beyond ICS: How should we govern complex disasters in the United States? *Journal of Homeland Security and Emergency Management*, 2019. **16**(2): p. 20180067. https://doi.org/10.1515/jhsem-2018-0067

17

Incident management practice

Marie Fredriksen, Gerry FitzGerald, and Colin Myers[1]

INTRODUCTION AND OBJECTIVES

Popular public imagery of the response phase of disasters has traditionally focussed on dramatic incidents such as cyclones, earthquakes, or train crashes. Such events are the bedrock of emergency response agencies. But if COVID-19 has taught us anything, it is that the response phase may be prolonged and evolutionary in nature. It will depend on the type and scale of the emergency, and the response required to manage the event. Consider the difference in response to a sudden onset earthquake vs. a prolonged and evolving drought or pandemic.

Nevertheless, the principles of the response to the disaster remain the same regardless of the event. As discussed in Chapter 16, best practice disaster response relies on a functional Incident Management System (IMS) that provides an organised and systematic framework for the management of the event. It also relies on the adoption of key principles that underpin the local arrangements in place.

For events with a clearly defined scene (e.g., a train crash) effective scene management and dispersal of the injured is critical to the optimal outcomes for those involved. It is vital that such processes are familiar to the emergency response agencies and therefore they should be based on routine operational approaches. Thus, disaster incident management should adopt the same principles as routine incident management, but with capacity to surge response capability to meet the needs of each individual event.

The aim of this chapter is to examine incident management and particularly scene management, so as to identify the core principles that underpin disaster response and the issues that need to be understood and prepared for. On completion of this chapter, you should have:

- An extensive understanding of the phases of a disaster response.
- An extensive understanding of the effective management of healthcare at the scene.
- An extensive understanding of the principles and practices that ensure effective scene management.
- The ability to identify obstacles to an effective disaster response and incident management and strategies to overcome these obstacles.

DOI: 10.4324/9781032626604-22

RESPONSE PHASES

We often conceptualise the response phase as starting with the event and for unexpected events this is likely to be so. However, for other events such as riverine flooding or cyclones there is time to prepare. For other events, it is only when the scale of the event has become clear that disaster response arrangements are put in place. For pandemics this may vary according to the stage of the pandemic and the local context. Every country has their own terms for these phases, and it is important to understand that not all disasters will follow all of the phases of activation.

- *Alert and alarm* is that time when it is anticipated a major event may occur either as a result of weather warnings or intelligence that may identify a potential threat exists. Public response is focussed on protection or evacuation.
- *Stand up* describes that period when the event is imminent, and the public messaging is focussed on taking shelter. Major services such as health services may use this period to preposition resources close to the potential impact site but out of harm's way. Or to take actions to prepare for any surge in demand.
- *Response* describes the period during which emergency and other response agencies focus on rescue and recovery of affected individuals and on the immediate recovery of vital infrastructure. This phase includes processes for defining the event and for notification of relevant authorities and initiation of systems and structures. It also involves the primary incident response from the emergency services such as Ambulance, Fire, and Police. Finally, it requires fast, automatic escalation of apparently trained personnel.

   In support of this response, coordination and communication centres will be established along with control and command structures. The authorities to act and the roles and responsibilities of different agencies will be determined including the identification of the lead agency if required.
- *Sustain* phase describes the period during which the response must be maintained, and the affected community provided with the necessities of life to prevent further injury.

The capacity to respond in any of these phases is dependent on the community and its infrastructure and on the nature and scale of the event.

Each country will have different triggers for activating their response arrangement and describing the scale of the event. For example, the United States of America have levels 5 – 1 with 5 being the least complex and the easiest to stabilise and/or mitigate while level 1 is the most complex requiring full-scale activation across multiple jurisdictions.

INCIDENT MANAGEMENT ISSUES

Within the broad strategic approach of an IMS, there are several issues that consistently challenge those responsible for the management of a disaster. There are no definitive answers to these issues; they all need to be addressed in the context of each jurisdiction.

Who is in charge?

There has been a surprisingly persistent debate regarding who is in charge underpinned by competing principles of familiarity and expertise. To over-simplify the debate, the police argue they should be in charge as they are in charge of other events (familiarity). Other agencies argue that the agency with relevant expertise (e.g., fire for fires, health for pandemics) should act as the *lead* agency. Each jurisdiction must resolve this debate and reach a determined position prior to any disaster. Regardless of which agency acts as the *lead,* this does not detract from the expertise and the roles and responsibilities of all other agencies involved.

Roles and responsibilities

The roles and responsibilities of various agencies and individuals must be determined either through negotiation or determination before the event. It is not appropriate to determine these at the time of an incident. These may evolve over time, but the initial response should be based on predetermined agreements. Disaster management should have its foundations on existing systems and practices. Disasters are larger events, but the skills used in responding to an incident cannot be easily scaled up to respond to a disaster. It is the scale required that needs well-exercised management to cope. Well-documented plans can be used to achieve outcomes in large-scale disasters. Incidents usually need careful application of complex operational procedures and standards.

Safety and security

Scene safety and security is a critical consideration, particularly where the danger is ongoing, such as a fire or terrorist attack. A highly disciplined approach to the safety of responders needs to be the first consideration. Examples where responders may be at risk include:

- Police responding to a mass shooting.
- Fire fighters responding into a chemically contaminated zone.
- Search and rescue squads responding into unstable buildings.

Additionally, spectators and helpers will be attracted to such events, and it may be difficult to distinguish these onlookers from the *walking wounded.* There is a tendency in developed countries for overwhelming responses, as all agencies seek to be involved. The media will seek immediate access and may impede access by emergency responders. There is also a risk that media could breach the privacy of those affected. This creates the very real danger of scene congestion while denuding the remaining community of its emergency coverage. There is a need to secure the site quickly and to restrict entry in the interests of safety and efficiency of response. Active management is critical to maintain access and egress.

Volunteers

It should also be recognised that the first responders to any event will be people in closest proximity including those involved. In almost all circumstances these individuals will render aid within the limits of their ability. It is important for response agencies to understand that such actions are appropriate and potentially lifesaving and to be respectful to those concerned.

CASE STUDY 17.1 – BYSTANDER FIRST AID

It has long been recognised that out-of-hospital CPR performed correctly is associated with greater patient survival. A study by Bakke et al. (2015) found trauma patients receiving bystander-provided first-aid treatment is also associated with reduced mortality and morbidity. The prospective study conducted over an 18-month period examined bystander first aid in the out-of-hospital setting. Of the trauma cases included in this study cohort, 97% were provided with correct airway management, 81% were provided with correct haemorrhage control, and 62% were provided with measures to prevent hypothermia. Of the bystanders providing out-of-hospital first aid, only 35% had some first-aid training (Bakke et al. 2015).

Source: Bakke, H.K., T. Steinvik, S.I. Eldissen, M. Gilbert, T. Wisborg, Bystander first aid in trauma – prevalence and quality: A prospective observational study. *Acts Anaesthesiologica Scandinavica.* 2015. **59**(2015): 1187–1193.

Other volunteer responders fall broadly into two categories. Those who form part of organised volunteer organisations, and those who spontaneously respond. The latter includes many well-meaning individuals who seek only to offer assistance; however, there are those whose enthusiasm for involvement in such events overwhelms not only their expertise, but also the need for safe and secure scene management. For this reason, incident managers need to consider how spontaneous volunteers can be utilised safely within the organised incident response.

Surge capacity

Surge capacity describes the ability of response agencies to expand capability at a time when there is a significant increase in demand. Regardless of the agency, surge capacity is a critical principle that needs to be planned for and addressed. With the demand for healthcare growing, especially in hospitals, access to healthcare globally is at crisis point. Research [1] has demonstrated that access to operating theatres, intensive care, and radiography would be severely compromised during a mass-casualty event. It is imperative for healthcare facilities and response agencies to develop preparedness plans and benchmarks to ensure they have the surge capacity in the event of a mass casualty incident. It is equally imperative for governments to provide the necessary funding and infrastructure to ensure these benchmarks are sustainable.

Healthcare at scene

Scene medical management is dependent on the availability of appropriate resources and expertise. Passing trained personnel will often offer help although there are debates regarding the expectations that they do so and their vulnerability. Organised medical responses to the scene should leverage off normal community-based emergency health

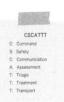

CSCATTT
C: Command
S: Safety
C: Communication
A: Assessment
T: Triage
T: Treatment
T: Transport

arrangements. Ambulance services will usually be the first health responders. It is critical that this be recognised and that any surge in health responses leverage up from, and be controlled by, those first medical responders. Additional assistance may be obtained from specialist retrieval and urban search and rescue teams.

The primary purpose of healthcare on scene of a disaster is to triage, treat, and transport patients to appropriate definitive care. The amount of care rendered will depend on the available resources, and the style of definitive care will depend on the local environment.

- *Triage* is the process of sorting patients according to their urgency and severity into categories to determine their immediate health needs. There are two elements for this triage: extrication priority and clinical triage.
  - *Extrication priority* determines the prioritisation of treatment and movement of patients from the scene to the causality-clearing post. Those who are alive and mobile should be directed to a place of safety. Patients who require assistance in extrication are the next priority, and those trapped and requiring extrication will be retrieved only when they can be released. There are formal triage systems (e.g., START or SIEVE). The principle of familiarity suggests conformity with normal practice is the most useful approach.
  - The second triage step involves the determination of *urgency for treatment*. This is usually based on a more thorough physiologic assessment (e.g., SORT). SORT triage provides each casualty is further assessed and provided with a score which will determine their priority and the most appropriate location they should be transported to.
- *Forward aid* involves stabilisation of the patient sufficiently to allow safe transport to a place of ongoing care. Healthcare on scene should be provided in a safe environment and minimised to that essential to preserve life and limb. The scene is not an appropriate location to undertake advanced medical procedures because of the lack of infrastructure, infection control, and the ongoing risk to the patient and responders.
- *Medical teams* responding to the scene should be trained and equipped, and act in liaison with first responding professional health services (ambulance/EMS).
- *Appropriate dispersal* of patients is critical to the optimal outcomes. A system-wide approach with central clinical coordination is necessary to ensure the health system is managed strategically, and that individual health facilities are not overwhelmed.

Rescue

In many countries search and rescue services have developed specialist programs to deal with particular hazards. These services are coordinated and directed through government agencies or NGOs and volunteer-based organisations. Their engagement and tasking must form an integrated part of an overall response. Some examples of specialist rescue programs include:

- Road rescue – trapped within a vehicle.
- Rail, air or industrial rescue (RAIR) – trapped in a complex environment involving special hazards.
- Urban search and rescue (USAR) – trapped within the collapsed buildings.
- Hazardous material response (HAZMAT) – located inside a contaminated area.
- Wilderness/alpine response – located in an extreme environment.

Incident management elements: the 11 'C's

The management of the response and relief phase is complex and contextualised by the nature and scope of the community and the nature and scale of the event. But within this complexity there are consistent issues to be determined and addressed. We propose these as the 11 'C's of disaster response management.

- **Community,** it is important to remember the primary goal of any emergency response is to preserve life and protect the community. It is also important to ensure that the community are engaged with the management of the incident.
- **Control** refers to the overall direction of emergency management activities in an emergency situation. Control arrangements operate horizontally across organisations and seek to ensure various organisations take a coordinated and collaborative approach to the response. Establishing command and control arrangements is a critical first step.
- **Command** refers to the direction that members of an organisation follow in the performance of roles and tasks. Command arrangements operate vertically within an organisation and ensure that the organisation's resources can be directed to the delivery of its roles and responsibilities.
- **Coordination** describes the bringing together of organisations and elements to ensure an effective response. Coordination is mainly concerned with the systematic acquisition and application of resources from various agencies and locations. Coordination operates both vertically and horizontally as an adjunct to the authority to command and control.

Command applies vertically to one agency.

Control applies horizontally across all agencies.

Coordination is assisted by clearly defined command and control arrangements.

- **Collaboration** refers to the required behaviour of all involved to work towards the mission in response to an emergency. It is not enough to simply control, command, or coordinate. It is essential that all responders collaborate with each other and the community in order to achieve a successful outcome.
- **Communication** refers to the provision of information, which facilitates an efficient and effective response. Communication refers to the design and development of the message, including its clarity, as well as the means of communication and its distribution. Most response personnel complain about breakdowns in communication in major incidents. In reality, communication is very difficult to maintain during a crisis. It is worth considering the vulnerability of normal means of communication and to have contingency plans in place. Many disasters have demonstrated the vulnerability of modern communications, with power failures affecting transmission towers, systems overload etc. Often non-technological means, such as runners, may prove more reliable and resilient. Web-based platforms to share information across multiple agencies in real-time are available, however they do require the technology and training to act as an enabler.

  Communication also implies information flow in two directions. Briefing upward is important to ensure that the key political players are aware of what is happening. Briefing downward ensures the strategic intent and strategic decisions are informed to those responsible for implementation.
- **Clinical** care addresses ongoing caring for the ill and injured as well as the people in the vicinity of the event. Disasters may directly affect the health and wellbeing of individuals as well as disrupting the health infrastructure. A major event may impact

on the capacity to provide ongoing clinical care. For example, chronically ill patients may lose access to specialised medical care or be unable to obtain ongoing supplies and prescriptions.

The key strategic management issues to be addressed include the following:

- Development of *clinical standards* preferably in advance of an emergency, or in response to any novel presentation.
- Clinical care in a disaster should be *based on the principles of maximum benefit*, so immediate interventions should be restricted to life and limb preservation, with deferred definitive care.
- *Clinical documentation* is essential. Field Triage tags can be useful as a method to identify, SIEVE and SORT patients as well as providing information to ongoing carers. Initial documentation is essential to ensure the safety of ongoing care.
- *Definitive diagnosis* of the nature and extent of injuries or illness is essential to defining the healthcare requirements, particularly during pandemics. Accurate diagnosis is essential to inform the development of clinical standards and disease control strategies. Equally important is determining the requirements for decontamination and isolation.
- It is also important to ensure *care for family and contacts* of those suffering directly from the event.
- **Capability** is the ability of the organisation to deliver a particular service or function including the protection of critical health infrastructure and personnel through enhanced infection control, PPE, isolation of patients, and anti-viral agents if indicated and other recommended immunisations.

CASE STUDY 17.2 – MANCHESTER ARENA BOMBING

Key lessons

- Consistent labelling of patients using triage tags numbers until their identity is confirmed.
- Major incidents also have a significant knock-on effect to all hospitals within a region.
- Routine surgical and medical emergencies continue to occur.
- Communication during major incidents is key. Hospital switchboards can be overwhelmed by both internal and external calls. Mobile phone signals can be poor or non-existent.
- Coordination of care is vital with regular trauma meetings where all involved must attend.
- Care of families is critical. Managing them as a unit and caring for the bereaved.
- The complex, and sometimes life-threatening, pattern of blast injuries requires a careful but quick radiological assessment. The experience of managing ballistic injuries by military surgeons is unmatched by any surgeon working in civilian practice.

Source: Craigie, R.J., P.J. Farrelly, R. Santos, S.R. Smith, J.S. Pollard, and D.J. Jones, Manchester Arena bombing: Lessons learnt from a mass casualty incident. *BMJ Military Health*, 2020. **166**. p. 72–75.

- **Capacity** addresses the organisation's resource needs and the ability to surge and maintain health services' capability. In order to maintain health services, attention must be given to a number of significant issues including:
  - *Maintaining access* to services; both physical access and service availability,
  - *Health business continuity* throughout an event that may be impaired by damage to physical infrastructure, the lack of key personnel or the availability of critical resources such as communications, water, power, and supplies including fuel.
  - There may be a need to create *additional capability*. There is value in taking a hierarchical approach to the mismatch of demand for healthcare and the capability available. A simplified approach to understanding the need for additional infrastructure involves four tiers of response:
    - *Tier 1* actions require concentration of expertise utilising existing infrastructure.
    - *Tier 2* actions require the preservation of infrastructure for the event by early discharge of patients and limiting non-urgent activity.
    - *Tier 3* requires the expansion of health infrastructure through system-wide management, growing capacity, and importing capacity (e.g., field hospitals).
    - *Tier 4* requires rationing of access to health infrastructure through triage of patients and escalation involving international assistance.

Containment refers to the strategies required to limit the scope and spread of an event. The concept has most relevance for pandemic management, whereby strategies seek to limit the spread of an infectious disease through quarantine, isolation, and containment. Containment in pandemic responses is achieved through isolation and quarantine, immunisation, and prophylactic use of antiviral or antibacterial agents. They may also include social distancing measures, such as school closure or banning of mass gatherings. Pandemics are covered in detail in Chapter 24.

However, the concept is also relevant to other events where limiting the extent and impact of the incident is desirable. People involved in a major traumatic incident often depart independently from the scene. This makes it difficult to determine the extent of the problem and to ensure appropriate care. Often the *walking wounded* will crowd the nearest hospital, limiting the hospital's capacity to deal with the critically ill and injured. This is also the case with patients injured or exposed to a major toxin. In these cases, their departure from the scene continues the spread of the exposure and places the safety of hospital staff and the general public at risk.

CASE STUDY 17.3 – SARIN NERVE GAS ATTACK, TOKYO 1995

Following the Sarin nerve gas attack on the Tokyo subway in 1995, emergency staff at St Luke's hospital, unaware they were dealing with a chemical contamination, did not wear appropriate PPE. As a result, 46% of staff later reported symptoms of acute chemical poisoning due to secondary exposure (Okumura et al., 1998).

Source: Okumura, T., K. Suzuki, A. Fukuda, A. Kohama, N. Takasu, S. Ishimatsu, et al., The Tokyo Subway Sarin attack: Disaster Management, Part 2: Hospital response. Tokyo. *Academic Emergency Management*, 1998. 5(6): p. 618–624.

- **Continuity** describes the strategies needed to maintain functionality. Generally, the three keys to continuity include people, facilities, and systems.

  People: When events are long-term, it is neither possible nor safe to maintain key personnel on duty. They need to be relieved, particularly if their own families are under threat, or they have suffered personally from the incident. Sometimes effort put into securing the safety of the families of key personnel will free them up to maintain activity. However, in addition to the workforce, continuity relies on other strategies including volunteers and the flexible use of other professional staff. Volunteer management is a critical aspect of maintaining functions as a complement and aid to expert staff. Flexible use of other professional staff will aid in concentrating expertise. General Practitioners may be useful as surgical assistants, to care for families or provide vaccinations and counselling. However, allocating tasks to a group that is outside their normal day-to-day functions requires consultation and pre-planning. This needs to be done prior to a disaster.

  Facilities: Facilities and buildings may be damaged by the incident, and planning should consider the loss of the building or facilities. Similarly supplies need to be maintained through a prolonged event and supply and distribution systems are necessary. Supplies must be secured, as the imbedded stockpile will be consumed first and in an uncoordinated manner.

  Systems: Data and information systems must be maintained. It is important to ensure that through sensible preparedness, facilities have access to documents needed to enable the response in the event of power failure, for example, staff lists are generally stored on computer systems, it is also essential to have a hard copy as well.

Obstacles to effective disaster response

There are many factors that impair the effectiveness of disaster response and the application of tried and tested principles including organisational, human and structural impediments.

Every organisation involved in a disaster response brings with them *their own organisational culture, language, policies, procedures, and expertise.* Large-scale events require a well-coordinated, multi-agency response. House et al. [2] contend response agencies

> 'become a collective whole by sharing cognitive aspects relating to agency-specific mental models (i.e., their knowledge and awareness of what the situation presents) and areas of expertise to produce a coherent and collaborative response.'

Many civil organisations operate through a chain of command model with *personnel in senior roles who may not be the most qualified person to undertake a leading role in a disaster response.* The success of any disaster response requires appropriately qualified personnel who have undertaken comprehensive all-hazards/all-agencies disaster management training to enable them to successfully undertake a senior role in a disaster response.

The disaster response will be strengthened when a *connectedness exists between organisations.* Implementing multiple bridging strategies as part of disaster preparedness is essential to linking organisations and creating diversity in disaster management networks. Vachette et al. [3] contend bonding, bridging, and linking social networks can be achieved through continuous relationship building within and across the diverse array of agencies and actors involved in all facets of disaster management. Networking mechanisms and communication pathways established, built upon, and maintained across all sectors through regular interactions and training exercises are often reinforced at times of disaster [3]. Nowell et al. [4] contend that the ability of response agencies to establish and maintain an effective disaster response in complex environments requires all actors and their established networks to be able to:

- rapidly adapt to evolving situations,
- undertake bilateral coordination,
- effectively manage and distribute information; and
- engage in emergent collective action.

The larger the scale, or number of levels within the disaster response and the IMS, the greater the need for there to **be flexibility at every level of action**, but sufficient order to hold and exchange information in real time. Whilst the design of hierarchical organisations is to improve efficiencies and decrease the transaction of information, Hugelius et al. [5] found the major challenges organisations face are the:

- Lack of conformity of contingency plans and the actual situation.
- Organisational inability to manage uncertainty.
- Ineffective information management.

The problem is intensified in larger organisations and in large-scale disasters where there exists a rapidly evolving disaster event with significant environmental variables. [5]

A multi-agency response to a disaster requires **a collaborative network of timely information exchange and coordination** within and between all the actors involved. Information can often be unreliable and information overload adds to the challenges faced by the tactical and operational response. To reduce the risk of confusion and loss of sense making in these conditions, it is imperative the interoperability of the response agencies is solid. Furthermore, the IMS requires robust intelligence and planning, and flexible adaptation to comprehend and respond to any situation [6].

Fatigue adds to the complexities of the response to a disaster, particularly if it is a protracted event where the coordination centre/s had been on standby in the lead-up to the impact. It is vital all staff in the IMS only be allowed to work short, maximum eight-hour shifts and be provided with enough down time to allow them to rest and recover before returning for another shift. Therefore, it is important each organisation have enough appropriately trained staff to undertake shifts throughout the duration of the disaster response.

CASE STUDY 17.4 – DECISION-MAKING ERRORS DURING MULTI-LEVEL, MULTI-TEAM PROTRACTED DISASTER RESPONSE

Brooks et al. (2018) employed the Human Factors Analysis and Classification System to analyse the frequency and distribution of human error at all levels of coordination during three Australian Bushfires. The study found that the more complex the disaster and the higher the levels of uncertainty, time constraints, fatigue and personal interactions all contributed to errors in decision-making. These errors were compounded when decisions were made without validation of information or information was fragmented and where there had been a limited discussion process.

Source: Brooks, B., S. Curnun, C. Bearman, C. Owen, Human error during the multilevel responses to three Australian bushfire disasters. *Journal of Contingencies and Crisis Management*. 2018. **26**: 440–452. https://doi.org/10.1111/1468-5973.12221

The success of any disaster response requires a diverse array of multi-faceted conditions to be in place prior to its use in a disaster and during the response phase if the system is to effectively achieve the desired outcomes [7].

ACTIVITY

Examine the Royal Commission report into the 2009 Black Saturday bushfires in Victoria, Australia. Discuss at the strategic, tactical, and operational levels:

1. How the rapidly changing event, the structure of the IMS, and a constantly changing lead agency impacted on the response?
2. How did other disasters in Australia that weekend, i.e., heatwave in South Australia and Western Australia and floods in Queensland impact on operations in Victoria?
3. Can you identify additional improvements beyond those of the recommendations of the Royal Commission report[2]?

KEY READINGS

Hardy, K., and L.K. Comfort, Dynamic decision processes in complex, high-risk operations: The Yarnell Hill Fire. *Safety Science*. 2015. **71**: p. 39–47.

House, A., N. Power, and L. Alison, A systematic review of the potential hurdles of interoperability to the emergency services in major incidents: Recommendations for solutions and alternatives. *Cognition, Technology & Work*. 2014. **16**(3): p. 319–335.

Jung, K., and M. Song, Linking emergency management networks to disaster resilience: Bonding and bridging strategy in hierarchical or horizontal collaboration networks. *Quality and Quanity*. 2015; **49**: p. 1465–1483.

Lockey, D., Pre-hospital critical care at major incidents. *British Journal of Anaesthesia*. 2022; **128**(2): p. e82–e85, ISSN 0007-0912, https://doi.org/10.1016/j.bja.2021.10.002.

Rimstad, R. and G.S. Braut, Literature review on medical incident command. *Prehospital and Disaster Medicine*. 2015; **30**(2): p. 205–215.

Notes

1. With acknowledgement to previous authors Justin Dunlop and Andrew Pearce
2. http://royalcommission.vic.gov.au/finaldocuments/summary/PF/VBRC_Summary_PF.pdf

References

1. Traub, M., D.A. Bradt, and A.P. Joseph, The surge capacity for people in emergencies (SCOPE) study in Australasian hospitals. *Medical Journal of Australia*, 2007. **186**(8): p. 394–398.
2. House, A., N. Power, and L. Alison, A systematic review of the potential hurdles of interoperability to the emergency services in major incidents: Recommendations for solutions and alternatives. *Cognition, Technology & Work*, 2014. **16**: p. 319–335.
3. Vachette, A., D. King, and A. Cottrell, Bonding, bridging and linking social networks: A qualitative study of the emergency management of Cyclone Pam, Vanuatu. *Asia Pacific Viewpoint*, 2017. **58**(3): p. 315–330.
4. Nowell, B., et al., The structure of effective governance of disaster response networks: Insights from the field. *The American Review of Public Administration*, 2018. **48**(7): p. 699–715.

5. Hugelius, K., J. Becker, and A. Adolfsson, Five challenges when managing mass casualty or disaster situations: A review study. *International Journal of Environmental Research and Public Health*, 2020. **17**(9): p. 3068.

6. Hardy, K. and L.K. Comfort, Dynamic decision processes in complex, high-risk operations: The Yarnell Hill Fire, June 30, 2013. *Safety Science*, 2015. **71**: p. 39–47.

7. Jensen, J. and W.L. Waugh Jr, The United States' experience with the incident command system: What we think we know and what we need to know more about. *Journal of Contingencies and Crisis Management*, 2014. **22**(1): p. 5–17.

18
External assistance in disasters

Peter Aitken, Gerry FitzGerald,
Colin Myers and Stacey Pizzino[1]

INTRODUCTION

The most immediate response to a community affected by a disaster is from the community itself; initially bystanders, rapidly supplemented by first responders, emergency services and health services within the affected area. As such, the resilience and preparedness of communities (including hazard reduction activities), response capacity and existing levels of care, are the principal factors in mitigating disaster morbidity and mortality. External assistance is available to assist communities in building resilience and preparedness.

However, these local first responders may be overwhelmed by the size of the disaster response required or find themselves and their families also impacted by the disaster so as to limit their capacity to mount and sustain responses, particularly during the acute phase of the incident. Therefore, communities often require external assistance which, in the first instance, will be provided by the emergency response agencies of neighbouring communities, cities or states. When these resources are also stretched external assistance may be provided by services or people not normally a part of the integrated emergency response model.

External assistance may be part of an organised response by distant response agencies or may take the form of spontaneous volunteers. In some circumstances external assistance may simply appear, creating many of its own challenges. External assistance may take many forms including economic aid, as well as both human and physical resources. Health support may include health supplies and equipment as well as medical care, best structured in the form of medical assistance teams.

In addition to formal reporting social connectedness and crowd-sourced information and social media coverage will increase the visibility of disasters to the global community and this may lead to further offers of assistance.

The aim of this chapter is to examine specific issues associated with the provision and organisation of external assistance. It reflects on the community's capacity to receive and organise external assistance or to provide that assistance to other communities. On completion of this chapter, you should have developed an understanding of:

1. The types and priorities for external assistance.
2. The core standards and guiding principles underpinning effective aid.

DOI: 10.4324/9781032626604-23

3. The challenges posed by external assistance and strategies required to minimise risk.
4. The international assistance coordination frameworks and in particular the composition and organisation of Emergency Medical Teams (EMTs).

PROVIDING EXTERNAL ASSISTANCE

Worldwide understanding of disaster management has changed over time with relief seen not as a charity but a right and a humanitarian obligation. Article 3 of the Universal Declaration of Human Rights states that *"Everyone has the right to life, liberty and security of person"* [1]. It is not just response however it is also built into the proactive international strategies that seek to build resilience. This is best articulated by the Millennium Development Goals and the Sendai Framework [2, 3].

External assistance is any aid provided from outside of the affected community. This may be from neighbouring communities, from distant communities within the same country or from other countries. Obviously the greater the distance involved, the longer it takes for assistance to arrive and often the greater risk of language or cultural differences. The longer the assistance takes to arrive the more the need changes from emergency aid to sustenance and then recovery.

However, external assistance must be respectful of the context in both the affected community and the community providing the assistance. Assistance needs to recognise the legislative and policy environment in both the receiving and sending jurisdictions, along with the social, political, and organisational context within which the event has occurred. There are many examples of inappropriate aid adding to the distress in the affected community and aggravating the economic and social impacts of the disaster. Thus, there is a need to better organise external assistance and match it to the needs of the community.

External assistance must also be subject to identification of actual need. Evaluating the need is often challenging as initial chaos and confusion along with the impact of the disaster on normal communication channels, may limit access to a detailed understanding of the needs of the community. Reliance on media reports, particularly social media is potentially of high risk. Mechanisms need to be in place to evaluate need and communicate that need to potential sources of external assistance.

External assistance may be provided as direct financial assistance as well as the provision of essential drugs, medical supplies, equipment, and personnel. Cash is often promoted as the best form of aid as it enables autonomy of the affected community, can be directed to meet locally determined needs, and stimulates the local economy. However, to be effective it is reliant on an intact economy, infrastructure and logistic support and sufficient numbers of locally available skilled personnel. There are many situations where this is not possible.

Resources may be provided from prepositioned stockpiles or acquired from suppliers. Personnel may also take the form of specially trained and prepared disaster services such as the military, Disaster Victim Identification, Urban Search and Rescue or EMTs, or in the form of specialist resources assigned to work within their area of expertise (e.g., specialist surgeons and anaesthetists).

Stockpiled resources

Prepositioned and pre-identified resources (stockpiles) are often available to be dispatched immediately to a crisis location. The construct of these supply caches is based on the likely need within the immediate vicinity and the capacity of the donors. Considering the delays in dispatch and arrival of such resources, it is likely that they will mostly need to address the ongoing survival needs of the population. An example is the 'Emergency Health Kit', which was first promoted by World Health Organisation (WHO) in 1984 and has been adopted by most relief organisations and national authorities [4].

However, such stockpiles are difficult to justify and maintain, consuming resources not only for the initial setup and stocking, but also for their maintenance and restocking. A rational approach to the pre-positioning of these resources is necessary. The challenge of these stockpiles is to ensure their appropriateness and accessibility.

Some nations seek not to stockpile resources but rather to identify where stockpiles would normally be held and have in place operational mechanisms to rapidly construct a resource cache based on a predetermined list of appropriate items. This approach has the potential to reduce the risk of 'out of date' stock. As an example, the WHO, under the auspices of the United Nations, is now coordinating the strategic placement of multiple stockpiles to serve the many small islands of the South Pacific such that resources are never too far removed from the area in which they might be required.

CASE STUDY 18.1 – STOCKPILING VENTILATORS

In the early days of COVID-19, the U.S. government announced orders for almost $3 billion of ventilators for a national stockpile (Reuters 2020). Almost half were basic breathing devices that don't meet the minimum requirements needed to treat Acute Respiratory Distress Syndrome (ARDS). Only about 10% were full intensive care unit ventilators.

Many countries followed suit, but stockpiling ventilators is not a trivial warehousing problem and may present a false sense of security.

- The ventilators need to be fit for purpose. Most ventilators purchased were transport ventilators that have a limited use in the treatment of ARDS.
- There is a limit to the number of ventilators that any hospital can absorb determined by the number of trained staff.
- The Ventilators need to be maintained to ensure functionality.
- Distribution mechanisms need to be identified to get the ventilators from a central storage facility to hospitals in need.
- Consumables need to be identified and supply ensured.

Sources: Reuters, 2020. The U.S. has spent billions stockpiling ventilators, but many won't save critically ill COVID-19 patients. Accessible at https://www.reuters.com/article/us-health-coronavirus-ventilators-insigh-idUSKBN28C1N6

Meltzer, M.I., A. Patel, Stockpiling ventilators for influenza pandemics. *Emerging Infectious Diseases*. 2017. **23**(6):1021–1022. doi: 10.3201/eid2306.170434. PMCID: PMC5443457

H.C. Huang, O.M. Araz, D.P. Morton, G.P. Johnson, P. Damien, B. Clements, L.A. Meyers, Stockpiling ventilators for influenza pandemics. *Emerging Infectious Diseases*. 2017 **23**(6):914–921. doi: 10.3201/eid2306.161417. PMID: 28518041; PMCID: PMC5443432

The donation of medical equipment and consumable needs also to follow ethical principles. Special considerations apply to the donation of unused or surplus medical supplies and pharmaceuticals at the end of a mission. These should follow relevant international standards (e.g., WHO) and be agreed with relevant authorities.

Logistics

Logistics is one of the most important elements of a relief operation. The ability to deliver the right supplies in the right amount in optimal condition, where and when required is critical for effective emergency operations. Logistics refers to the mechanisms by which resources and personnel are able to be delivered to, and sustained within, an affected community. It also refers to the provision of resources required to sustain the response including food, shelter, and water for the responding personnel. Logistics also refers to moving bulk items required for the response.

Pre-existing logistics infrastructure, political factors, the number of humanitarian actors, damage caused and security will limit or have an impact on logistics. Effective planning for logistics must also attend to the information and control systems required to track and sustain the response. Tracking the logistics is important. A computer system has been developed by the Pan American Health Organisation (PAHO) called SUMA (Supply Management) which sorts, classifies and makes an inventory of relief supplies at ports of entry to ensure appropriate distribution occurs [5].

The logistic support of Search and Rescue or medical teams is a significant and challenging issue. Teams should be completely self-sufficient as imposing the support of foreign teams onto a devastated community with insufficient resources for its own support is unethical. Teams need not only accommodation but also sufficient food and water to sustain their deployment and this requires transportation. They also require security as well-resourced foreign teams with adequate supplies, food and clean water are understandably attractive targets to devastated communities who have lost everything. Teams also need to respect local medical standards and integrate with and not supplant local medical care services with a plan to transition care back to local services as soon as it is sustainable.

EXTERNAL MEDICAL ASSISTANCE

The need for medical care varies according to the community context, the nature and impact of the event and the time since the disaster. von Schreeb [6] describes a conceptual model for the burden of medical needs following a disaster

- The immediate reaction is that the *elective surgical need* and *utilisation of hospital resources* drop to zero when a disaster occurs.
- At the same time *trauma resource need and use* spikes before eventually declining to baseline.
- *Need and utilisation* arising from the event has a long tail as result of secondary cases, delayed presentations, and complications.
- Subsequently a second spike of secondary non-trauma emergency demand, driven by infectious diseases may also occur.

The relationship and scale of the disease burden will depend on the community context, hazard type and the effectiveness of the multi-sectoral response. Many communities will respond as a network, therefore *use and demand* for elective cases may be absorbed by other parts of the system unaffected by the disaster.

External medical assistance usually arrives only after immediate assistance and lifesaving trauma surgery, has been provided by the local community and functioning health providers [6–8]. Thus, the medical needs may have shifted to repair and recovery and the provision of routine healthcare.

For example, a review of the Foreign Field Hospital (FFH) response to disasters in Iran, Haiti, Indonesia and Pakistan found that none of the 43 FFHs reviewed were operational early enough to provide life-saving emergency trauma care. Findings suggest that deployed hospitals are better suited to meeting the ongoing medical needs of a community and substituting for existing damaged facilities than to meet immediate trauma needs [6].

Nonetheless the speed of deployment and time to becoming operational for responding EMTs does appear to be improving. For example, the international response to the 2015 Nepal Earthquake was extensive. Camacho et al [9] identified a total of 136 international medical teams with various degrees of compliance with international standards and reporting. Due to the limited airport capacity in Nepal, the arrival of these teams restricted access by EMTs and supplies in general [10]. The government of Nepal requested a standdown for non-deployed International USAR teams two days after the earthquake yet a further 54 teams, including 12 classified under the UN system arrived.

CASE STUDY 18.2 – INTERNATIONAL MEDICAL TEAMS RESPONDING TO THE 2015 NEPAL EARTHQUAKE

Overall, 137 I-EMTs were deployed from 36 countries.

- They were classified as Type I (65%), Type II (15%), Type III (1%) and specialised cells (19%).
- Provided 28,372 out-patient consultations, 1,499 in-patient admissions and 440 major surgeries.
- The activities were significantly lower than the capacities they offered at arrival.
- Over 80% of I-EMTs registered through WHO or national registration mechanisms, but daily reporting of activities was low.

There remains a need to improve I-EMT coordination, reporting, and quality assurance while strengthening national EMT capacity.

Source: Amat Camacho, N., K. Karki, S. Subedi, J. von Schreeb, International Emergency Medical Teams in the Aftermath of the 2015 Nepal Earthquake. *Prehospital and Disaster Medicine*, 2019. **34**(3): p. 260–264. doi: 10.1017/S1049023X19004291. Epub 2019 May 6. PMID: 31057142.

COORDINATION OF ASSISTANCE

Emergency managers should be cognisant of both national and international coordination frameworks for external assistance. These include the processes within a jurisdiction to request assistance, and the mechanism by which the relevant national authorities will

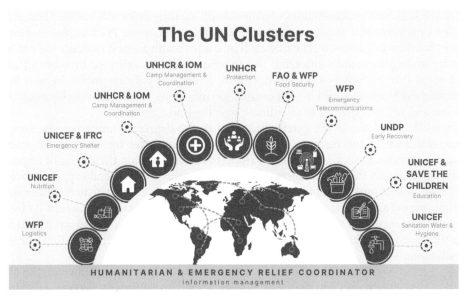

Figure 18.1 UN Humanitarian Clusters (adapted from The UN and Disaster Management at https://www.un-spider.org/risks-and-disasters/the-un-and-disaster-management)

determine whether this can be resourced domestically, or international assistance may be required. Emergency managers need to be familiar with the process by which the relevant national authority will request and accept offers of external assistance, and specifically how medical assistance will be requested and coordinated. This includes assistance from unaffected domestic resources or facilitating the transfer of patients to unaffected parts of the country.

The humanitarian and disaster-relief efforts of the UN system are overseen and facilitated by the Office for the Coordination of Humanitarian Affairs, led by the UN Emergency Response Coordinator. The UN cluster system is one of the outcomes of the humanitarian reform of 2005 aimed at improving capacity, predictability, accountability, leadership, and partnership (Figure 18.1). They provide a common mechanism for national agencies to meet clear humanitarian needs by supporting coordination across numerous actors and identifying leading actors in each of the clusters.

Other than in limited circumstances of a failed state or complex emergencies, the responsibility for managing the request, or accepting international assistance is that of the affected country. UN General Assembly Resolution 46/182 – *Strengthening of the coordination of humanitarian emergency assistance of the United Nations* [11] was adopted on 19 December 1991. This resolution outlines an enhanced framework for humanitarian assistance and specifies 12 guiding principles, including those related to the responsibilities and authorities of the States, these include

- Humanitarian assistance should be provided with the consent of the affected country.
- Each state has the responsibility first and foremost to take care of the victims of natural disasters and other emergencies occurring on its territory.
- States whose populations are in need of humanitarian assistance are called upon to facilitate the work of these organisations in implementing humanitarian assistance.

Often the roles and responsibilities of national and local agencies will be described in legislation or government mandates such as a *National Civil Defence Plan*, or *National Emergency Plan*. Most disasters will be managed by a non-health agency, typically the national disaster management authorities, but this function could be delivered by other agencies such as the Prime Minister or President's office, defence, or police agencies. In most jurisdictions health agencies will be responsible for managing the health consequences of a disaster and will be expected to coordinate with the lead agencies.

In seeking and deploying external assistance, the degree of autonomy for support agencies will vary. Some disasters may see a wide mandate given by the executive government for agencies to seek and manage external assistance within their areas of responsibility. For example, the NZ Canterbury 2011 earthquake saw bi-lateral support provided to USAR, police, health, and defence agencies from international partners. Other jurisdictions may require all accepted offers of international assistance to be *signed-off* by the executive government or lead agency. Emergency managers should understand and exercise the decision-making and approval frameworks that would apply within their own jurisdictions.

In the 2005 South Asia earthquake, despite decades of ongoing violence and tension in Kashmir, India and Pakistan eased cross-border travel restrictions & 'no-fly' zones to allow each other's governments & citizens to provide region-wide assistance in the disputed territory.

The national disaster authorities will likely be working with the Ministry or Department of Foreign Affairs or equivalent. Foreign Affairs will have a critical role in managing the political risks and implications for foreign policy in accepting or rejecting offers of assistance and managing issues on the ground. They may also provide advice to ensure teams from countries with historical conflict are deployed in either different areas of operation or used in such a way as to avoid conflict between themselves and the affected country.

Foreign affairs will also be working to ensure the diplomatic corps within the affected country is kept informed of the situation, including any general or targeted requests for assistance. Requests for assistance may be communicated through embassies or overseas missions in donor countries. Foreign affairs will also be working with external countries to manage the response to foreign citizens affected by the disaster. There is a risk that international assistance may be targeted to affected foreign citizens. Whilst there is a legitimate role in facilitating medical evacuation of expatriates in order to free up hospital capacity, the role and function of these teams need to be clearly understood and accepted.

Regardless of the authorising agency, it is vitally important the lead agency is engaged in the coordination of the international response. International assistance may be entering the affected country through international airports and will be drawing on the same national resources to *move forward* to its area of operation. Incoming teams, regardless of function, will be competing for the same logistics resources including airport landing and apron space, customs and immigration clearance, freight forwarding, local transport providers and translation services. Even a fully self-sufficient team will require local support.

External assistance will need to prioritise and allocate support across a range of different types of assistance. High-profile rescue teams may be competing for support against primary care teams that may have a much greater impact but do not make as compelling a media story. Support from law enforcement may be necessary for ensuring a safe operating environment. Other assistance, such as food distribution may be assessed as more strategically important in terms of maintaining security and governance.

STANDARDS

Methodologies for quality management have been slowly developed [12], but there is still a need for agencies and governments to agree to benchmarks, standards and codes of practice for the provision of external assistance.

The International Red Cross/Red Crescent has established Guidelines for the Domestic Facilitation of International Disaster Relief [13].

The Sphere Project has been one of the first systematic efforts to improve accountability [14]. The Sphere standards have been adopted by the UNHCR as the humanitarian charter and minimum standards for disaster response (UNHCR 2022). Sphere addresses key indicators for five sectors: water supply and sanitation, nutrition, food aid, shelter and site management and health services Reluctance in accepting these standards has arisen due to concerns about levels of flexibility and the potential use of minimum standards as a punitive tool.

The other development that arose at approximately the same time was the 1994 voluntary Code of Conduct, with ten underpinning principles, which promote the impartial character of aid, respect of local cultures, building on local capacities, involvement of beneficiaries and respect for local dignity [15].

The lack of quality enforcement mechanisms means the same problems keep reappearing. Telford (2006) suggests that this is due to the lack of external pressure for improvement in the humanitarian sector. Normally market forces lead to quality improvement in a consumer-driven market. This does not apply to humanitarian aid and the failure of agencies to meet their formal commitments to Sphere or Good Humanitarian Donorship principles suggests that the various quality initiatives are not having sufficient impact [16]. The Tsunami Evaluation Coalition feels that, if improvement is to occur, there is a need for a regulatory system to ensure agencies put the affected population at the centre of measures of effectiveness, and to provide detailed and accurate information to the donor public on assistance outcomes, including the affected populations' views of that assistance [16].

In 2012, the Humanitarian Accountability Partnership International, People In Aid and Sphere joined forces as the Joint Standards Initiative to promote greater coherence for users of humanitarian standards. The Core Humanitarian Standards (CHS) is now managed by Sphere, the CHS Alliance and Groupe URD, and is integrated in the 2018 edition of the Sphere Handbook. The CHS reaffirms a rights-based approach and alignment with international law and declarations. The latest versions of the Sphere handbook include the Humanitarian Charter, the CHS, the Protection Principles and the four sets of technical standards covering water supply, sanitation and hygiene, food security and nutrition, shelter and settlement and health. The Humanitarian Charter describes the right to life with dignity. It builds on the Code of Conduct of the International Red Cross and Red Crescent and NGOs in Disaster Relief. Sphere also hosts the Humanitarian Standards Partnership (HSP) that strives to harmonise and promote the quality and accountability of humanitarian work.

INTERNATIONAL MEDICAL ASSISTANCE TEAMS

Perhaps the most prominent example of international assistance for health is in the form of Internal Medical Assistance Teams. International medical assistance can come in the form of physical resources and/or medical personnel. The latter may be ad hoc and provided by individual volunteers or it may be organised and highly structured. The term EMTs is now used as a collective descriptor of structured and organised medical assistance known previously as FFHs, Disaster Medical Assistance Teams, and Foreign Medical Teams.

The number of medical teams responding to disaster-affected countries continues to increase which poses challenges for coordination and the delivery of effective and timely assistance. The deployment of EMTs has occurred globally in both high- and low-resource settings. In previous instances, a lack of formalised coordination of arriving international FFHs and EMTs occurred along with a lack of integration with the existing national health systems and authorities. The following case studies reflect on these issues.

A review of the health response to the 2010 Haiti earthquake found that

> if the impact was unprecedented, the organisation of the response was not. It followed the same chaotic pattern as in past disasters… the humanitarian community failed to put in practice the lessons learned.
>
> [17]

The Haiti review set clear expectations that WHO establish a Global Registry for Foreign Medical Teams[2] and FFHs, jointly now known as EMTs, as a basis for international accreditation.

The WHO has now promoted international standards for the Classification and minimum standards for EMTss [18]. These standards are intended as informative guidance for Member States, to build capability and better understand requirements. It is complemented by information and technical guidance documents.

The core guiding principles include coordination, training, mechanism to ensure staff are recruited, screened, keep clinical records, self-sufficiency, managing safety and security and liaison with relevant local authorities and media, support affected health services, professional licensing and support wider public health response.

The EMT standards note that international EMTs should expect to register with relevant national authorities, and only deploy on request of the affected government. They are to maintain and provide clinical records to the patient and relevant national authorities and operate as part of the health network receiving and referring where appropriate. All staff must be licensed and registered in their own country and have temporary permissions to practice in the affected country. They must be appropriately trained and operate within their *scope of practice*. Teams are to be self-sufficient in all regards [19].

Each classification is further supported by corresponding technical standards for key component, service delivery areas. Teams should strive to adhere to and meet all relevant operational qualifiers such as the ratio of post-operative inpatient beds to operating theatres.

It was the medical response to the Philippines after Typhoon Yolanda devastated the region in 2013 that signified an important milestone in the development of coordination and management mechanisms for EMTs. Over 150 teams deployed to the region during the response [20]. The Philippines Ministry of Health, supported by the WHO Country Office, utilised for the first time the WHO Classification and Minimum Standards for Foreign Medical Teams in Sudden Onset disasters (published three months prior to September 2013). The standard provides reporting and a registration template to register 88 teams prior to their arrival, and to manage other teams already in country. A similar number of national teams deployed domestically were also concurrently managed.

A 2019 review of the response of EMTs to the 2015 Nepal Earthquake found that 137 teams responded from 36 countries. While the response was quicker with improved coordination, registration and follow-up, there remained a need to improve coordination, reporting and quality assurance [9].

Key issues to ensure the effectiveness of external assistance teams include understanding, respecting, and working with local customs & beliefs, clear mission selection to provide agreed outcomes, selection and training of team members, international coordination and close liaison with host health services to ensure healthcare is appropriate to local standards and thus able to be transitioned back to local care upon denature of the EMT.

Coordination will extend from the national to the local level. Ideally teams will be accepted and allocated to areas of operation at the national level based on local reporting of *need*. This is particularly important where a disaster has impacted more than one location. Typhoon Yolanda in the Philippines impacted nine government regions and approximately 14 million people, however many international teams were focussed and concentrated solely in Tacloban. Whilst this regional city was directly under the path of the cyclone and affected by geography and tidal surge, these factors together with a functioning regional airport drew international media. This amplified the impact on the immediate area making it the focus for responding teams.

Support from Foreign affairs will also be critical in managing deployed teams where the host nation's Ministry of Health determines that a team should not be operating, either as they have self-deployed and refuse to be registered or are not meeting minimum standards. Options for what to do with such a team already on the ground are limited. Key questions would be:

1. Does the team meet the relevant standards for teams that have been requested or accepted?
2. Is it performing a required function?
3. Is the team willing to operate within the established coordination framework?

If the team is to remain operating, they will need to be integrated into the reporting structure and EMT coordination mechanisms and steps taken to ensure all staff are appropriately registered and operating within their scope of practice. This could involve re-tasking or allocating tasks better suited to their skills. Alternatively, facilitating a dignified exit of the team may be required. Such issues occurred during the response to the Nepal Earthquake 2015 when medical capability within International USAR teams attempted to register and deploy as *type 1-outpatient* teams.

Where external medical assistance is required, the 2015 Global EMT meeting endorsed three options in order of preference, these are:

- Host Government has a pre-existing mechanism for EMT coordination at their (Health) emergency operations centre.
- Host Government will be supported to create a reception and departure centre and EMT coordination cell by WHO/PAHO.
- EMTs will be coordinated externally in the case of host government capacity limitations.

Many of the elements that had been developed to facilitate the rapid and effective deployment of EMTs to disasters were re-purposed for the international response to the Ebola

Virus Disease outbreak in 2014. This included establishing coordination functions in partnership with the affected Ministries of Health, and ensuring deployed teams met reporting and registration requirements. Notably, rather than teams _deploying with their own self-sufficient healthcare facilities, a range of government and NGO donors built and established the supply chain to establish the Ebola Treatment Centres [21].

Experience with the Ebola outbreak led to *emergency reform* to address shortcomings identified internally and externally during the response. One of the themes of this reform is development of a *Global Health Emergency Workforce* and a key element is EMTs.

The COVID-19 response demonstrated the contrary effect. Domestic challenges and freezes on international movements reduced the capacity of international assistance and the vulnerabilities of the international assistance frameworks.

CONCLUSION

External assistance should meet the needs of the affected population rather than being driven only by the desires of the donor, no matter how well-intentioned these are. Any assistance should also be safe, efficient, effective, appropriate and ethical and not pose an additional burden on that community. These principles need to be considered by both donor and host country and by those involved directly in the deployment. Those funding external assistance frameworks must ensure their response is based on the request and is *needs-led* and appropriately resourced.

The scope, composition and timeliness of external assistance should also meet ethical, cultural, and operational principles and be directed towards the real need and respectful of the recipient community's autonomy.

External assistance should recognise that the deployment of self-sufficient medical support is complex and requires detailed planning and preparedness and must incorporate expertise not only in the clinical care to be offered but also in regard to the logistical and support needs of the community and of those providing the assistance.

ACTIVITIES

Familiarise yourself with the WHO Classification and Minimum Standards for EMTs (WHO 2021)

1. A small island nation has been devastated by a cyclone.
   a. What might be the priorities for external assistance?
   b. How would you determine this?
   c. Identify the construct of an EMT that may be required to respond immediately.
   d. How would you ensure the team was suitably prepared to deploy at short notice?
2. Identify how you would integrate international and national EMTs from outside your jurisdiction into your area following a disaster. How would you:
   a. Coordinate with relevant national authorities to request assistance?
   b. Manage their activity within your jurisdiction? How would you expect them to refer patients and report their activity?
   c. What information and process would you expect them to follow when they exit?

KEY READINGS

The Sphere Handbook 2018 accessible at https://spherestandards.org/wp-content/uploads/
Sphere-Handbook-2018-EN.pdf
Classification and minimum standards for emergency medical teams. Geneva: World
Health Organisation 2021. Licence: CC BY-NC-SA 3.0. IGO

Notes

1. *With acknowledgement to previous authors Charles Blanch, Ian Norton, and Bronte Martin.*
2. The December 2015 WHO Global Meeting endorsed the use of *Emergency Medical Teams*,
   including National and International (N-EMT, I-EMT) recognising that *Foreign* was an outdated
   concept. Both terms are used in this section, FMT where it refers to a quoted source.

References

1. United Nations. *Universal declaration of human rights*. 1948; Available from: https://www.
   un.org/en/about-us/universal-declaration-of-human-rights.
2. United Nations, *Sendai framework for disaster risk reduction 2015–2030*. 2015, Geneva: United
   Nations.
3. World Health Organisation. *Millennium development goals (MDGs)* 2018 [November 22,
   2022]; Available from: https://www.who.int/news-room/fact-sheets/detail/millennium-
   development-goals-(mdgs).
4. Organisation, W.H. *Emergency health kits*. n.d.; Available from: https://www.who.int/
   emergencies/emergency-health-kits.
5. De Ville de Goyet, C., et al., SUMA (Supply Management Project), a management tool for post-
   disaster relief supplies. *World Health Statistics Quarterly*, 1996. **49**(3–4): p. 189–194.
6. von Schreeb, J., et al., Foreign field hospitals in the recent sudden-onset disasters in Iran, Haiti,
   Indonesia, and Pakistan. *Prehospital and Disaster Medicine*, 2008. **23**(2): p. 144–151.
7. Bremer, R., Policy development in disaster preparedness and management: Lessons learned
   from the January 2001 earthquake in Gujarat, India. *Prehospital and Disaster Medicine*, 2003.
   18(4): p. 372–384.
8. Roy, N., et al., The Gujarat earthquake (2001) experience in a seismically unprepared area: Community hospital medical response. *Prehospital and Disaster Medicine*, 2002. **17**(4): p. 186–195.
9. Camacho, N.A., et al., International emergency medical teams in the aftermath of the 2015
   Nepal earthquake. *Prehospital and Disaster Medicine*, 2019. **34**(3): p. 260–264.
10. Alistair D.B. Cook, Maxim Shrestha, Zin Bo Htet. An assessment of international emergency
    disaster response to the 2015 Nepal earthquakes. *International Journal of Disaster Risk Reduc-
    tion*, 2018. **31**: p. 535–547.
11. United Nations. General Assembly Resolution 46/182. Strengthening of the coordination of
    emergency humanitarian assistance of the United Nations, in *78th Plenary meeting*. 1991, New
    York (NY): United Nations.
12. Sondorp, E., T. Kaiser, and A. Zwi, *Beyond emergency care: Challenges to health planning in
    complex emergencies*. 2001, Oxford (UK): Blackwell Science Ltd. p. 965–970.
13. International Committee of the Red Cross. *Guidelines for the domestic facilitation and regu-
    lation of international disaster relief and initial recovery assistance*. [December 12, 2022];
    Available from: https://www.icrc.org/en/doc/assets/files/red-cross-crescent-movement/31st-
    international-conference/idrl-guidelines-en.pdf.
14. Sphere Association, *The Sphere handbook*, in *Humanitarian charter and minimum standards in
    humanitarian response* 2018, Geneva (CH): Sphere Handbook (spherestandards.org).
15. International Committee of the Red Cross. *Code of conduct for the movement and NGOs in
    disaster relief*. Available from: https://www.ifrc.org/our-promise/do-good/code-conduct-
    movement-ngos.

16. Telford, J. and J. Cosgrave, *Joint evaluation of the international response to the Indian Ocean tsunami: Synthesis report.* 2006, London: Tsunami Evaluation Coalition (TEC). ISBN 0 85003 807 3.
17. De Ville de Goyet, C., F. Grünewald, and J.P. Sarmiento, *Health responses to the earthquake in haiti january 2010: Lessons to be learned for the next massive sudden-onset disaster.* 2011, Washington DC: Pan American Health Organization (PAHO).
18. World Health Organisation. *Classification and minimum standards for emergency medical teams.* 2021, Geneva (CH): World Health Organisation.
19. Norton I, et al., *Classification and minimum standards for foreign medical teams in sudden onset disasters.* 2013, Geneva (CH): World Health Organisation.
20. Peiris, S., J. Buenaventura, and N. Zagaria, Is registration of foreign medical teams needed for disaster response? Findings from the response to Typhoon Haiyan. *Western Pacific Surveillance and Response Journal: WPSAR*, 2015. **6**(Suppl 1): p. 29.
21. Gulland, A., UK built Ebola treatment centre opens in Sierra Leone. *BMJ: British Medical Journal*, 2014. **349**: p. g6704.

Part 6

Recovering

19
Community recovery

Bob Lonne and Rose Henderson[1]

INTRODUCTION AND OBJECTIVES

It is in the recovery phase that the most assistance is required by the community. Disaster recovery is the most complex and often least understood of all the phases in the disaster management cycle. In Chapter 1 we outlined the discursive nature and lack of consensus of the definition of 'disaster'; similarly, agreement is not assured concerning definitions of 'recovery', or when the actual recovery has been reached. One useful definition is:

> The restoring or improving of livelihoods and health, as well as economic, physical, social, cultural, and environmental assets, systems and activities, of a disaster-affected community or society, aligning with the principles of sustainable development and 'build back better', to avoid or reduce future disaster risk.
>
> [1]

Recovery is a developmental and a remedial process encompassing:

- Minimising the escalation of the consequences of the disaster.
- Coordinating efforts towards mitigating the diverse impacts.
- Regeneration of the social, emotional, economic and physical wellbeing of individuals and communities.
- Adapting to meet the social, economic, natural and built environment needs.
- Reducing future exposure to hazards and their associated risks.

The nature and type of disasters are major shapers of the recovery process, which is a complex, multifaceted process involving many individuals, groups and organisations. Each may have different understandings of what is involved, and varying priorities as to what exactly should be done. In circumstances where social systems are severely impacted and everyday routines disrupted, coordination of recovery tasks is imperative. The development of a shared discourse is foundational to understanding the impacts of the disaster, ensuring effective communication and making sound decisions that enable the community to cope and adjust. It enables those with a stake in recovery to participate in the

DOI: 10.4324/9781032626604-25

development of shared understandings of the diverse needs, expectations and aspirations concerning recovery goals and ambitions and the complexity that abounds.

The aim of this chapter is to examine the recovery phase and to identify the principles and processes required to successfully manage recovery and restore functionality. On completion of this chapter, you should be able to:

1. Demonstrate an advanced understanding of the factors that need to be addressed to achieve improved social resilience during recovery.
2. Evaluate community development processes and the role of non-governmental organisations (NGOs), and the community and community-based agencies in prevention, preparedness and management of major health incidents.
3. Describe the role of the community and strategies to strengthen community resilience.
4. Evaluate evidence of altered mental health and identify prevention strategies suitable for individuals, the community and organisations.
5. Identify the range of evaluation tools used after an incident, and review plans.
6. Analyse the components and understand the purpose of the audit cycle (systematic critical analysis of medical care) in disaster response.
7. Discuss the importance of evaluating the effectiveness of aid.

UNDERSTANDING RECOVERY

Communities have the potential to function effectively and adapt successfully in the aftermath of disasters. Community resilience emerges from four primary sets of adaptive capacities: economic development, social capital, information and communication technologies and community capabilities and competence. Together these provide a strategy for disaster readiness. The disaster recovery phase begins with the incident that caused the disaster and may continue for many months or years. Recovery begins

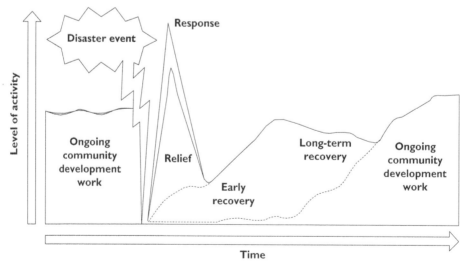

Figure 19.1 Effect of disaster on ongoing community development and interface with relief and recovery (adapted from AIDR [2], p. 32)

**The Pauses in the Comprehensive Emergency
Management Cycle**

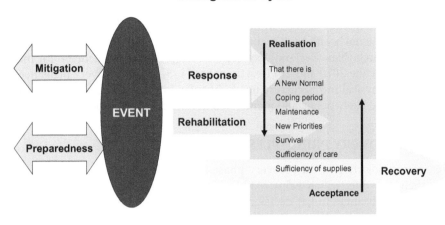

Figure 19.2 The pause in the emergency management cycle between response and recovery (adapted from McColl and Burkle [3])

with preparedness and continues until recovery transforms into ongoing community development. Figure 19.1 summarises these disaster recovery phases.

Depending on the scale and scope of the disaster, recovery entails immediate rehabilitation. Individuals and organisations assess their situations and commence the survival process by gaining the necessities for life (i.e., water, food and shelter). Most people require some time to process events and accept that a disaster has happened. This then enables a sustained movement into the recovery phase. Figure 19.2 outlines this pause in the emergency management cycle.

The language used to describe this period is important. The term 'recovery' implies a return to the prior state with a new equilibrium achieved and a *new normal* evident. 'Rehabilitation' suggests restoration of normal function. 'Resilience' is important when the outcome is the re-establishment of pre-disaster levels of functioning. Resilience itself is not transformation or reformulation, but rather a facilitative capacity for achieving positive change. Some use terms such as 'development' to emphasise the search for improvement. However, in the same way that disaster can be defined by individuals relative to their own conceptions of community functioning, so too can recovery. Whilst this variation in definition matters little in many circumstances, some disasters are on such a high scale and scope of impact that consensus about terminology quickly ensues.

However, defined, the objective of the recovery phase is to restore the community to a level that implies some degree of *normal* community function and control. A 'new normal' entails a transition to altered living situations, lifestyles and routines. Where possible, this assumes reconstruction or redevelopment will find, and build on, a reasonable balance of what the community previously had, what is left and what can now be achieved. For example, recovery can require complex planning and decisions early in the recovery phase whether to repair and restore, or whether to 'build back better'. Building back better typically involves difficult decisions to abandon housing areas because of continuing danger from fires, earthquakes or floods and revised building codes for greater future protection. However, many people are deeply connected to the place and for some, the suggestion of relocating is unacceptable. These decisions should be communicated widely, with clear reasoning, and individuals likely to be affected given an opportunity to engage in a genuine community consultative process.

As an integral part of the Prevention Planning Response and Recovery (PPRR) cycle, recovery plans often include actions to mitigate the impact of a disaster or future risks. Public health and mental health are key challenges to recovery and recovery processes. For example, Christchurch (New Zealand) experienced steep rises in the demand for mental health services after the 2010 and 2011 earthquakes [4, 5]. Thus, recovery plans need to not only address physical infrastructure needs, but also to incorporate processes to mitigate and address the likely public and mental health impacts of disaster.

DISASTER RECOVERY PRINCIPLES

The overarching objective of the recovery phase is a restoration of an individual's control over their own life, which helps reduce dependency and encourages self-efficacy. Thus, genuine involvement in key decision-making processes, as in the build back better example above, is essential. The main principles of disaster recovery designed to achieve this objective have been summarised by the (Australian Institute for Disaster Resilience (AIDR) in their Community Recovery Handbook [2]) as:

- Understanding the community context.
- Recognising the complex and dynamic nature of emergencies and communities.
- Using community-led approaches that are responsive, flexible, engaging communities and empowering them to move forward.
- A planned, coordinated and adaptive approach based on continuing assessment of impacts and needs.
- Effective communication with affected communities and other stakeholders.
- Recognising, supporting and building on community, individual and organisational capacity.

The 2016 US National Disaster Recovery Framework (NDRF) highlights the importance of pre-disaster planning. Opportunities for successful recovery are optimised with an understanding of each affected community's historical, cultural, economic and institutional context, and the complexities arising from the disaster's impacts upon the various groups, their relationships and interactions. Based on this, community and support services will be most effective when:

- Provided in a *coordinated, timely and culturally safe* manner. This is achieved by establishing a dialogue with community representatives, coordinating activities within the community to support structure, and developing common goals with recovery agencies utilising local expertise.
- *Available for all those affected* including individuals, families, communities, groups/organisations, emergency services and volunteers. An inclusive approach should be adopted, through a service delivery process that is relevant and responsive to changing and variable individual needs.
- *They engage the affected community* in the key decisions to maximise participation and self-determination. Key community members and cultural leaders should be identified to facilitate this process.
- They *facilitate sharing of information* within and between agencies. This is foundational to the cooperative and collaborative provision of services.

- *Open and effective communication* is used across all areas to ensure that people can access and receive accurate and current information about their situation and where these services are accessible.
- *Integrated with all other recovery services*, especially financial assistance. Interagency understanding of overall service provision and responsibilities should be facilitated where possible to ensure maximum integration of all service delivery. This should include ensuring that the affected community is aware of the eligibility criteria governing grants, loans and gifts.
- Assistance and resources are provided to create, enhance and support community infrastructure.
- An *integrated and cooperative approach* is used to support and promote the economic base of the affected community.
- They recognise that *cultural and spiritual rituals provide an important dimension* to the community recovery process and should be encouraged and facilitated.
- They utilise *personnel with the appropriate capacities, personal skills and knowledge.* Personnel must have an awareness of the full range of services they provide as well as all the assistance available, appropriate referral processes and the ability to identify individual and community needs.

DISASTER RECOVERY PROCESSES

The purpose of providing disaster recovery services is to assist the disaster-affected community to 'more effectively manage and enable recovery' [6]. The primary method is through community development, which strives to facilitate community change and advancement. Community development draws on a range of strategies and approaches that build social capital and community resilience, and which are consistent with the principles and processes of community-led recovery outlined below [7].

The major processes in successful disaster recovery include: community involvement; management at a local level (community or affected area) that recognises differing impacts or needs; a developmental approach that promotes empowerment, recognition of resourcefulness, planned/timely withdrawal and minimising over-intervention; and accountability, flexibility, adaptability and responsiveness coupled with coordination and integration of services.

Community involvement in all aspects of the recovery process is vital; however, capacity may be limited. The government and broader community may need to supplement local recovery initiatives and resources. This may come from unexpected sources or spontaneous initiatives from far away, for example, online philanthropic fundraising. It is important to shape and influence spontaneous giving from others so that this meets local community needs. Community recovery committees, incorporating local and external representatives, can be very useful for facilitating connections and communication with community members and stimulating their involvement. Advantages include a reinforcement of local and community orientation, recognition of common interests, ensuring equitable application of resources and services, identification and prioritisation of needs which can and cannot be met and overall monitoring of progress. Beneficial approaches:

- Centre on the community and enable those affected to actively participate in their own recovery.
- Seek to address the needs of all affected groups and communities, and consider their values, culture and priorities.
- Allow individuals, families and communities to manage their own recovery.

- Use and develop community knowledge, leadership and resilience.
- Recognise that communities may choose different paths to recovery.
- Utilise adaptive policies, plans and services to build strong partnerships between communities and those involved in the recovery process.
- Ensure that their specific and changing needs are flexibly met.

Management at a local level should take on as much responsibility as possible. Past experience has shown that locally based recovery programs tend to have greater success with increased community input and capacity for self-management. The local level is where state, national and international disaster recovery policies are interpreted and actioned. Disasters will often affect more than one government area and may sometimes affect people from multiple geographic areas (e.g., a mass gathering incident or events in a tourist region with foreign visitors). Depending on the disaster and its physical and emotional impacts, the capacity to restore losses and establish normal living patterns will vary greatly depending on the person's or community's capacity. However, outside assistance should not overwhelm those affected, detracting from their participation or preventing them from making their own decisions. Decisions not focused in this way can be seen as dictatorial and unacceptable; the ensuing tensions and conflict can drain the emotional energy that is required for recovery and collaborative efforts. *The management approach taken should supplement local involvement rather than supplant it.*

A *development approach* draws and builds on the resources within the community. Resourcefulness within the community during recovery is tantamount to a continued improvement once external resources are withdrawn. This withdrawal must occur at the appropriate time to ensure a void is not left. For example, where post-disaster specialist services have been provided, their withdrawal must occur following planning for local services to take responsibility for ongoing care. Such planning may require training locals or arranging long-term specialist support.

Accountability, flexibility, adaptability and responsiveness are vital aspects of effective recovery management. Events unfold at vastly different speeds with the various elements accentuated by public, media and political reactions. Organisations need to be able to adapt and respond quickly to deal with these multiple pressures. Inattention to these aspects can lead to unnecessary delays in decision-making and the provision of required support. Central to much of the criticism received about recovery processes are *communication, coordination and integration* issues. Response and recovery activities should run parallel, requiring an integration of all services. This requires appropriate planning and effective liaison arrangements and networks.

It is usually most effective when one single agency coordinates the provision of recovery services. The roles, responsibilities and processes of this coordinating agency must be clearly identified and articulated. The agency facilitates the regular involvement of individuals and groups in the community, and government organisations and NGOs to address the physical, environmental and economic aspects, along with psychosocial wellbeing.

PREVENTING AND MANAGING MENTAL HEALTH RISK IN THE COMMUNITY

Increased demand for mental health services following a disaster is well documented across cultures and disaster types [8–10] with people often impacted by stress, anxiety and/or depression, sometimes well after the event. Children and young people can be disproportionally and severely affected [11]. Beyond the usually identified 'vulnerable' populations (e.g., age, disability, disadvantaged populations) it is important to identify those newly 'vulnerable' as the result of the disaster. Even those usually regarded as independent and self-reliant can become very vulnerable if loved ones, their home or livelihood are suddenly taken away from them during the disaster. Attention must be given to all of the known and new vulnerable populations when planning the short-, medium- and long-term community recovery.

Service provision and public health approaches to prevention are essential, including providing information concerning the recognition of mental health issues and encouraging the use of existing informal supports by family, friends and community members. For example, the often-cited response – 'I'm ok, there are people worse off than me' provides an opportunity to normalise the stress levels experienced and gently reassure the person that this event has impacted all in various ways. It is important to capture the range of impacts in order to facilitate recovery for everyone. Public health messaging can assist all to be very mindful of changes in people's general presentation and pay attention to friends and family members who may be experiencing these changes themselves or with a loved one. People may confide in trusted health or support agencies rather than worry about their loved ones with how they are feeling. Removing all financial and other barriers to primary health care and other health or support services, including culturally based services, is essential for improving accessibility to timely help.

How decisions about recovery planning are communicated immediately following an event can have profound impacts on the community's short- and long-term recovery. Sometimes it is not what has to be done that is at issue, but rather how and when these decisions are conveyed to the community. Public communication strategies need to include an easily understood rationale, explanation for what has to be done, together with an outline of supports available to assist in navigating the recovery journey. Requiring information to be delivered with sign language and in a number of different languages is also very important. Leaders in disaster work should bear this in mind from the earliest point in managing the response and recovery efforts.

Being well prepared individually, as a family and a community is one of the best strategies to mitigate challenges to our psychosocial recovery. Ideally 'everyday' aligned public health and NGO messaging related to building resilience and maintaining wellbeing is widely promoted. These campaigns should be based on evidence such as the Aked and Thompson's [12] 'Five Ways to Wellbeing'. They need to include adaptations for diversity such as culture, language, ability, age, orientation, locality, etc. and to be promoted using multiple forms of media. This messaging needs to not only target what an individual can do but also how community connectedness can be strengthened and maintained and foster a sense of community wellbeing. For example, actions can build public morale and sustain smart collective efforts through public health strategies that emphasise 'if we stick together, we can get through this'. Hickie [13] supported this and noted that one clear lesson of the Covid pandemic has been that a cohesive society is 'more likely to build public morale, engender hope and guide a path to a safer and more mentally wealthy nation'.

Such campaigns need ongoing investment to maintain 'freshness' and relevance and avoid fading into the 'background noise' of communities undergoing dynamic recovery processes. Following a disaster, these campaigns can then be adapted for bespoke responses and promoted as needed, taking into account the specific context, demographics and other context characteristics to optimise outcomes. An example of this is the 'All Right?' campaign which had its genesis in New Zealand after the Christchurch Earthquakes of

2010-11. Based on the Five Ways of Wellbeing, this campaign had a number of different phases from awareness raising at the beginning through to messaging aimed at maintaining wellbeing throughout the long haul of recovery. It has since been adapted for more rural messaging following the Kaikoura and North Canterbury Earthquakes in 2016, and then again following the Christchurch Mosque Shootings in 2019, and maintains relevance for general wellbeing messaging in the current pandemic.

If this messaging is widespread, relevant and able to be translated into everyday actions for people and communities, it acts as a type of insurance against mental ill-health at times of distress, be that distress of personal, family, community, regional or national significance.

Following the New Zealand Kaikoura and North Canterbury earthquakes a small team of mainly social workers and nurses from secondary mental health services developed bespoke 'Recovery and Wellbeing' services. This team had no barriers to accessing them, met people in the places of their choice (including school barbecues and various farming events), provided individual, couple and family sessions, undertook community liaison and education sessions, and provided consult and liaison services to support agencies already engaged with families. There was a culture of not saying 'no' but rather 'how can we help'. One of the consequences of this service along with other response efforts was a significant reduction in the pre-existing trajectory of referrals to the secondary mental health services from this region following the event.

PREVENTING AND MANAGING MENTAL HEALTH RISK IN EMERGENCY AND HEALTHCARE WORKERS

When assigning staff to work in a disaster recovery environment it is important that they are able to work well together so that the potential for interpersonal conflicts is minimised. The team on the frontline will often be isolated from their usual networks and need to quickly form constructive and professional peer support relationships. They will need to have the necessary support from their personal/family situation to be freely able to travel and engage in this work without the distraction of personal pressures. Screening for this is essential as the post-disaster environment is dynamic and often plans such as returning home are changed at the last minute, and unforeseen impacts emerge, and all parties need to be aware of, and comfortable with, these realities.

As well as their qualifications, the selection of staff for deployment into a disaster area, should also consider their other skills and attributes such as their empathic ability to engage with diverse community members, without thinking that they already have the solutions. The ability to listen, communicate ideas and suggestions sensitively, and with an open mind to adapting these as needed, is critical as the affected community may well be in varying degrees of shock and distress. The flexibility to work alongside others in caring and sensitive ways and in contexts outside of the usual worker's experience is essential and potentially more important than their professional qualification or experience. Staff who are 'disciplinary bound' can be out of place in dynamic recovery contexts.

Frontline staff need to be supported by a leader who

- Understands the community recovery context within which they are working.
- Is ideally co-located with them.
- Can ensure the team take regular breaks, are able to talk through any issues that arise and feel supported to do the work asked of them.
- Possesses an appropriate sense of humour, including the ability to laugh at oneself.

Because of connectivity issues or difficulties with usual supports, the team leader may be the team's on-site wellbeing support person and work supervisor, as well as managing the logistics of rosters, etc. Team leaders need to be clear about personal-professional boundaries within such competing and complex situations. Ensuring staff can access the usual workplace support as needed is critical.

Psychological First Aid (PFA) is another strategy that can be promoted widely across health and social service agencies as a 'mandatory' basic level training to equip workers. Most workers will find opportunities to put into practice the learnings from PFA in their everyday work as they support their colleagues to cope with adverse events in their lives. Despite the best preparation there may be times when deployed personnel may need to be withdrawn due to a personal or professional challenge, and agencies should be checking regularly if any changes are needed.

Building on public messaging a bespoke multi-agency collaborative partnership can be developed that includes governmental agencies, NGOs and relevant community groups such as cultural, inter-faith and other community leaders. This needs to occur quickly and those leading the work need to be aware of the challenges in doing so, and be prepared to evolve as new information and needs emerge. Multiple diverse agencies need to be able to work together and focus on the shared goal of meeting the identified needs of those affected and be willing to think and act innovatively outside of 'business as usual'. Agency executives should back their frontline leaders to be creative and collaborative.

Following the completion of the recovery work both a reflection on the learnings from the experience and having a group celebration to acknowledge the achievements are important. It is also important to acknowledge the contributions of staff who have not been deployed and are 'holding the fort'. This should be completed both within each agency as well as across the collaborative agency partnerships.

ELEMENTS FOR SUCCESSFUL DISASTER RECOVERY

Effective recovery processes result in greater community resilience by improving previous conditions through the enhancement of social and natural environments, infrastructure and economies. The elements of successful recovery rely on understanding the context; recognising the complexity of the situation; using community-led approaches; ensuring coordination of all activities; and acknowledging and building capacity, which must be underpinned by effective communication (as discussed in Chapter 7). These concepts are explained as follows.

Understanding the context of the disaster community is important for the recovery process because it enables appreciation of the risks faced by individuals, groups and communities. There is a particular need to identify those who are vulnerable, impoverished or face significant disadvantages. It requires developing an understanding of the social, economic, geographic, cultural and religious dimensions of the disaster community. Understanding the context requires recognition of and respect for differences, including people's culture, strengths, capacities, resources and experiences.

Recognising the complexity of the individual and community experiences of disaster is essential to facilitating a smoother transition to the recovery process. This entails the type, nature, scope and scale of the disaster, including how it is similar and different to what has been previously experienced. Information on impacts is limited at first and changes over time. Affected individuals and communities have diverse needs, wants and expectations that are immediate and rapidly evolving. Quick action to respond to, and address, immediate needs is crucial. However, conflicting knowledge, values and priorities among individuals, communities and organisations may create tensions. Emergencies create stressful environments, and grief or blame may also affect those involved. Comprehending the complexities helps us to acknowledge that the achievement of recovery is often long and challenging, and existing community knowledge and values may challenge our own assumptions.

Community development and recovery processes utilise *community-led approaches* to ensure engagement and involvement of the community and to facilitate restoration of local control. This element centres on 'bottom–up' strategies that help to rebuild community capacity and ownership of the recovery decision-making processes. Facilitating community-led approaches necessitates that those involved in the recovery, particularly those outside the affected area, embrace power-sharing methods that aim to enable those affected to actively participate in, and manage, their own recovery. Such approaches use and develop community knowledge and capacity, leadership and resilience, thereby building community capacity.

In addition to the coordination and integration between recovery and response activities mentioned previously, the *coordination of all activities* constituting the recovery phase is required. This is to ensure effectiveness and avoid duplication, waste and inefficiency. This element should be guided by those with experience and expertise, using skilled and trusted leadership who undertake well-developed planning and detailed information gathering. As noted earlier, an understanding of the roles, responsibilities and authority of other organisations is necessary to coordinate across agencies and ensure minimal service disruption. Such approaches integrate responses and contribute to future prevention and preparedness. They require staff to be inclusive while using relationships created before and after the emergency. Clearly articulated and shared goals based on desired outcomes are essential, along with clear decision-making and reporting structures. This element enables staff to incorporate the planned introduction to, and transition from, recovery-specific actions and services.

Effective communication in any complex circumstance such as in disasters requires a range of strategies to address multiple communication needs, priorities and audiences (see Chapter 7). Consistency, collaboration and coordination must exist between all responding agencies over the content of messages and the right to deliver, and the means of delivery. Message/information formats and key means of delivery must be identified in the planning process to ensure that they can become functional immediately following a disaster. Language and narratives are important considerations for leadership in recovery as they influence the ways in which individuals and communities perceive and respond to the adversity they face.

Importantly, various groups within the community often utilise different forms of communication, so communication strategies need to employ a variety of methods and platforms (e.g., social media, radio, online and websites, printed materials, word of mouth, etc.). Importantly, social media postings and questions need to be monitored and responded to quickly. Social media postings can go viral – for better or worse. Select community leaders and respected personalities can be used to deliver keynote messages and information. A 2022 systematic review by Ogie and colleagues [14] identified that social media during recovery is important for:

- Donations and financial support.
- Solidarity and social cohesion.
- Post-disaster reconstruction and infrastructure services.

- Socio-economic and physical wellbeing.
- Information support.
- Mental health and emotional support.
- Business and economic activities.

Communication planning is critical to provide for the diversity of information needs, which will change over time. Unfortunately, as the Covid pandemic has shown, social media can also be open to the spreading of misinformation, fear and angst but this makes it critical to have effective communication of fact-based guidance and support messaging.

Finally, the recovery phase should *acknowledge and build capacity* through respecting the community's resilience and capacity (no matter how depleted it may be) and identifying the gaps and working towards closing these. Although it can be a slow process, supporting the development of self-efficacy through identifying and mobilising the community skills, strengths and resources that are provided by a range of stakeholders helps to build community ownership and autonomy. This process needs to accommodate the reality that existing resources will be stretched and additional resources may only be available for a limited period. Sustainability needs to be addressed through approaches that share, transfer and develop knowledge, skills and training, and facilitate networks and partnerships to strengthen capacity.

LEADERSHIP FOR COMMUNITY RECOVERY

It is clear that leadership in disaster and community recovery roles and organisations is an inherently difficult and complex task (see Chapter 26). On the one hand there may be immense pressure to 'take charge' and make decisions unilaterally and quickly in order to get things done. On the other hand, there will likely be resistance to approaches that disempower others and restrict their involvement in decision-making which directly affects them. To follow the principles and processes of disaster recovery requires a leadership approach that is inclusive, open to feedback and visionary about the necessary destination and journey. This must be provided while also attending to the operational and management aspects required to ensure that people's needs and expectations are met within reasonable timeframes. A 'command and control' approach to leadership will generally be counterproductive in the recovery phase. The approaches to leadership we advocate (see Chapter 26) are necessary at all strategic and operational levels if community confidence is to be gained and maintained.

ROLE OF RECOVERY MANAGER

It is important to establish an interim management structure to coordinate recovery measures for the participating organisations and agencies. This needs to be established in consultation with the relevant authorities. Goals and aims for the recovery process need to be determined (e.g., repair or enhance services and infrastructure). Essentially, the role of the recovery manager is to:

- Enable the operation of agencies engaged in the recovery operation and coordinate their involvement.
- Facilitate the involvement of all affected parties in the development of long-term solutions that address priority issues.

- Disseminate relevant information so that all parties are aware of the scope and nature of the recovery process, including critical steps.
- Regularly report on the progress of recovery operations to national, state and local government organisations and agencies involved in the recovery process.
- Highlight important issues where required decisions go beyond current policies and procedures and advise on recommended options.
- Provide a final evaluation report detailing the resources committed, actions taken, lessons learnt and any recommendations for future operations.

RECOVERY GUIDELINES

The AIDR has developed guidelines to inform all government departments, agencies and individuals involved in the disaster recovery process in the Emergency Management Arrangements handbook (2019). There are detailed guidelines outlined across more than 20 handbooks that are invaluable for disaster preparation and recovery planning and service delivery, providing information on the desired community outcomes, indicators of need, funding and personnel and specific initiatives and activities. Integration with broader recovery systems is also vital for all parties to understand.

Recovery organisational structure

Like all phases of disaster management, recovery requires an organised approach assigning roles and responsibilities to ensure all needs are managed. The organisational structure must be based on the structure principles described in Chapter 4. It should be modular,

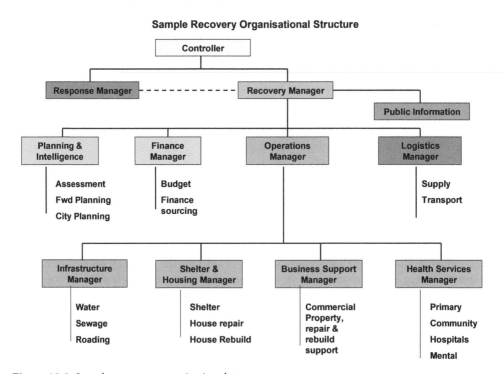

Figure 19.3 Sample recovery organisational structure

flexible and adaptable so that it can respond to rapidly changing circumstances as well as differences in need and expectations. Roles in the structure are activated, or not, according to the needs, amount of damage and activity required, or staff available. Lines of accountability must be clear. The structural arrangements need to be fit for purpose and congruent with the local community context. The recovery manager must work closely with the overall controller and the response manager to ensure continuity and collaboration of roles and responsibilities. Figure 19.3 is an example of a recovery organisational structure adaptable for general use.

Essential for the success of any organisational structure is the need for communication, coordination and collaboration between all levels and positions, particularly in assessment and planning. The realities, however, are that significant tensions are often evident in intra- and inter-organisational interactions. Operational and relational effectiveness is impacted by alliances, rivalries and boundary and role issues. Leaders must devote attention to ensuring that these do not thwart the achievement of desired outcomes.

COMMUNITY RECOVERY OUTCOMES

Disaster recovery processes are usually highly political due to the significant disruption to lives and community expectations of rapid improvement. Hence, managers, agencies and individuals need clear aims and scope of activity. While measures and outcomes are not usually the same across events, a common vision should be evident for an enhanced future addressing sustainability, social justice, the economic environment and equity [2, 15]. Key benchmarks include:

- An informed and engaged community.
- Equitable access to services and facilities.
- A sense of community safety.
- Wide participation in community life through cooperative partnerships.
- Strong community identity incorporating tradition and history.
- Economic recovery through capacity development.

Utilisation of existing community resources enables the achievement of the outcomes of recovery management. Recovery managers need to accurately assess the disaster's impact upon the affected community's needs and the level of resources required to support necessary community development. Five areas indicate the level of need for community development activity and resources:

1. *Event profile/scale* is the disaster's overall scale and public profile. This may entail national and international media attention potentially complicating the recovery process. Indicators of scale include: the type of disaster; its unexpectedness and the extent of community preparation; the number of deaths/injuries; coordination of the range of responses required; and a high media profile, with associated requests for information from many people and groups.
2. *Physical effects* of the disaster significantly impact upon the capacity of the affected community and often require community development activities. Indicators of this need include: the scale of the disaster and loss of infrastructure; the proportion of the community displaced and for how long; increased requests for material aid and financial assistance; and time needed to restore services.

3. *Psychosocial/emotional effects* are usually more difficult to measure than physical ones. Importantly, service responses should be cognisant that people cope in a variety of ways. Indicators were outlined above and also in Chapter 12.
4. *Service capacity* is the capacity of existing services to meet the additional demands generated by the disaster. Indicators include: disrupted communication systems; how well the available workforce can meet increased service complexity and demands; increased need for information on health and safety issues; and service disruptions.
5. *General indicators of need* for community development include: rising unemployment, and the relative disadvantage and impoverishment of the community pre-event; increased community tensions and exacerbation of pre-existing community rifts; increased residential sales and relocations; increased attendance at religious services; and a rising need for child health services and medical services.

RESOURCING OF RECOVERY ACTIVITIES

The timing of the disaster, along with political and media interest, has an impact on the availability and willingness to commit funds. Therefore, assessment of the need for additional resources should occur as early as possible and cover an extended period of 12 months or typically longer. Assessment should include statistical analysis of service demand and use, as well as intuitive assessment of experienced staff and community members. For example, domestic and family violence may increase post-disaster. Local knowledge, experts and outreach programs should be the focus of consultations to assist in identifying which groups are vulnerable and why, if the disaster exacerbated this, and in which ways.

Recovery managers and staff should be employed as close as possible to the affected community. Funds can be sourced from governments, the community, corporate sources, or international aid and development organisations. Funding submissions need to include detailed assessments of need, political and community expectations and the benefits of expenditure. Submissions should also address likely activities and programs, and the integration of the community in recovery processes. There is often pressure to quickly appoint appropriate people so that the recovery process benefits from effective partnerships forming rapidly within the community.

The recovery period requires continued funding and support, often for years, to address all aspects of infrastructure reconstruction, and public and mental health. This can be a significant issue. Financial aid is at its most abundant immediately following the disaster, but through the recovery phases there is usually less media and political attention with a consequent decrease in support and donations. Similarly, different types of disasters can be more or less attractive to benevolent support.

EVALUATION

Evaluation is vital to assess the performance, effectiveness and value of community recovery programs. Evaluation acts as a learning tool, gives credibility to and validates previous work, and shapes the ongoing development of recovery processes. It is necessary for continued or new funding. Evaluation seeks to identify the actual outcomes with respect to desired goals, objectives and expectations; how operations have been conducted; and where improvements are required. The focus is on achievements, processes and problem-solving.

Quantitative measures include existing community capacity and activity, measuring the scope, utility and quantifiable outcomes of recovery initiatives and community participation. Qualitative measures include a range of person-centred satisfaction and other assessments of how people are responding to, and perceiving, the recovery. Desired outcomes vary for different disaster types and community contexts, and will change over time, requiring re-evaluation. Remember, it is often difficult to define an end to the recovery phase: it tends to transform into a new reality.

Evaluation reports should address: contextual issues; desired outcomes of the recovery process; strategies used; performance indicators; adherence to recovery principles and processes; data sources; findings and recommendations. Key considerations in evaluations are: community participation, feedback and ownership; quantitative and qualitative approaches; appropriateness of evaluation tools; flexibility; opinions of stakeholders; and independence in evaluation. The evidence-based prevention and intervention strategies for disaster relief and recovery are based on the 'medical audit cycle' and epidemiological research on disasters as outlined in Chapter 18. For example, the World Health Organisation and international aid agencies have a longstanding involvement and commitment to the evaluation of disaster relief and recovery programs. The Sphere movement [16] has provided a critical framework for assessing the operationalisation of the Humanitarian Charter, the Protection Principles and the Core and Minimum Standards for disaster recovery interventions.

The analysis of responses to disasters identifies valuable *lessons to be learnt* which underpin the development of more efficient and effective evidence-based recovery strategies. With the dignity of people threatened by disasters and subsequent recovery measures, those coordinating the recovery need to ensure collective efforts are achieving desired outcomes and building the community's own capacity to manage its recovery and resilience.

CASE STUDY 19.1 – ASIAN TSUNAMI, 2004

The scale of the 2004 Asian tsunami overwhelmed the international community and challenged their capacity to manage the huge surge of money and resources and to deal with problems of coordination associated with agency proliferation. The Tsunami Evaluation Coalition undertook analysis of the recovery interventions 11 months after the disaster (Telford et al. 2006). The findings demonstrated *patchy* funding arrangements of response agencies prevented them from having an adequate *standing capacity*, resulting in a shortage of trained staff on standby, and a lack of necessary financial tracking systems and working relationships. While funding was unprecedented, the standing capacity was not in place to deliver aid to the greatest effect (Telford et al. 2006).

Telford et al. (2006) also concluded donor governments and international agencies:

- Often overlooked the contribution of local communities and organisations.
- Failed to understand the local context and demonstrated a reluctance and/or inability to consult with, and work through and with, local communities, groups and organisations.

- Did not adequately consult with, or even inform, the affected population about projects.
- Initiated inappropriate and poor-quality programs and poorly executed aid projects, which in some cases acted against the best interests of affected people and even undermined the progress of local initiatives.
- Rarely allocated funds based on need or used formal assessments of the needs of affected people, and did not undertake assessments jointly or share information.
- Failed to ensure adequate tracking of funds.
- Missed opportunities to strengthen and build local capacity.
- Did not establish firm foundations for building appropriate local capacity and longer-term recovery.

Source: Telford, J., J. Cosgrave, *Joint evaluation of the international response to the Indian Ocean Tsunami: Synthesis report.* Tsunami Evaluation Coalition (TEC); 2006.

ACTIVITIES

- How might you assess the community context and the complexity of the impacts of a major storm and flood disaster?
- Identify and briefly describe the key principles and processes required for community recovery.
- How would you evaluate the effectiveness of the community development processes and the organisations providing services during the recovery phase of a major earthquake?
- What are the particular issues and challenges associated with leadership and communication in disaster recovery processes?

KEY READINGS

Australian Institute for Disaster Resilience (AIDR). *Community recovery handbook.* 2018, Canberra: Australian Government.

Department of Homeland Security. *The Federal response to Hurricane Katrina: Lessons learned.* 2006, Washington, DC: US Government. Read Chapter 5.

Homeland Security. *National disaster recovery framework*, 2nd ed. 2016. https://www.fema.gov/emergency-managers/national-preparedness/frameworks/recovery

Kenny, S., and P. Connors, *Developing communities for the future.* 5th ed. 2017, Melbourne: Cengage Learning.

Ministry of Health. *Framework for psychosocial support in emergencies.* 2016, Wellington: Ministry of Health. https://www.health.govt.nz/publication/framework-psychosocial-support-emergencies

Examine the following websites and explore relevant information that they can add to your understanding of incident management and disaster recovery.

Australian Disaster Resilience – *Knowledge hub handbook collection.* https://knowledge.aidr.org.au/collections/handbook-collection/

Australian Disaster Resilience – *Knowledge hub manual series.* https://knowledge.aidr.org.au/resources/manual-series/

Centers for Disease Control and Prevention – *Emergency response and recovery*. https://www.cdc.gov/globalhealth/healthprotection/errb/index.html

Department of Homeland Security USA – *Disasters*. http://www.dhs.gov/index.shtm

European Commission – *Recovery and peacebuilding assessments, post-disaster needs assessments and COVID recovery needs assessments*. https://ec.europa.eu/fpi/what-we-do/recovery-and-peacebuilding-assessments-post-disaster-needs-assessments-and-covid-recovery-needs_en

HM Government – *Emergency response and recovery 2013*. https://www.gov.uk/government/publications/emergency-response-and-recovery

National Emergency Management Agency – *Co-ordinated incident management system (CIMS)* (3rd ed.), 2019, Wellington: New Zealand Government. https://www.civildefence.govt.nz/resources/coordinated-incident-management-system-cims-third-edition/

SPHERE – *Humanitarian standards*. http://www.spherestandards.org/

Torrens Resilience Institute – *Resources*. https://www.flinders.edu.au/torrens-resilience-initiative/resources

UNICEF Australia and Royal Far West – *After the disaster: Recovery for Australia's children*. 2021. https://www.unicef.org.au/our-work/unicef-in-australia/bushfire-response/after-the-disaster

United Nations Development Programme – *Recovery: Challenges and lessons 2019*. https://www.undp.org/publications/recovery-challenges-and-lessons

United Nations Office for Disaster Risk Reduction – *Recovery*, 2022. https://www.undrr.org/terminology/recovery

U.S. Department of the Interior – *Selected restoration and recovery guidelines* https://www.doi.gov/recovery/reference-materials/guidelines

Note

1. With acknowledgement to previous authors Graeme McColl & Greg Marston.

References

1. UN Office for Disaster Risk Reducation. *Recovery*. 2022; Available from: https://www.undrr.org/terminology/recovery
2. Australian Institute for Disaster Resilience (AIDR), *Community recovery handbook*. 2018, Canberra: Australian Government.
3. McColl, G.J. and F.M. Burkle, The new normal: Twelve months of resiliency and recovery in Christchurch. *Disaster Medicine and Public Health Preparedness*, 2012. **6**(1): p. 33–43.
4. Hogg, D. et al., Geographic variation of clinically diagnosed mood and anxiety disorders in Christchurch after the 2010/11 earthquakes. *Health & Place*, 2014. **30**: p. 270–278.
5. Osborne, D. and C. G. Sibley, After the disaster: Using the Big-Five to predict changes in mental health among survivors of the 2011 Christchurch Earthquake. *Disaster Prevention and Management*, 2013. **22**(5): p. 456–466.
6. Homeland Security, *National disaster recovery framework*. 2016.
7. Kenny, S. and P. Connors, *Developing communities for the future*. 5th ed. 2017, Melbourne: Cengage Learning.
8. Phillips, B.D. (2015). Disaster Recovery (2nd ed.). CRC Press. https://doi.org/10.1201/b19328
9. Prewitt Diaz, J. and S. Agarwal, Theoretical building blocks for community-based psychological support, in *Disaster recovery: Community-based psychological support in the aftermath*, J.P. Diaz, Editor. 2018, Florida: Apple Academic Press.
10. van der Velden, P.G., et al., Persistent mental health disturbances during the 10 years after a disaster: Four-wave longitudinal comparative study. *Psychiatry and Clinical Neurosciences*, 2013. **67**(2): p. 110–118.

11. Danese, A., et al., Child and adolescent mental health amidst emergencies and disasters. *The British Journal of Psychiatry*, 2020. **216**(3): p. 159–162.
12. Aked, J. and S. Thompson. *Five ways to wellbeing: New applications, new ways of thinking.* 2011; Available from: https://neweconomics.org/2011/07/five-ways-well-new-applications-new-ways-thinking.
13. Hickie, I. *A drop in morale as Australians urged to 'sink or swim' in the Omicron wave.* Crikey, 2022.
14. Ogie, R., et al., Social media use in disaster recovery: A systematic literature review. *International Journal of Disaster Risk Reduction*, 2022. **70**: p. 102783.
15. Joseph, J., S.M. Irshad, and A.M. Alex, Disaster recovery and structural inequalities: A case study of community assertion for justice. *International Journal of Disaster Risk Reduction*, 2021. **66**: p. 102555.
16. Sphere Association, The Sphere handbook, in *Humanitarian charter and minimum standards in humanitarian response*. 2018, Geneva (CH): The Sphere Association

20

Recovery of physical and social infrastructure

Rebuilding a stronger community

Marie Fredriksen, Gerry FitzGerald, Mike Tarrant,
Colin Myers, and Stacey Pizzino

INTRODUCTION AND OBJECTIVES

Chapter 19 explored the principles and practices of community recovery. This Chapter explores how those principles may be applied to the recovery of the physical and social infrastructure that support communities. Disaster recovery will often involve multiple actors, each with competing priorities and expectations which in turn adds to the complexities in what is already a highly complex and stressful environment [1, 2]. These multiple actors have differing perspectives that result in a contestable political landscape which further challenges the recovery process.

Every community is unique in terms of its risks and vulnerabilities to disasters and the social and physical structures that support it. But one thing remains constant, and that is, no one knows the community better than its citizens. While the recovery principles remain the same, the management of the recovery process must be led by the community. Community-led recovery, supported by governments and agencies provides communities with an opportunity to reduce vulnerabilities by ensuring recovery activities mitigate future disaster risk and to rebuild the physical and social infrastructure in accordance with the community needs.

Sustainable recovery involves restoring or improving the community's physical and social infrastructure and the population's psychosocial health and wellbeing. The aim of this chapter is to explore the ways in which the recovery needs are assessed and the infrastructure that supports community functioning is restored or improved. On completion of this chapter, you should have:

1. An extensive understanding of the recovery principles and how these can be applied in rebuilding disaster-devastated communities.
2. A detailed understanding of the process of assessment of recovery needs.
3. An understanding of how the recovery process is managed.

DOI: 10.4324/9781032626604-26

ASSESSING THE NEED

In Chapter 16, we explored the methods used in assessing the impact of an event on the community and its infrastructure. However, as we enter the recovery phase, it is important to assess the future needs of the community. Those needs are not only informed by the damage caused to existing infrastructure but also by the aspirations of the community. The assessment can be categorised into immediate, short term and long term.

During the initial stages of the disaster, assessments determine the most immediate needs of the community to protect life and limb and to restore essential services and infrastructure. As the disaster response comes to an end and recovery operations develop momentum, it will be important to complete a more detailed assessment of the future community needs that may inform reconstruction. Thus, the focus on the longer-term recovery and reconstruction is not only on the replacement of infrastructure that was designed for past needs but rather on meeting the future needs of the community in a sustainable manner.

The international humanitarian community has a highly structured approach to this needs assessment which is dealt with in Chapter 18. However the principles and key elements of any such assessment are applicable to any scale of incident or community.

This assessment may be done at a whole of community level facilitated by agencies assigned to that purpose. It may also be done by specific purpose agencies set up to manage the recovery of a particular event. However, it must also be done at all layers including the local government, organisational and community level.

The assessment must identify the needs and the risks and vulnerabilities of communities but also the capacities and capabilities of local communities and thus the resource gaps that need to be filled.

RECOVERY PRINCIPLES

Chapter 19 introduced the principles of disaster recovery including the understanding of the context and complexity of the disaster recovery processes and the use of community-led, planned, coordinated and adaptive approaches based on effective communication. These principles apply equally to the recovery of physical and social infrastructure. However, there is also a widely accepted principle that the focus should be on the concept of "Build Back Better". The principle of building back better encompasses more than just the replacement of physical and social infrastructure but rather ensuring where possible that the infrastructure is appropriate to the future needs of the community. Build back better is a process that allows communities to become more resilient and sustainable in the long term [3, 4].

Reducing disaster risk

Mannakkara et al. [3] contend that using the recovery process to reduce risk often requires a combination of strategies. These strategies need to be contextualised to the local community and often involve multiple levels. For example:

- *Improving structural resilience* – ensuring the built environment can withstand the impact of future natural disasters. Reconstruction may permit the upgrading to more modern building codes relevant to the risks the community faces and current regulations. Mannakkara et al. [3] suggest structural resilience will be improved through investment to upgrade existing public infrastructure, and incentives for homeowners and businesses to improve and maintain their own buildings to bring them into line with current standards.

- *Multi-hazard land use planning* – Land use planning is an integral component of DRR in a post-disaster community that has *built back better*. Risk-based land use planning and zoning will identify high-risk zones relevant to the risks each community faces. Detailed mapping of high-, medium- and low-risk zones will identify areas where building and development should never be allowed or where resettlement ought to be considered. It will also identify areas where risks can be mitigated with appropriate structural engineering and building codes [5].
- *Risk-based zoning* allows authorities to regulate how the land will be used. High-risk zones where mitigation strategies do not significantly reduce the risks will often be used for parks and green spaces. Medium- and low-risk zones may be developed with appropriate building codes and standards.
- *Resettlement* away from high-risk zones where development has already taken place will separate communities from the hazards. In some cases, communities in high-risk zones that have endured repeated natural disasters have been the drivers of change, compelling their respective governments to introduce buy-back schemes [6] or to relocate the entire community to an area of lower risk [7].

  After the 2004 Indian Ocean Tsunami entire islands in the Maldives which had been decimated were left deserted and the populations relocated to other "safer"islands.

- However, resettlement can be difficult in communities where cultural beliefs and customs hold significant importance to the people and the land on which they live. If resettlement is not planned and implemented correctly in consultation with the people, it will have a negative impact on the survivors [8]. Research that has focused on individuals and communities who have been forced to relocate [8–10], or voluntarily choose to resettle after a natural disaster [11–15] reveals a process that is both complex and multi-dimensional. The success of relocation in the post-disaster context primarily depends upon the structure and state of the community prior to the disaster. This will determine the intensity of the emotions and feelings of dislocation and isolation relocated communities can experience [7].
- *Building early warning* systems strives to inform people of the potential and imminent threats and advise them of the actions they ought to take to reduce their risk of injury or loss. Effective early warning systems require technology and procedures that will allow real-time monitoring, data collection, analysis and interpretation and information sharing across agencies and jurisdictions. This will enable authorities to generate and disseminate meaningful warnings about potential and imminent threats in a timely and effective format that will encourage people to prepare and act before the disaster [16, 17].
- *Disaster risk reduction education* raises awareness about the types and scale of disasters the community encounters and the actions the people ought to take to reduce their risk of injury or loss. Disaster risk reduction education and training programs must build on lessons identified from previous disasters and the local knowledge of the people in the community. Stakeholders ought to receive education that addresses their disaster risks and hazards [3], the practical measures households, businesses and individuals can take to prepare for a disaster, and the actions to take both during the disaster and in the immediate aftermath. Education materials must be in a user-friendly language and format specific to the community to ensure it is targeted at the intended audience.

Restoring and redeveloping social infrastructure

Infrastructure Australia defines social infrastructure as the "facilities, spaces, services and networks that support the quality of life and wellbeing of our communities". It identifies examples of social infrastructure including the physical and human capital associated with health and aged care, education, recreation, arts and culture, social housing and justice and emergency services. In the context of the build back better strategy, community recovery requires attention to the redevelopment of this social infrastructure to reinforce the restoration of a sense of community functioning and adaptation to a new normality. The scope and nature of actions required are necessarily dependent on the nature and scope of the damage but also on the nature of the community and its future aspirations. Some examples of the importance of social infrastructure are discussed below [18].

- *Restoring education* is critical to avoid the potential for generational adverse impacts of a disaster and the impact on the psychological and intellectual development of children. Additionally, there are practical considerations. Children returning to school restore a sense of normality and also help parents attend to recovery and restore economic activity essential to community functionality.
- *Restoring health services* is essential to reduce the risk of further injury or illness, sustain those injured in the event and reduce long-term adverse health outcomes including poor mental health by addressing risk factors.
- *Returning sport and recreation* helps communities restore a sense of normality and offers distractions from the challenges faced in the recovery phase and also allows opportunities for community consolidation and mutual support.
- *Similarly, restoring entertainment* provides communities with an opportunity to come together, offering mutual support and distraction from the recovery challenges.

Recovery of the social infrastructure requires a range of measures which primarily rely on recovery organisations and agencies listening to the community to ensure they have a comprehensive understanding of the local context. This includes the social environment, cultural beliefs and customs, religious and ethnic factors which exist in each community [3]. Authorities and recovery groups can develop an understanding of the community by engaging with local community leaders, respected citizens and representatives from existing community groups. By first understanding the community, recovery strategies including the rebuilding of infrastructure and psychological and social support programs can be designed and implemented in ways that empower the people and meet the specific needs of the community [3].

Economic recovery

Economic recovery is a critical component of assisting a community. It encompasses not only attention to the financial costs of recovery and reconstruction but also to restoring individual and community confidence in their financial future. Disasters adversely impact on the economy and on businesses and thus employment. The cascading impact of personal injury, damaged homes and lost employment has significant adverse impacts on the health and wellbeing of those affected by disasters. Previous experience has shown that detrimental economic impacts may be compounded by the well-intended actions of generous outsiders whose donations and actions may deprive local businesses of their involvement in the recovery.

Thus, economic recovery programs must support local businesses to re-establish as quickly as possible and protect the livelihood of the people in the disaster-affected community long after the disaster recovery operations have ceased. Strategies for economic recovery should include financial support in the short to mid-term and sustainable activity and employment in the long term. Local businesses and tradespeople ought to be given the first opportunity to provide the resources required for the recovery efforts. Programs could also include fast-tracking building approvals and insurance claims, business support and advice as well as incentives for tradespeople to employ and train residents to help with the skilled workforce required to rebuild the community [3].

Recovery of the environment

The environment in which people live is critical to the wellbeing of a community after a disaster. It supports the economy through tourism and agriculture and supports community confidence and recreation.

- Cleaning debris permits access to the community for essential supplies and for the return of employment and other community activities.
- Cleaning up contaminated material may be an essential component of restoring the environment and of reducing the potential risk to health and wellbeing.
- Restoring the productive capacity of the landscape particularly agricultural activities.

ENGAGING LOCAL COMMUNITIES IN RECOVERY AND RECONSTRUCTION

A fundamental component of a person's identity is informed by their culture and customs and their religious and spiritual beliefs and these have significant importance to these individuals, and in many cases, to their wider community. These beliefs often form the basis for their values and the way they behave, their view of the world and how they prepare, respond and recover from disasters [19–21].

When disaster strikes in these communities, the world is often quick to respond, and rightly so. In the haste to restore the community, recovery efforts, especially those delivered by external organisations and humanitarian agencies have often been undertaken without consultation with the community or consideration of the culture and customs, religious and spiritual beliefs of the local people. Examples of culturally insensitive disaster recovery operations [22, 23] and loss of livelihood due to forced resettlement [24, 25] were seen following the 2004 Indian Ocean Tsunami.

Gianisa & Le De [20] found that cultural and religious beliefs have the potential to reduce vulnerability while increasing resilience in many of these communities and as such, they should be seen as a resource on which external recovery agencies can build on.

In some societies, culture shapes human resilience in disasters [26]. Disaster recovery undertaken without consideration of the culture, customs, religious and spiritual beliefs of the people and their community has the potential to impede the long-term recovery in communities where these beliefs form a major part of their identity.

EFFECTIVE IMPLEMENTATION

A key component to the effective implementation of any disaster recovery program is for authorities and recovery agencies to have a robust relationship with the stakeholders and local partners [27]. A strong relationship with key community members and clearly defined roles and responsibilities of all actors will help to eliminate duplication and ensure recovery activities remain sensitive to the needs of the community. Successful implementation of all build back better programs requires institutional mechanisms, legislation and regulation and continued monitoring and evaluation [3].

- *Institutional mechanisms* that are not wholly centralised, adopt, foster and maintain multi-stakeholder engagement, and have robust coordination and role allocation between stakeholders. This is the preferred model for successful build back better programs [3]. The recovery program may be managed by an existing government authority or a new recovery authority which has formed because of the disaster. The appropriate institutional mechanism that will lead recovery efforts will again be informed by the characteristics and context of the local community [3].
- *Legislation and regulation* facilitate the recovery process, but it must be designed in a way that prevents the pre-disaster vulnerabilities from being repeated, but with enough flexibility to allow the residents to get back into their own homes as quickly as possible. Rules, regulations and red tape that are excessive add to the time and costs of rebuilding [3] and is an impediment to the psychosocial recovery of the people. Apart from regulations governing the reconstruction of the built environment, the local government will also need to have in place legislation, regulations and a management plan to oversee the recovery of the natural environment and areas of cultural and natural heritage [28].
- *Monitoring and evaluation* must be ongoing throughout the recovery process to ensure that rebuilding complies with the relevant legislation and regulations and to evaluate the recovery plan so that it can be modified and improved upon as the recovery progresses. Monitoring and evaluation must allow for the collection of data that captures both the positive and the negative aspects of the recovery process so that lessons can be identified. While every recovery operation will be different, sharing data obtained during recovery operations with the community as well as national and international organisations involved in disaster recovery enhances knowledge what can be applied during successive disasters [3].

MANAGING THE RECOVERY PROCESS

The process of recovery requires the management of many challenges. Competing priorities will need to be assessed and managed. Achieving sustainable well-thought-out rebuilding and recovery operations will need to be balanced against the pressure to return to normal as quickly as possible. The interests of multiple agencies need to be balanced. Long-term approaches will need to be balanced against strategic short- and medium-term interventions. The process will need to ensure that vulnerable individuals and communities are not overlooked, particularly those who may lack the advocacy of more influential people. The focus should be sustained on building resilient capacities and avoiding the development of dependence or learned helplessness.

Inevitably communities will implement organisational arrangements and identify strategies designed to help the community recovery and rebuild. The process requires all of the normal elements of strategy including policies, guidelines, planning, implementation, monitoring and evaluation.

From all the details noted above, the involvement of the local community is essential, and the recovery process should be designed around building local capacity and engagement through communication and the provision of information to all stakeholders.

Proposals will be required to be developed to help acquire the funding required for reconstruction. The process of recovery will require the maintenance of transparency, accountability and governance.

ACTIVITIES – SELF-ASSESSMENT AGAINST LEARNING OUTCOMES

1. Imagine you are a key member of a community recovery team in a small rural town that has been the subject of a major natural disasters which has destroyed community infrastructure. Make a list of the top ten strategies you consider need to be implemented to help get the community back on its feet.
2. Consider that you are trying to engage local stakeholders in the task of reconstruction. Craft a letter inviting them to participate and in doing so, craft the argument for the importance of local engagement.

KEY READINGS

1. UN World Conference on Disaster Risk Reduction. Issue brief. Reconstructing after disasters: Build back better. Ministerial Roundtable 2015; Available from: https://www.wcdrr.org/uploads/Reconstructing-after-disasters-Build-back-better.pdf
2. *Australian disaster resilience handbook collection community recovery handbook 2.* Available from: https://knowledge.aidr.org.au/media/5634/community-recovery-handbook.pdf

References

1. Mooney, M.F., et al., *Psychosocial recovery from disasters: A framework informed by evidence. New Zealand Journal of Psychology*, 2011. **40** (4): p. 26–38.
2. Ryan, R., L. Wortley, and É. Ní Shé, Evaluations of post-disaster recovery: A review of practice material. *Evidence Base: A Journal of Evidence Reviews in Key Policy Areas*, 2016. **4**: p. 1–33.
3. Mannakkara, S., S. Wilkinson, and R. Potangaroa, *Resilient post disaster recovery through building back better*. 2018, London: Routledge.
4. United Nations International Strategy for Disaster Reduction, *The Sendai Framework for Disaster Risk Reduction 2015–2030*, U. Nations, Editor. 2015, Geneva: United Nations.
5. Davis, I., K. Yanagisawa, and K. Georgieva, *Disaster risk reduction for economic growth and livelihood: Investing in resilience and development*. 2015, London: Routledge.
6. Binder, S.B., C.K. Baker, and J.P. Barile, Rebuild or relocate? Resilience and postdisaster decision-making after Hurricane Sandy. *American Journal of Community Psychology*, 2015. **56**: p. 180–196.
7. Iuchi, K., Planning resettlement after disasters. *Journal of the American Planning Association*, 2014. **80**(4): p. 413–425.
8. Bang, H.N. and R. Few, Social risks and challenges in post-disaster resettlement: The case of Lake Nyos, Cameroon. *Journal of Risk Research*, 2012. **15**(9): p. 1141–1157.
9. Likuwa, K.M., Flooding and its impacts on Nkondo community in Rundu, Kavango east region of Namibia, 1950s. *Jàmbá: Journal of Disaster Risk Studies*, 2016. **8**(2): p. 1–5.
10. Ranque, L. and M. Quetulio-Navarra, 'One Safe Future' in the Philippines. *Forced Migration Review*, 2015. **49**: p. 50–52.
11. Adams-Hutcheson, G., Voices from the margins of recovery: Relocated Cantabrians in Waikato. *Kōtuitui: New Zealand Journal of Social Sciences Online*, 2015. **10**(2): p. 135–143.
12. Alaniz, R., *From strangers to neighbors: Post-disaster resettlement and community building in honduras*. 2017, Austin, TX: University of Texas Press.
13. Chen, Y., Tan, Y. and Luo, Y., Post-disaster resettlement and livelihood vulnerability in rural China. *Disaster Prevention and Management*, 2017. **26**(1): p. 65–78. https://doi.org/10.1108/DPM-07-2016-0130

14. Hogg, D., et al., The effects of relocation and level of affectedness on mood and anxiety symptom treatments after the 2011 Christchurch earthquake. *Social Science & Medicine*, 2016. **152**: p. 18–26.

15. Mordeno, I.G. and B.J. Hall, DSM-5-based latent PTSD models: Assessing structural relations with GAD in Filipino post-relocatees. *Psychiatry Research*, 2017. **258**: p. 1–8.

16. United Nations Office for Disaster Risk Reduction. *UNISDR terminology on disaster risk reduction*. 2009.

17. Basher, R., Global early warning systems for natural hazards: Systematic and people-centred. *Philosophical Transactions of the Royal Society A: Mathematical, Physical and Engineering Sciences*, 2006. **364**(1845): p. 2167–2182.

18. Infrastructure Australia. *Social infrastructure*. 2019; Available from: https://www.infrastructureaustralia.gov.au/sites/default/files/2019-08/Australian%20Infrastructure%20Audit%202019%20-%206.%20Social%20Infrastructure.pdf.

19. Ayeb-Karlsson, S., et al., I will not go, I cannot go: Cultural and social limitations of disaster preparedness in Asia, Africa, and Oceania. *Disasters*, 2019. **43**(4): p. 752–770.

20. Gianisa, A. and L. Le De, The role of religious beliefs and practices in disaster: The case study of 2009 earthquake in Padang city, Indonesia. *Disaster Prevention and Management*, 2018. **27**(1): p. 74–86.

21. Joakim, E.P. and R.S. White, Exploring the impact of religious beliefs, leadership, and networks on response and recovery of disaster-affected populations: A case study from Indonesia. *Journal of Contemporary Religion*, 2015. **30**(2): p. 193–212.

22. Ruwanpura, K.N., Putting houses in place: 1 rebuilding communities in post-tsunami Sri Lanka. *Disasters*, 2009. **33**(3): p. 436–456.

23. Telford, J. and J. Cosgrave, *Joint evaluation of the international response to the Indian Ocean tsunami: Synthesis report*. 2006, Tsunami Evaluation Coalition (TEC).

24. Frerks, G. and B. Klem, *Tsunami response in Sri Lanka*. report on a field visit from, 2005. **6**.

25. Spence, R., Palmer, J, Potangaroa, R., *Eyewitness reports of the 2004 Indian Ocean Tsunami from Sri Lanka, Thailand and Indonesia*, in *The 1755 Lisbon Earthquake: Revisited. Geotechnical, Geological, and Earthquake Engineering*. 2009, Dordrecht: Springer.

26. Mori, M., et al., Sinabung volcano: How culture shapes community resilience. *Disaster Prevention and Management: An International Journal*, 2019. **28**(3): p. 290–303.

27. Francis, T.R., et al., Post-disaster reconstruction in Christchurch: A "build back better" perspective. *International Journal of Disaster Resilience in the Built Environment*, 2018. **9**(3): p. 239–248.

28. Duyne, J.E., et al., *Safer homes, stronger communities*. 2010, Washington (DC): World Bank.

Part 7
Unique challenges of particular disasters

21

Natural disasters

Weiwei Du and Penelope Burns[1]

INTRODUCTION & OBJECTIVES

Natural disasters are a major adverse event due to natural hazards, resulting from environmental or natural earthly processes. These include: bushfires, floods, earthquakes, tsunamis, and storms. Globally, hundreds of natural disasters occur annually affecting millions of people. Severity is usually measured in terms of human impact: lives lost, illness and injury, social disruption, economic losses, and the ability of affected communities to adapt and recover. In previous chapters, disaster risk reduction was discussed as a cornerstone of disaster management. This is particularly important for natural disasters. If communities develop in a coastal tropical region prone to cyclones, near rivers that could flood, forests where bushfires could occur, or in regions prone to earthquakes; governance, capacity building, planning, mitigation strategies, and enhancing disaster preparedness will reduce the impact of natural disaster on those communities.

The aim of this chapter is to identify the particular considerations of disasters due to natural hazards and their overall impact on the health of a population. This chapter is not intended to be comprehensive, as the range and scope of events exceed imagination. However, it is intended to provide observations around common impacts of common natural hazards. On completion of this chapter, you should be able to:

1. Discuss the health impacts of particular natural disasters.
2. Identify and discuss the issues for consideration when preparing for, and mitigating, the health impacts of natural disasters.
3. Understand disaster warning complacency, and strategies to address this.

A CHANGING CLIMATE AND THE EFFECTS OF A WARMING PLANET

The world's average surface temperature increased by approximately 1°C above pre-industrial levels in 2017, and is predicted to increase 0.2°C per decade [1]. Changes in climate not only affect average temperatures, but also extreme temperatures, and temperature difference between the poles and the equator, increasing the extent and frequency

DOI: 10.4324/9781032626604-28

of climate-related natural disasters. These may include droughts, heatwaves, wildfires, cyclones, storms, floods, landslides, outbreaks of insect vectors, and infestations.

Droughts, heatwaves, and wildfires are becoming more extensive due to the increased evapotranspiration associated with the extra heat added to the climate system. Earth's hydrologic cycle shifts as warmer air retains more moisture than cooler air, and water vapor is the fuel to storms [2]. In addition, decrease in temperature difference between the poles and the equator can affect storm formulation. These may result in tropical cyclones with higher wind speeds, a wetter Asian monsoon, more intense mid-latitude storms, and more frequent, intense, prolonged floods [3].

Global warming has also caused acceleration of melting snowpack and glaciers [4]. Sea level may rise, exacerbating coastal flooding when a storm comes ashore. Glacial retreat may also trigger earthquakes as the crust rebounds when the load lightens.

HEALTHCARE IN NATURAL DISASTERS

Disaster response planning must consider the pre-disaster background health status of the affected population. Although initial response efforts focus on assisting persons injured as a direct result of the natural disaster, the largest demand for health services is for day-to-day medical issues. Planning should include not only those directly affected by the disaster, but the entire population.

This includes healthcare for chronic illnesses such as diabetes, cardiovascular, renal, or respiratory disease, for replacement of lost medications, for those requiring medical equipment and power for nebulizers, home oxygen, and dialysis. Routine healthcare needs will continue. Pregnant women will still deliver babies, children will still develop childhood infections, and the daily caseload of myocardial infarctions, strokes, and non-disaster related fractures will continue.

Sustaining existing health centers is vital. If they are damaged or destroyed, access is limited and the burden on other health services increases. During non-disaster periods, health services have a daily elective caseload to manage. Immediately after a disaster the elective demand may decrease temporarily, however, it is important to predict and plan for increased demand in the months post-disaster.

CASE STUDY 21.1 – TYPHOON HAIYAN, NOVEMBER 2013

After Typhoon Haiyan in the Philippines in 2013, the AusMAT field hospital performed 222 procedures in 21 days. Of these, 74 procedures (33%) were performed on 30 patients presenting with chronic foot wounds resulting from type-2 diabetes (Read et al., 2016).

Canadian Military level 1 mobile medical teams treated 6,596 patients. Only 3.6% of these presentations had a disaster-related injury or illness, whereas 65.5% had an acute post-disaster medical illness and 30.9% presented for care for a chronic health issue (Savage et al. 2015).

Sources: Read, D.J., A. Holian, C.C. Moller, and V. Poutawera, Surgical workload of a foreign medical team after Typhoon Haiyan. *ANZ Journal of Surgery*, 2016. **86**(5): p. 361–365. doi: 10.1111/ans.13175.

Savage, E., M.D. Christian, S. Smith et al. The Canadian Armed Forces medical response to Typhoon Haiyan. *Candian Journal of Surgery*, 2015. **58**(3 Suppl 3): s146–s152.

A Medicin Sans Frontieres surveillance system following the 2010 Haiti earthquake showed that 25% of 102,054 consultations were acute respiratory infections. These accounted for half the consultations for children < 5 years. Other leading consultations were acute watery diarrhea and malaria/fever of unknown origin [5].

Predicting health impacts according to type of natural disaster

The general health needs of a community affected by a natural disaster are largely predictable [6]. Common experiences can be used to plan mitigation strategies to manage the expected health effects of affected communities. The following discussion focuses on the health impacts of common natural disasters.

Cyclones, storms, and floods

Cyclones, hurricanes, and typhoons are rapidly rotating storm systems with a low-pressure center and are associated with strong winds, storm surge, and heavy rainfall. Cyclones develop, primarily in the tropics, over large bodies of warm water. The extent of death and injury caused by a cyclone is directly related to the degree of physical protection available to withstand the storm [7].

Flood refers to water overflowing the natural or artificial confines of a river or other body of water or accumulating by drainage over low-lying areas. Floods account for 44% of all natural disasters and 41% of the total people affected by natural disasters [8]. The main causes of flooding include

FACT

Cyclones, tornados, and hurricanes rarely form within five degrees of the equator.

- Precipitation (rain and snow)
- Rising water levels (due to tidal waves, tsunamis, or global warming)
- Structural failure (dam, sea defenses)
- Reduced natural draining (reduced absorption, blocked drainage)

The speed of flood onset is the main factor determining the number of flood-related deaths. This can be related to the local geography. Flash flood implies sudden onset, and may be associated with tsunamis, sudden downpour, or breach of reservoirs, whereas, gradual inundation or riverine flooding is slower, more predictable, and less likely to cause drowning and injury.

Drowning can occur when individuals underestimate the power of the current or the depth of the water. In many cases, drowning is associated with people choosing to enter the water on foot or by motor vehicle.

Storm and flood-related injuries may occur as individuals attempt to escape from danger, collapsing buildings, or other structures. Orthopedic injuries, puncture wounds, lacerations, blunt trauma, and falls commonly result from fast-moving water containing debris, or during clean-up. Electrical injuries and burns may be caused as floodwaters disrupt power lines, propane and natural gas lines, and chemical storage tanks. Carbon monoxide poisoning can result from the use of petrol-powered machinery in closed environments (e.g., indoors). Hypothermia, with or without submersion, is seen in some floods, and occurs in any season. Respiratory problems account for a significant proportion of morbidity associated with floods, and mold is a particular hazard for persons with impaired host defenses or allergies.

Communicable diseases including *Escherichia coli*, *Shigella*, *Salmonella*, and *hepatitis A* virus can occur if floodwaters contaminate the local water and food supply and damage the sewage system. Stagnant water provides a breeding ground for vectors such as mosquitoes resulting in diseases including *malaria* and *dengue*.

Displacement of domesticated animals, rats, insects, snakes, and other reptiles during storms and flooding can result in an increased incidence of bites. Diseases transmitted by rodents or sick animals may increase because of altered patterns of contact.

MORTALITY FROM
CYCLONES

Of the 1080 cyclones recorded
during 1980-2009, two thirds
of all deaths have occurred in
two cyclones:

TC Gorky, Bangladesh 1991,
138,866 deaths
TC Nargis, Myanmar 2008,
138,366 deaths

In developing nations, the rate of mortality is highest during the immediate impact phase, caused by drowning, structural collapse, and wind-borne debris [7]. In developed nations, the highest rate of mortality and morbidity occurs in the post-impact period attributed to electrocution and penetrating and blunt force trauma caused by fallen trees, and power lines, chainsaws, falls, and motor vehicle accidents.

Earthquakes and tsunamis

Earthquakes are due to a sudden release of energy from the earth's crust resulting in seismic activity. The magnitude of the energy released is ranked according to the Richter scale. Earthquakes with a magnitude of 3 are rarely felt and those with a magnitude > 7 often result in serious damage. In addition to ground shaking, earthquakes can cause tsunamis, landslides, fires from disruption of gas and power lines, soil liquefaction, and floods. These may result in significant injury and death, and damage to infrastructure.

Tsunamis are usually generated by movements in the sea floor creating a surge of water inundating land in coastal areas. A significant earthquake off the coast of Indonesia in 2004 generated a major tsunami. Fourteen countries were affected with an estimated death toll of 250,000 people. Large tsunamis can be incredibly destructive to the coastal zone, especially if the shape of the land funnels the water. For example, in Japan in 2011 the tsunami reached 40 meters above sea level on land after 10-metre-high waves struck the coast.

CASE STUDY 21.2 – GREAT EASTERN JAPAN EARTHQUAKE AND TSUNAMI, 11 MARCH 2011

Japan has a long history of earthquakes and tsunamis. With a multi-tier sophisticated earthquake and tsunami defense system and a well-educated population, Japan is well prepared to deal with the threat.

In March 2011, warnings were issued for a tremor predicted to be magnitude of 7.2. The earthquake was 100 times more severe measuring magnitude 9. Despite this, defenses held and damage was minimal.

Further warnings were issued for a tsunami. People were encouraged to get to higher ground or move to designated purpose-built evacuation centers. Japan's tsunami defenses were designed to withstand a mega-thrust event up to 12 meters: however, the 2011 tsunami was 40 meters. Evacuation centers were inundated, the multi-tiered defense system had failed catastrophically, due in part to the way the defenses funneled the flow of water.

Earthquakes tend to cause high mortality and numerous injuries associated with buildings and infrastructure collapse. In the 20th Century 1.87 million deaths occurred due to earthquakes [9], while the EM-DAT international disasters database reports 760,000 earthquake deaths from 2001 to March 2023 [10]. More deadly earthquakes occur at night, in densely populated areas, where residential housing is structurally weak.

EARTHQUAKES

The Pacific rim has experienced 81% of the world's largest earthquakes.

Major injuries from earthquakes include limb and spinal fractures, dislocations, crush injuries and head injuries. There are significantly more cases of minor injuries and wounds. The 2011 earthquake in Christchurch, New Zealand, caused 6,659 injuries and 182 deaths. Of those injured, the majority had soft tissue injuries and limb wounds. Christchurch Hospital and local general practices were overwhelmed with casualties immediately after the earthquake [11].

Earthquakes occur with little warning. Critical warning times for moving people to higher ground during tsunamis vary from minutes to hours. Casualties may present for treatment and overwhelm health services. If an earthquake or tsunami is large, health facility damage and disruption are likely. Damage to water and sewerage systems may increase the risk of **endemic** waterborne diseases including gastroenteritis. Surveillance for infectious disease outbreaks with pneumonia, diarrhea, and measles, is necessary, especially in densely populated regions of developing countries with lower vaccination rates and limited public health capacity. Sea-based tsunami early warning systems have been developed since the 2004 Indian Ocean tsunami in many countries.

Volcanic eruptions

A volcano is an opening or rupture in the earth's surface, that allows magma, volcanic ash, and gases to escape. A volcanic eruption occurs when lava, ash, gases, and ballistic projectiles are ejected, sometimes explosively. Volcanic ash is composed of fine particles of fragmented volcanic rock (< 2 mm diameter). The most common volcanic gas is water vapor. Other volcanic gases include carbon dioxide, sulfur dioxide, hydrogen chloride, carbon monoxide, and hydrogen fluoride. An estimated 1,500 potentially active volcanoes exist globally, with around 20 actively erupting on any day. Large-scale volcanic activity may last only a few days, but the massive outpouring of gases and ash can influence weather and land in the surrounding areas including contamination of air and water supplies resulting in displacement of populations for many years.

Health concerns after a volcanic eruption include respiratory illness, infectious disease, burns, injuries from volcanic projectiles, falls, trauma, death from roof collapse due to ash accumulation, and vehicle accidents due to the slippery, hazy conditions caused by ash. Effects depend on the distance from a volcano, magma viscosity, and gas concentrations. Although gases usually dissipate rapidly, people close to the volcano, or in low-lying areas downwind, may be exposed to levels that affect health, including irritation of the eyes, nose, throat, and skin, and may lead to dizziness, headache, or difficulty breathing. In a worst-case scenario (such as Pompei in 79AD) the population was overrun and suffocated by a "pyroclastic flow" of hot gas and ash traveling at high speed down the mountain.

Volcanic eruptions can result in secondary health threats, such as floods, landslides, thunderstorms, tsunamis, power outages, drinking water contamination, and wildfires. Management strategies include early warning and evacuation, public safety advice (e.g., provision of volcano hazard maps, and advice to avoid driving and protect eyes and lungs with goggles and masks), evacuation shelters, and prevention of excessive ash accumulation on roofs and roads.

Landslide/avalanches

A landslide is a rapid down-slope movement of rocks or soil mass under the force of gravity, often occurring when water seeps through the earth under a loose surface of unstable material, such as clay. An avalanche is a type of landslide involving a large mass of snow, ice, and rock debris, often initiated by an overload of fresh snowfall, vibrations from an earthquake, or even loud sounds. Landslides and avalanches are usually natural, but human activities like deforestation, mining, use of explosions, and vibrations from the traffic and machinery can induce landslides. Skiing can also trigger an avalanche.

Landslides and avalanches tend to grow in volume and mass as they accelerate downhill. The effects include uprooted trees and degraded soil, buried buildings and settlements, damage to crops and infrastructure such as roads, and injury and death of humans and animals. The impact is defined by the underlying geology, speed of flow, distance traveled, and generated debris.

The health effects include injury, illness, and death caused by rapidly moving water and debris; broken electrical, water, gas, and sewage lines; road accidents; and limited access to health care due to transport disruption.

Mitigating the risk of landslide and avalanche, in areas with steep slopes, destroyed vegetation, steep river channels, or where previous landslides have occurred, includes landslide hazard zonation mapping and landslide remediation (protecting forests and planting more trees to improve soil structure). Ski-cutting and boot-packing can help stabilize snow. Other management procedures include monitoring and early warning, enhancing awareness and education, and developing emergency and evacuation plans.

Drought

A drought is a period of below-average precipitation in a given region, resulting in prolonged shortages of water supply. Although drought accounts for around 5% of disaster occurrences, it affects 35% of disaster-affected populations worldwide. Between 2000 and 2019, an estimated 1.43 billion people were affected by drought [8]. The impact of drought and famine is compounded by issues of armed conflict and refugee forced displacement, often referred to as societal "fragility". See Chapter 25 – Complex Health Emergencies.

Droughts can last years and have extensive, long-term economic impacts resulting in negative health impacts and displacement of large sections of affected populations. The health effects from drought are difficult to document and quantify, with both direct and indirect effects that impact over time. The start and end dates of droughts are difficult to define. Drought morbidity and mortality are however thought to be high, particularly in developing countries, due to increased famine, poverty, and perpetuation of underdevelopment. Nutrition-related health effects of general malnutrition, micronutrient malnutrition, and anti-nutrient consumption, are some of the most prominent effects, due to agricultural failures, loss of livestock, and shortages of safe drinking water.

Dry soils and wildfires during a drought can cause dusty, dry air, which can exacerbate asthma, chronic airway disease, and cardiac failure. In developing countries an increased risk of communicable diseases may occur during drought. This may include water, air- and vector-borne diseases: water-related disease due to *salmonella*, *Escherichia coli*, *cholera*, and algal bloom; airborne infectious respiratory disease due to bacterial pathogens, fungal pathogens such as coccidioidomycosis, and poor air quality; and vector-borne disease, including malaria, dengue, West Nile virus, and St. Louis encephalitis, due to changing wildlife habitats and stagnant water reserves [12]. Psychological impacts of drought can also be significant, aggravated by financial hardship and resulting in increased rates of stress, depression, anxiety, and suicide.

The probability of drought-related health impacts varies widely and depends upon drought severity, baseline population vulnerability including conflict, existing health and sanitation infrastructure, and available resources [13]. Health management strategies include sanitation and hygiene education to reduce contamination and disease transmission, better monitoring of indirect health effects, and early warning systems to allow people to prepare better for water shortages. Risk reduction strategies to decrease the impact of drought could include building dams and canals, desalination of seawater, and redirecting rivers. Water management could be improved by promoting green buildings, capturing rainwater, and recycling water.

Bushfires

Bushfire, also known as wildfire, grassfire, or forest fire, is an uncontrolled, often rapidly spreading fire. Bushfires are a particularly dangerous hazardous at the wildland-urban interface. Causes of bushfires vary, including natural reasons such as lightning, or human activities such as campfires or controlled burns that escape. In rural areas, windstorm-damaged power cables can cause bushfires.

Major bushfires can result in severe loss of life as fast-moving fires isolate and trap people, as well as destroy power lines, communications, and other infrastructure. Fires can cause extensive damage to property, crops, domestic and wild animal stocks, and vegetation, increasing the financial and psychological burden on affected populations.

Bushfires produce copious quantities of smoke that may disperse over hundreds of kilometers and persist for months, depending on climatic conditions, topography, and vegetation sources. The most common health effects from bushfires are due to exposure to particulate matter in smoke causing an increased incidence of respiratory and cardiovascular ill-health (e.g., shortness of breath, itchy eyes, sore throat, runny nose, and coughing), and increased hospital presentations for asthma and chronic respiratory disease [14]. Bushfires may pose occupational health and safety risks for emergency responders. Anxiety, depression, and poorer sleep can occur in people affected by bushfires [15].

Management strategies for bushfires are directed at mitigation, early detection, and suppression. Mitigation focuses on appropriate land use planning and on fuel load reduction using controlled burning. Preparedness strategies include proper building design, construction of fire refuges, preparation of water storage, firefighting equipment, and personal protective kits. Early detection and warning, evacuation, controlled back burning, clearing of firebreaks, and suppression, are important during the response. Education and self-reliance are critical to strengthen individuals' ability to prevent harm and protect personal health.

CASE STUDY 21.3 – BUSHFIRES IN VICTORIA, FEBRUARY 2009

Tibbits et al. (2007) found that 78% of bushfire fatalities in Australia occurred outside or in an indefensible space.

However, in a bushfire in Victoria, Australia, in 2009, only 22 of the 173 deaths occurred when people were attempting to evacuate. The remaining 151 people died in houses or other buildings close to their homes. Seventeen of the deaths were people older than 80 years, with 23 deaths of people under 17 years old.

These fires caused a rethink of the concept of defensible space and the need to consider early evacuation for children, the elderly and frail, and pets at times of catastrophic fire conditions.

Source: Tibbits, A., J. Handmer, K. Haynes, T. Lowe, and J. Whittaker, Prepare, stay and defend or leave early: Evidence for the Australian approach, in *Community bushfire safety,* J. Handmer, and K. Haynes, Editors. Melbourne: CSIRO Publishing.

Heatwaves

The Australian Bureau of Meteorology defines a heatwave as three or more days in a row when both daytime and night-time temperatures are unusually high based on previous local climate. There is no single temperature level in the literature as a heatwave in one region, may be a normal temperature in another (e.g., an unusually hot 35°C day in London is a regular summer day in northern Australia). This is largely attributed to the adaptions inherent in the lived environment including the design of houses, buildings, and transport, the provision of air conditioning, and the adaption of the population. Heatwaves are considered the deadliest of natural disasters affecting thousands of people annually.

Those at the highest risk of death in heatwaves are the elderly, and those with cardio-respiratory disease, diabetes, or obesity. Heat impairs core body temperature regulation which is aggravated by dehydration [16]. Persons with psychiatric illness are another high-risk group during heatwaves. This is thought due to an inability to self-care, or the effects of neuroleptic drugs.

Heatwaves tend to be more predictable than other disasters, with governments developing strategies to mitigate the adverse effects. These revolve around early warning systems, public announcements with specific education on increasing hydration, maintaining a tolerable environmental temperature, and encouraging community support.

HEATWAVE
In a heatwave, the elderly are arguably the most vulnerable group.

During a heatwave, conduct daily welfare checks on elderly friends and neighbours, especially if they live alone.

Cadavers

Natural disasters are highly likely to result in increased mortality whether at the time of the disaster or in the aftermath. It is important that health-care personnel work closely with local communities to observe not only local customs but also to follow the correct legal processes, especially important when dealing with the deceased.

INFECTIOUS DISEASE MYTHS

Deaths caused by the traumatic forces of natural disasters, as opposed to deaths caused by contagious disease, do not lead to epidemics of infectious diseases.

There are unsubstantiated beliefs about health risks to the public in areas where there exist large numbers of deceased. Other than a few exceptional circumstances, dead bodies do not present an increased risk for infection. They do however present logistical and legal challenges.

Disaster warning complacency

Disaster warning complacency is people's tendency to ignore disaster warnings. People tend to believe a "low-probability high-impact" disaster won't happen, and so ignore the threat and fail to prepare. Complacency is different from poor awareness where people don't understand the risk or disaster warning. It is also different from poor preparedness.

Disaster warning complacency may be influenced by many factors, including an individual's capacity to prepare, their expectation of the level of damages, and their demographic status in gender, ethnicity, parenthood status, family connection, and possession of pets. Repeated threat warnings are another influencing factor as people who have already taken protective measures feel no need to undertake additional preparation.

Complacency needs to be managed because a complacent public is less prepared for emergencies. Government plays an important role in developing effective communication strategies to reduce this. Timely, accurate, authoritative, and reliable information is the key. It is preferably delivered through television, radio, and social media, with tailored messages to more vulnerable groups such as elders or children. Monitoring complacency is important to allow early management.

Developing a global response to natural disasters

The world is now more interconnected than ever, interdependent with flows of goods, capital, people, and ideas. In this globalized world, the impact of natural disasters goes far beyond directly affected regions, and a timely global response is often required.

Global response to natural disasters means mobilizing global efforts to tackle a natural disaster in an individual nation or region and requires alliances that bring together different perspectives, organizations, and skills. There are a number of existing international organizations working in the field of disaster response including the U.N. International Strategy for Disaster Reduction, the World Meteorological Organization, the International Federation of the Red Cross and Red Crescent Societies, Médecins Sans Frontières, and the International Tsunami Society. However, there is a need for better coordination and distribution of resources. It is an increasingly urgent global priority to develop the tools, processes, and best practices to manage natural disasters more effectively.

There are several key considerations to be considered while developing the global response and relief mechanisms to manage natural disasters. Firstly, information sharing among all countries, and establishment and dissemination of a standardized base of emergency management knowledge adaptable to local context. Secondly, establishing a global disaster surveillance and warning system, which will improve the capability of individual nations in disaster prevention and risk control. Thirdly, carrying out disaster prevention education and international emergency drills to improve the disaster-relief capabilities of individual nations and international organizations. Fourthly, setting up a long-term and effective international relief foundation and funding mechanism, such as the establishment of a global natural disaster insurance system.

CONCLUSION

When responding to a natural disaster it is important to understand not only the epidemiology of the injuries that are associated with specific disaster types, but also the pre-disaster health status of the affected population. This includes understanding the endemic disease patterns that already existed in the affected region and the known chronic health issues. Health responders should plan to treat the day-to-day health needs of the community that existed before the disaster.

Injuries suffered in natural disasters are often partially predictable. When these are considered with the pre-disaster health status of the population, a focused and more targeted health response can occur, which will not only avoid waste, but more importantly be directed toward benefitting those in greatest need of health services.

In developing countries, there is a likely increase in endemic communicable illnesses following natural disasters. Management of vaccine-preventable diseases requires the early establishment of surveillance systems to monitor and treat disease outbreaks, prompt population vaccination programs, and effective public health interventions such as restoration of clean water and sanitation services. These measures are likely to have the most impact on overall morbidity and mortality.

ACTIVITIES

1. Identify the natural disasters that affect your community and their risks. How would those risks vary in a less developed nation?
2. How should health services be reconfigured during a natural disaster to ensure the ongoing risks to the community are reduced?

KEY READINGS

Stanke, C., M. Kerac, C. Prudhomme, J. Medlock, V. Murray, Health effects of drought: A systematic review of the evidence. *Plos Currents*, 2013. 5(5):1–32.

Rydberg, H., G. Marrone, S. Stromdahl, and J. von Schreeb, A promising tool to assess long term public health effects of natural disasters: Combining routine health survey data and geographic information systems to assess stunting after the 2001 earthquake in Peru. *PLoS ONE,* 10(6): e0130889. http://dx.doi.org/10.1371/journal.pone.0130889

Dancause, K., D. Laplante, D. Hart, M. O'Hara, G. Elgbeili, A. Brunet, and S. King, Prenatal stress due to a natural disaster predicts adiposity in childhood: The Iowa flood study. Hindawi Publishing Corporation *Journal of Obesity,* **2015**, Article ID 570541, 10 pp. http://dx.doi.org/10.1155/2015/570541

Murray, V., A. Aitsi-Selmi, and K. Blanchard, The role of public health within the United Nations post 2015 framework for disaster risk reduction. *International Journal of Disaster Risk Science,* 2015. **6**:28–37. http://dx.doi.org/10.1007/s13753-015-0036-7

Note

1. With acknowledgment to previous authors Mark Little & Angie Jackson

References

1. Masson-Delmotte, V., et al., Global warming of 1.5 C. *An IPCC Special Report on the Impacts of Global Warming of,* 2018. **1**(5): p. 43–50.
2. Huntington, T.G., Climate warming-induced intensification of the hydrologic cycle: An assessment of the published record and potential impacts on agriculture. *Advances in Agronomy,* 2010. **109**: p. 1–53.
3. The Earth Observatory. *The impact of climate change on natural disasters.* 2005; Available from: https://earthobservatory.nasa.gov/features/RisingCost/rising_cost5.php.
4. Shannon, S., et al., Global glacier volume projections under high-end climate change scenarios. *The Cryosphere,* 2019. **13**(1): p. 325–350.

5. Polonsky J, Luquero F, Francois G, Rousseau C, Caleo G, Ciglenecki I, Delacre C, Siddiqui MR, Terzian M, Verhenne L, Porten K, Checchi F. Public health surveillance after the 2010 haiti earthquake: the experience of médecins sans frontières. *PLoS Currents*. 2013 Jan 7.5:ecurrents. dis.6aec18e84816c055b8c2a06456811c7a. doi: 10.1371/currents.dis.6aec18e84816c055b8c2a0 6456811c7a. PMID: 23330069; PMCID: PMC3544554

6. Pan American Health Organization. *Natural disasters: Protecting the public's health.* 2000, Washington DC: PAHO/WHO.

7. Shultz, J.M., J. Russell, and Z. Espinel, Epidemiology of tropical cyclones: The dynamics of disaster, disease, and development. *Epidemiologic Reviews*, 2005. **27**(1): p. 21–35.

8. Centre for Research on the Epidemiology of Disasters. *Human cost of disasters: An overview of the last 20 years (2000–2019).* 2020, Brussels (BE): Centre for Research on the Epidemiology of Disasters (CRED) and UN Office for Disaster Risk Reduction.

9. Doocy S, Daniels A, Packer C, Dick A, Kirsch TD. The human impact of earthquakes: a historical review of events 1980-2009 and systematic literature review. PLoS Curr. 2013 Apr 16;5:ecurrents.dis.67bd14fe457f1db0b5433a8ee20fb833. doi: 10.1371/currents.dis.67bd14fe457f1db0b5 433a8ee20fb833. PMID: 23857161; PMCID: PMC3644288

10. Guha-Sapir, D., R. Below, and P.H. Hoyois, *EM-DAT: The CRED/OFDA international disaster database.* Available from: www.emdat.be

11. Ardagh, M.W., et al., The initial health-system response to the earthquake in Christchurch, New Zealand, in February, 2011. *The Lancet*, 2012. **379**(9831): p. 2109–2115.

12. Yang, L., D. Han, and B. Jiang, Drought and human health: A review of recent studies. *Journal of Environmental Health*, 2013. **30**(5): p. 453–455.

13. Stanke, C., et al., Health effects of drought: A systematic review of the evidence. *PLoS Currents*, 2013. 5.

14. Johnston, F.H., et al., Unprecedented health costs of smoke-related PM2. 5 from the 2019–20 Australian megafires. *Nature Sustainability*, 2021. **4**(1): p. 42–47.

15. Rodney, R.M., et al., Physical and mental health effects of bushfire and smoke in the Australian Capital Territory 2019–20. *Frontiers in Public Health*, 2021. **9**: p. 682402.

16. Kovats, R.S., S. Hajat, and P. Wilkinson, Contrasting patterns of mortality and hospital admissions during hot weather and heat waves in Greater London, UK. *Occupational and Environmental Medicine*, 2004. **61**(11): p. 893–898.

22

Manmade (technological) disasters

Carissa Oh, Stefan M. Mazur, and Peter Logan

INTRODUCTION AND OBJECTIVES

The terminology of natural versus manmade disasters generates considerable debate. Natural disasters, for example, earthquakes, cyclones, and floods, imply unavoidable occurrences, but effects can be mitigated with preparation and planning. Manmade or technological disasters are events caused by system failures, which may include human negligence, and, as a consequence should be preventable through legislation and regulation. These often affect large numbers of people.

On completion of this chapter, you should be able to:

1. Identify the risks posed by manmade disasters.
2. Demonstrate an understanding of the particular clinical and logistic issues associated with different types of manmade events.
3. Discuss the particular management strategies required to prepare for, and respond to, such events.

INDUSTRIAL DISASTERS

An industrial disaster can be defined as the release or spill of a hazardous material (hazmat) from an industrial source that results in an abrupt and serious disruption of the functioning of a society, causing widespread human, material, or environmental losses that exceed the ability of the affected society to cope using only its own resources [1]. It includes fires, accidental emissions, and explosions due to chemical mixtures or gas, with resultant release of radiation or toxic substances.

Industrial disasters may be the consequence of system failure, mechanical failure, negligence, incompetence, or a deliberate act of sabotage. Irrespective of the cause, the outcome may result in significant morbidity and mortality, often accompanied by significant damage to both property and the environment. These disasters may result in economic and social consequences for individuals and the community, in both the short and long term. For example, the Exxon Valdez oil spill in 1989 killed thousands of birds, marine life,

DOI: 10.4324/9781032626604-29

and wildlife. Three decades on, not all species have completely recovered and there are still remnants of crude oil on some Alaskan beaches.

Advances in technology and engineering, combined with occupational health and safety legislation, have created safer work environments and reduced risk for communities living near industrial facilities. However, in some developing countries, production costs (including labour costs) are cheap, attracting foreign companies to establish hazardous industry there. Unfortunately, these countries often have less developed occupational health and safety systems, and operations may occur far below the standards found in places with more stringent safety regulations.

Prevention and preparedness

All industrial sites must have an incident management plan for dealing with emergencies. Plans need to address all conceivable incidents, including those considered low probability [2]. Arrangements for incident management and response need to include both the site operator and external agencies. If decontamination is required, for example, due to a chemical, biological, radiological, or nuclear incident, the logistics of how, where and when this will be performed, and who will be responsible, must be pre-planned.

All organisations are required to keep a safety data sheet (SDS) for chemicals used, stored, or manufactured in the workplace. This is an international legislative requirement. The SDS is often prepared by the manufacturer and provides information such as the physical data, safe handling, potential hazards, and emergency procedures for dealing with each substance on site. This can be a useful source of information following an incident involving chemicals especially where decontamination needs to be considered. The SDS should be easily and immediately available for any responding resource.

For large-scale industries manufacturing hazardous chemicals, or for nuclear facilities, emergency plans may need to incorporate guidance from international agencies. This guidance may include the criteria and policies for immediate actions, longer-term actions, and plans for returning to normal.

Response and recovery

Following an industrial accident there needs to be a clear understanding of who will be responsible for implementing the emergency response, and what this response will be. This is necessary not only for the safety of the emergency responders but also for the well-being of the public. Confusing and contradictory public statements will erode public trust and may result in further harm, especially to those living in areas around the industrial site who may need to be evacuated.

The environmental risks and hazards associated with certain industries (e.g., nuclear) may mean that it is unsafe for untrained external rescue personnel to enter such an environment following an incident. It may be the responsibility of the site operator familiar with the environment to manage the hazards and extricate the injured. Arrangements for command and control of the site need to be determined well in advance of any incident.

Industrial disasters may have both immediate and long-term consequences. While fires and explosions may cause immediate traumatic injuries, in some situations, the consequences of an incident may only become apparent following increased deaths of local livestock or wildlife, as occurred with the 1976 Seveso (Italy) dioxin release. The effects of chemical and radiation exposure on humans may not become evident for many years. This may affect not only those living around the site but also emergency response workers and receiving healthcare facility staff who may be exposed.

Following large-scale industrial disasters, it is important that long-term health surveillance is conducted for all those potentially exposed. The aim is to monitor the long-term effects and to address complications which may arise. This includes a higher risk of haematological and solid organ malignancies (such as leukaemia and thyroid cancer). The mental health impact of an industrial disaster must also be considered.

Industrial disasters can have socioeconomic consequences. Companies may attempt to cover up or dissociate themselves from any legal or ethical responsibility (Bhopal, India 1984). A critical incident may result in the closure of the affected industry. This can be a double blow to the local community affected by the physical and environmental consequences of the initial disaster as well as the economic and social consequences that the closure of a major industry brings.

STRUCTURAL DISASTERS

Structural integrity is a vital consideration in the design and construction of any structure. It is the ability of a structure (and its individual components) to withstand and operate under the pressure of a load, for which it was designed and intended, without breaking or deforming. Structural failure (for example, building collapse, dam failure, bridge, and road collapse) results from loss of structural integrity. This will lead to injuries, fatalities, and economic loss in addition to the consequences of the absence of the structure and any environmental impact associated with its collapse.

Structural failures usually occur as a result of:

- Structural and design deficiencies
- Structural deterioration – corrosion, fatigue, wear, rot, creep
- Substandard or defective construction materials
- Human error or accident during construction
- Maintenance failure
- Overload or impact
- Effects of a natural disaster or act of terrorism

Prevention and preparedness

Advances in design, engineering and technology have resulted in the construction of structures which have evolved with the times. Reminiscent of the Olympic motto Citius, Altius, Fortius, these structures have been constructed to longer lengths, greater heights and are capable of bearing heavier loads than what has been previously possible. Legislation has ensured that these structures are required to comply with strict regulations, making them safer and reducing the possibility of collapse or failure. For example, buildings constructed in earthquake-prone areas of New Zealand, whilst constructed according to the relevant building codes at the time, have been identified as requiring further works to reinforce them and reduce the risk of collapse if an earthquake were to occur.

CASE STUDY 22.1 – CHRISTCHURCH, NEW ZEALAND

The Pyne Gould Corporation (PGC) Building in Christchurch, New Zealand was designed in 1963 and constructed to meet the seismic design loadings applicable at the time [Beca 2011]. In 1997, an assessment of the building's earthquake resilience was undertaken which demonstrated significant shortfalls with respect to the loading standards current at that time. In 1998, major refurbishment occurred to enhance the building's vertical load-carrying capacity but no additional horizontal resistance was added. While no structural damage occurred following smaller earthquakes, the PGC building suffered a pancake collapse in a 6.3 magnitude earthquake on 22 February 2011, killing 18 people in that building alone (Figure 22.1).

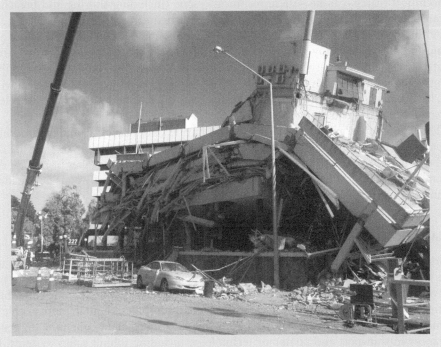

Figure 22.1 PGC building Photo by Carissa Oh

While structural failure may be unpredictable, the risk can be mitigated by routine inspections and preventative maintenance. Regular inspections are less expensive than major repairs and may detect small problems at an early stage. Unattended, minor issues may cumulatively result in greater, more costly problems which can lead to greater disruption when urgent repairs are required, or the structure fails altogether. This does not include the impact of injuries or fatalities that may occur, nor the impact on the community. Unfortunately, there may be a reluctance to allocate funds for preventative maintenance due to competing priorities.

Response and recovery

The collapse of any major structure, whether it be a building, road, bridge, or dam, will potentially result in many casualties. Many of these casualties will be crushed by the collapsed materials, although some may be trapped in voids and take some time to access. Depending on the nature of the incident, the initial response phase may be protracted. Safety concerns and the potential for further collapse may delay casualty access. If critical infrastructure is affected (for example, a bridge or major road), this may limit emergency service personnel, including Urban Search and Rescue (USAR) teams from responding to the scene.

Whilst beyond the scope of this chapter, USAR teams play a key role in dealing with the immediate consequences of a structural collapse, irrespective of the cause. USAR teams may be accredited regionally, nationally, or internationally. They can operate remotely in austere conditions and be self-sufficient. Team members may provide specialist expertise in technical search, canine search, technical rescue (including shoring and breaching), hazardous materials, emergency medical skills and engineering.

At the scene of any major incident, safety is paramount. This includes the safety of the scene and the safety of any survivors. A safety officer should be designated to ensure the safety of responding emergency personnel. This person will be responsible not only for identifying hazards (which may include smoke, airborne dust, exposed electrical wiring, gas, hazardous materials, and fire) but also for ensuring that responders have the relevant personal protective equipment.

The failure or collapse of any structure will have economic, social, and environmental impacts for some time afterwards. Investigations and a detailed analysis into the cause of the structural failure will need to occur to prevent the same mistakes from happening again. The design of the new structure will need to be very carefully considered and the rebuilding and recovery phase may be protracted.

TRANSPORT DISASTERS (MARINE, RAIL, ROAD, AND AIR)

Worldwide population growth, coupled with increasing population mobility, primarily due to advances in transport technology and capabilities has increased the total number of people exposed to the risk of a transport-related disaster at any one time. Bigger planes, faster trains, busier roads, cheaper cars, and motorbikes, result in more people (not to mention increased amounts of dangerous freight) mobile at any one time. In general, advances in transport and computer technology, including inbuilt safety systems, have made most modes of transport in the developed world intrinsically safer but when a significant incident does occur it can be catastrophic in its consequences due to the size and speed of the transport platform involved.

In developing economies where safety regulations may be less stringent and maintenance requirements less regulated, overcrowding, particularly on public mass transport platforms remains a problem. This, combined with inadequate safety equipment (such as insufficient life jackets on ferries) and poorly maintained infrastructure (roads and railways) all contributes to preventable mortality from major transport incidents.

Prevention and preparedness

Terrorism-inspired targeting of mass transport services (e.g., the Lockerbie disaster in 1988, the Twin Towers and Pentagon on 11 September 2001, the Madrid train bombings in 2004, the London underground bombings in 2005) have resulted in increased transport security vigilance, most notably at airports with increased passenger and luggage screening. The same security processes are less apparent on rail and bus services as the cost would cripple commuter systems worldwide, which leaves them as softer potential targets.

Commercial airports have rehearsed mass casualty plans and undertake real-time major incident scenarios regularly as dictated by legislation (e.g., Federal Aviation Administration Certification requirements Part 139). This will invariably involve the scenario of a catastrophic aeroplane failure somewhere in the boundaries of the airport and the use of emergency services in a real-time response involving infrastructure damage and simulated casualties. However, this type of mandated simulated major incident is much less likely to occur with other passenger transport modalities and dangerous freight transport.

Response and recovery

Transport disasters are often the result of environmental factors such as inclement weather or rugged geography. A consequence of this is that the conditions that contribute to incident causation can play a major role in the effectiveness of incident response. Poor environmental road conditions (i.e., snow, ice, flood) and challenging topography (i.e., tunnels, twisting narrow mountainous roads) will result in difficult access for emergency services in response to a major traffic incident. The 1999 Mont Blanc Tunnel fire is a classic example [3, 4]. This incident resulted in significant tunnel construction legislation change. Similarly, water transport based major incidents will often have significant adverse environmental conditions, which along with the added difficulty of sourcing appropriate rescue resources (rescue capable helicopters and boats) make adequate emergency response difficult. Extreme weather conditions, such as storm weather in the Yangtze Ferry disaster in 2015 (over 400 dead) and freezing water in the Zeebrugge Ferry disaster [5] in 1987 (193 dead) add significantly to rescue and response difficulties, and undoubtedly contribute to fatality rates. Compare the mortality rates of these incidents with that of the Costa Concordia Cruise ship incident (13 January 2012) which occurred in relatively benign environmental conditions resulting in a proportionally lesser loss of 34 lives of the over 4000 people onboard.

Transport disaster management can also be compromised by conflicts around accountability and responsibility for incident response. When is it the responsibility of the transport operator to manage the incident and its consequences versus when do externally designated rescue services have responsibility? Business and financial interests can create potential for conflict of interest with regards to incident management and communication. Often the size of the incident and complexity of the incident (or alternatively pre-ordained legislation or government regulation) will dictate where responsibilities lie. In transport-related incidents managed by external rescue and response services, the transport operator will be required to fit into the command-and-control structure for the incident management. This can create problems around conflict of interest and willingness to submit to an externally dictated hierarchy.

MASS GATHERINGS

The World Health Organisation defines a mass gathering as "an organised or unplanned event where the number of people attending is sufficient to strain the planning and response resources of the community, state or nation holding the event". A mass gathering may be of a sporting, religious, political, or cultural nature.

While some definitions specify the size of the crowd, this is simply a number and does not reflect a myriad of other factors that influence the impact of an event on the community or the capability to manage the number of people present.

Most mass gatherings are planned events. This allows for pre-event planning which is crucial to facilitating good crowd management, ensuring timely treatment and transport of the ill or injured and minimising the impact of the gathering on local health facilities.

Without prior event preparation and planning, any adverse incident, whether it be for an individual or a crowd, will result in significantly worse outcomes for those affected.

Prevention and preparedness

To fail to plan is to plan to fail and mass gatherings are no exception. When a large group of people gather, there is always the potential for the occurrence of a catastrophic event, including acts of terrorism.

While it may be difficult to predict if, what, or when, a major incident may occur, a risk assessment must be performed prior to the event to identify and mitigate risks and develop a response plan. This should involve extensive collaboration with key stakeholders, including government agencies, non-government organisations, emergency services, health organisations (including the public health authority) and the organisers of the event. Box 22.1 provides an overview of the issues to be considered as part of the risk assessment during the planning phase of a mass gathering event.

Risk assessment considerations for mass gathering planning

Type of event

- Sporting/religious/cultural/political
- Single or recurrent event
- Ticketed or unticketed
- Duration

Location

- Size and capacity of the site
- Temporary or permanent structure
- Indoors or outdoors
- Static (either seated or standing) or mobile
- Contained (fenced) or unbounded
- Access to the site (including clearly marked ingress and egress routes)
- Accessibility and topography within the site

Population

- Expected size of the crowd
- Demographics – age, potential for pre-existing health problems, socioeconomic status

- Presence of high-profile figures
- Mood, motives and behaviour of the crowd
- Availability of alcohol and illicit drugs

Environmental factors

- Day, time of day and season
- Weather – temperature, humidity, precipitation
- Toilets, sanitation and hand-washing facilities
- Local infrastructure – transport, health resources and facilities

Public health

- Surveillance for communicable diseases
- Potential for imported diseases
- Food and water safety
- Health messaging including pre-event health requirements such as vaccinations

Other factors to consider

- Command and control
- Communication
- Security
- Mass Casualty response plan

Each mass gathering will be different in terms of purpose, size, and population attending however an emergency management plan may already exist for high-risk venues or for recurring events. Examples of these include plans for sporting and concert venues and events such as religious gatherings (for example, pilgrimage to the Hajj, World Youth Day) and mass community events such as fun runs and New Year's Eve celebrations. It is important to ensure that all personnel on-site are aware of the emergency management plan and that the plan has been tested and exercised as part of the continuous quality improvement cycle for each event. This includes testing emergency evacuation procedures (Figure 22.2).

Figure 22.2 The plan do act check cycle

Response and recovery

Most mass gathering events have encountered 0.5–2 casualties per 1,000 attendees [6]. The provision of medical services at a mass gathering needs to be tailored to the type and complexity of the event as well as the number of attendees and the predicted medical problems that may be encountered. This will determine the resources required. Staff may range from first-aid providers and paramedics at mobile or static first-aid posts to nurses and doctors running a medical centre or field hospital.

Approximately 80% of patient presentations to healthcare services at mass gatherings consist of respiratory illnesses, minor injuries, heat-related injuries, and minor problems (such as headache, blisters, and sunburn) [7]. More than 95% of presentations are classified as mild and do not require transport to hospital [8]. Without prior planning, local health facilities may be burdened by increased presentations, which could effectively be managed on-site, largely by first aid personnel.

All health personnel employed at a mass gathering must be aware of their primary healthcare role, as well as how their role may change should the situation rapidly evolve from normal operations to a major incident. A catastrophic event may incite panic and will rapidly overwhelm on-site medical resources, the local health facilities, and emergency services. Plans for evacuating and managing the uninjured as well as the injured need to be established before the event. An all-hazards approach needs to be adopted for dealing with mass gatherings. The response to such an event may require the activation of disaster plans and the mobilisation of state and national resources.

MASS TRAUMA AND BURNS EVENTS

Mass trauma events involving mass burns place unique challenges on clinicians and trauma systems and are a classic example of the requirements for a whole of system approach. A mass casualty trauma and burns event is often the result of fire in a high-density urban dwelling or explosion at a mass gathering, mining site or off-shore oil rig. In terrorism-related improvised explosive device (IED) events, up to 15% of live casualties have severe burn injuries. The nature of severe burns-related injury dictates their management in specialist burns centres (generally located in major metropolitan centres), especially if there is accompanying respiratory or ventilatory compromise. The relatively low frequency of significant burn injuries in most developed economies means any individual institution's capacity to manage large numbers of burn patients is limited. For example, following the 2002 Bali bombing nearly all of Australia's adult burn beds were occupied.

Prevention and preparedness

Any detailed mass casualty plan should include specific details relating to the management of casualties with severe burns. Given the capacity limitations of individual burns centres, the matching of patient requirements to burns resources may see the need for patients to be distributed across regional, national or potentially international burns capabilities. This will have a significant impact on retrieval resources for those patients requiring critical care level support and this should be considered in any planning undertaken in preparation for a mass burns event.

Response and recovery

Management of mass trauma events with mass burns must factor in the mechanism of the burn injury. The incident could be explosion with concomitant blunt or penetrating trauma injuries, chemical burns with need for decontamination, enclosed space incident increasing the risk of carbon monoxide toxicity, or hydrogen cyanide exposure.

Whilst classical management of patients with potential airway burns dictates early definitive airway management with intubation and ventilation, this may not be feasible or desirable in a mass burns event with limited availability of transport ventilators and increased demand for ventilation gas (pressurised oxygen cylinders). In these circumstances, delaying or limiting initial fluid resuscitation to limit initial airway and facial swelling should be considered, with the clinical trade-off of increased incidence of renal failure and/or gut ischaemia downstream.

Traditional burns fluid resuscitation teaching (modified Parkland Formula) requires a significant amount of fluid resuscitation particularly in the first eight hours depending on the percentage of body surface area affected. This volume of fluid may be unavailable initially due to the number of patients affected and transport limitations. Receiving centres will find themselves having to play catch-up depending on transport times from the scene to receiving hospitals.

Although full-thickness burns are generally painless, associated partial-thickness burns will require high doses of analgesia. Any patients who are intubated and ventilated for impending airway or respiratory failure will also have high analgesic requirements as invariably they have a normal underlying conscious state. These analgesic and fluid requirements should be factored into resource requirements for responding teams. In patients with ventilatory compromise as the result of full-thickness chest burns or compromised limb perfusion due to circumferential burns, medical response teams will need to have the equipment and clinical expertise to undertake emergent escharotomies, particularly if transport time will be prolonged.

As age and the percentage of body surface area burn involvement increase, so too does mortality, both short-term and long-term. Whilst the expectant category is not generally used in civilian triage, it is worth considering how patients with severe burns (both nature and extent) will be managed when resources are limited and the number of casualties overwhelming.

CONCLUSION

Manmade or technological disasters are events that particularly suggest the need for a systems approach to disaster management due to the potential contribution of human negligence in some incidents. Morbidity and mortality from some incidents may be reducible through careful planning and preparedness, including through legislation and regulation.

ACTIVITIES

The Beirut Port Disaster in 2020 occurred when a stockpile of ammonium nitrate stored in a warehouse at Beirut Port exploded. The explosion killed more than 200 people, injured 7000, and displaced over 300,000 people.

1. How would you categorise this disaster?
2. Can you identify actions that could have been undertaken from a prevention and preparedness approach to reduce morbidity and mortality from this incident?

KEY READINGS

Public health for mass gatherings: Key considerations 2015. Available at: https://www.who.int/publications/i/item/public-health-for-mass-gatherings-key-considerations

United Nations Office for the Coordination of Humanitarian Affairs (OCHA). INSARAG guidelines 2020. https://www.insarag.org/methodology/insarag-guidelines/

References

1. Keim, M.E., The public health impact of industrial disasters. American Journal of Disaster Medicine, 2011. 6(5): p. 265–274.
2. McKenna, T., E. Buglova, and V. Kutkov, Lessons learned from Chernobyl and other emergencies: Establishing international requirements and guidance. Health Physics, 2007. 93(5): p. 527–537.
3. Fraser-Mitchell, J. and D. Charters, Human behaviour in tunnel fire incidents. Fire Safety Science, 2005. 8: p. 543–554.
4. Duffe, P. and M. Marec, M. and Cialdini, P., Joint report of the Italian and French administrative commissions of enquiry into the disaster that occurred on 24 March 1999 in the Mont Blanc Tunnel. République Française, Ministère de l'intérieur et Ministère de l'Equipment, du Transport et du Logement, Repubblica Italiana, Ministero dei Lavori Pubblici, 6 July 1999.
5. United Kingdom Government, The Merchant Shipping Act 1894, mv Herald of Free Enterprise, D.o. Transport, Editor. 1987, London: HMSO.
6. De Lorenzo, R.A., Mass gathering medicine: A review. Prehospital and Disaster Medicine, 1997. 12(1): p. 68–72.
7. Arbon, P., Mass-gathering medicine: A review of the evidence and future directions for research. Prehospital and Disaster Medicine, 2007. 22(2): p. 131–135.
8. Locoh-Donou, S., et al., Mass-gathering medicine: A descriptive analysis of a range of mass-gathering event types. The American Journal of Emergency Medicine, 2013. 31(5): p. 843–846.

23

Conflict, terrorism, and CBRNE

David Heslop and Sarah Hockaday

CONFLICT, TERRORISM AND CBRNE WEAPONS

Military operations involving risk from chemical, biological, radiological, nuclear and explosive (CBRNE) weapons, hazardous materials, or industrial activities, require special categorisation systems. Toxic hazards that fall into the highest risks to humans are identified in the CBRNE classification system. The system has evolved historically from systems used to operate in extreme environments. Equally, alternate systems of classification have replaced nuclear considerations with incendiary devices (CBRIE – chemical, biological, radiological, incendiary, and explosive). Such modifications are helpful in focusing on planning, preparation, and operational response in specific contexts.

CBRNE threats are a subset of the wider group of hazards that include Toxic Industrial Chemicals and Materials, physical hazards, biological hazards, and psychosocial hazards (see Figure 23.1). The CBRNE classification system also includes various types of explosive or special dissemination devices, often used together with CBRNE agents. The key hazards of concern within the CBRNE classification system share the following characteristics:

i. the ability to be utilised deliberately for terrorist, military, political, or strategic purposes,
ii. exert their negative effects on humans via toxic exposure, often coupled with other hazardous effects, and
iii. fall outside conventional weaponry classification systems.

CBRNE agents were progressively grouped across the early 20th century as they were researched and then employed in the field. Some CBRNE agents have a legitimate use in economic, industrial, or military contexts. An example of legitimate industrial use is the chemical Phosgene, used to manufacture polyurethane and polycarbonate plastics.

DOI: 10.4324/9781032626604-30

On completion of this chapter you should be able to:

1. Understand how CBRNE weapons fit within the broader context of human hazards with a special focus on conflicts and terrorism.
2. Understand how CBRNE weapons relate to conventional and unconventional warfare.
3. Identify examples of and special features of major CBRN weapons.
4. Reflect on the various psychological factors involved in terrorism.

CBRNE AND MODERN WARFARE

While the use of hazardous substances in warfare is not new, the scale of use of CBRNE agents against populations and the environment is a relatively new development. Chemical and biological agents have been employed for millennia – the use of burning pitch, catapulting infected corpses into citadels, and assassination through poison were commonplace but affected small numbers. With industrialisation, mass production, and large-scale manufacturing of chemical substances, cheaper and larger quantities of CBRNE agents became accessible. The First World War saw the first mass use of these weapons, with subsequent international condemnation and prohibition. This led to the conceptual distinction between historical (conventional) warfare, defined as the use of kinetic methods (ballistic) and direct inter-personal combat, compared with unconventional warfare, employing special tactics falling outside historical norms or acceptable conduct in warfare such as the use of CBRNE weapons. The use of CBRNE agents in warfare has been universally declared in various international fora as an atrocity (war crime) and in certain circumstances a crime against humanity.

Consequently, international agreements impose strict requirements, accountabilities, and punitive sanctions on nation states who either possess, seek to proliferate, or use CBRNE agents. Some of the key international agreements are the Chemical Weapons Convention, Biological Weapons Convention, Australia Group, Cartagena Protocol, and various regional non-proliferation arrangements. In the Chemical and Nuclear domains there has been significant success in promoting disarmament and de-proliferation, reducing the risk of accidental or deliberate escalation into unconventional conflict. This has been the focus of intensive diplomatic efforts over many years and the establishment of key agreements such as the Nuclear Non-Proliferation Treaty. Other agreements have focused on safeguarding barriers to proliferation such as controls on the export of technology, know-how, and personnel, critical to establishing the industrial base required to develop and manufacture CBRNE agents. This includes limitations on enabling technologies to deliver and disperse CBRNE agents "in the field" such as missile, packaging, dispersal, and explosive technologies. Recently, non-State actors, such as individuals or terrorist organisations, with no interest or knowledge of the historical norms and agreements of modern warfare, have utilised CBRNE agents to achieve their military or political aims. These emerging risks present new challenges to the international community for regulation and strategic CBRNE risk management.

CBRNE weapons and dissemination

CBRNE weapons require a form of dissemination to expose individuals or populations. The 1978 assassination of Georgi Markov with the biological toxin ricin was

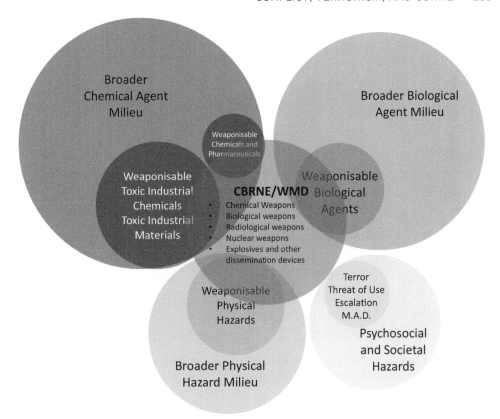

Figure 23.1 Relationships between physical hazards, weaponizable hazards, and CBRNE hazards. Mutually Assured Destruction (M.A.D.)

disseminated utilising an umbrella concealed injection system. Alternatively, chemical agents are often combined with explosive ordnance to disperse the hazardous substance over a population, such as seen since 2012 in the Syrian conflict. Explosive effects such as trauma may also be seen as desirable to increase the lethality and effect of a CBRNE weapon. However, in other cases, dissemination of agents can occur through environmental processes (e.g., wind) as seen in the Sverdlovsk anthrax accident in 1979. Improvised dissemination, using plastic bags pierced with umbrella tips containing Sarin (GB) was utilised in the Tokyo Subway attacks. Highly sophisticated methods, such as concealed perfume bottle sprayers, were used for Novichok nerve agent attacks in Salisbury, UK in 2018 (see Figure 23.2).

Explosives generate localised areas of pressure, usually through the compression of reacting substances. This can be achieved through pure chemical (e.g., TNT), mixed chemical and mechanical (e.g., thermobaric device), mechanical (e.g., motorised spray dispersal device) or nuclear (e.g., a two-stage thermonuclear device). Thus, the selection of method of dispersal is an important consideration when developing CBRNE weapons, and many nations have spent considerable resources on perfecting these systems.

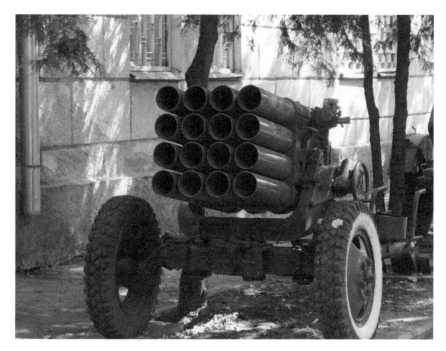

Figure 23.2 Example of a CBRNE agent dissemination: an artillery rocket launcher similar to the one used in Syria to launch Sarin-loaded rockets at civilian targets in Damascus (Vlad/CC By 3.0)

CBRNE: CHEMICAL, BIOLOGICAL, RADIOLOGICAL AGENTS IN WEAPONS OF MASS DESTRUCTION

The following section outlines the broad categories of CBRNE agents seen in Weapons of Mass Destruction. Examples of more prominent agents are provided with their NATO abbreviations provided in brackets. Further details about the agents presented and other CBR agents can be found in the references outlined in the bibliography.

CHEMICAL WEAPONS

During World War I chemical weapons were mass-produced and utilised *en masse* as weapons of war. On April 22 1915 Germany released 150 tons of chlorine gas (CL) on the battlefront at Ypres, Belgium killing an estimated 800 allied soldiers. It is estimated that mustard (HN) utilisation during WWI caused 400,000 injuries, 8,000 deaths, and innumerable long-term disabilities such as blindness, scarring, and respiratory dysfunction. Since that time chemical weapons have been used on populations many times. The Tokyo subway Sarin attack in 1995 by the terrorist group, Aum Shinrikyo, marked the first use of a chemical warfare agent by a terrorist organisation and resulted in 5,500 injuries and 11 deaths. On August 21 2013, during the Syrian conflict, Volcano missiles carrying Sarin were deployed upon the city of Ghouta killing an estimated 1,017 civilians. This section serves as a brief introduction to notable chemical weapons. Table 23.1 outlines the categories of chemical warfare agents.

Exemplar CBRNE Agent

Table 23.1 Categories of chemical warfare agents and exemplar agents, some of which have specific medical countermeasures or antidotes

Chemical warfare agent category	Well known examples	NATO abbreviation of examples	Specific medical countermeasure or antidote
Nerve agents			
	Sarin	GB	Oxime, atropine
	Soman	GD	Oxime, atropine
	VX	VX	Oxime, atropine
	Novichok	various	None
Vesicants or "blister agents"			
	Mustard	HN, HD	
	Lewisite	L	Dimercaprol
Cyanide like agents or "blood agents"			
	Hydrogen Cyanide	AC	Thiosulfate, nitrite, Hydroxycobalamin
Pulmonary agents or "choking agents" and irritants			
	Phosgene	CG	None
	Chlorine	CL	None
Incapacitants and sedatives			
	Fentanyl derivatives		Naloxone
	Inhaled anesthetics		None
	3-Quinuclidinyl benzilate	BZ	None
Riot control agents			
	Tear Gas	CS	None
	Pepper Spray	OC	None

NERVE AGENTS

Nerve agents are potent organophosphate chemicals, that work by binding to special enzymes within nerve synapses leading to an excess of the neurotransmitter acetylcholine. The resulting cholinergic syndrome causes neurological, cardiac, and respiratory effects. Without treatment symptoms rapidly progress, over minutes, to seizures, paralysis, coma, and death. **"G" series agents** are generally volatile, or easily dispersed, and include examples such as Sarin (GB) and Soman (GD). **"V" series and Novichok** agents are a more recently developed class of nerve agents. VX is the most well-known of these agents and is referred to as a "persistent agent" due to its ability to linger for long periods in the environment.

Exemplar CBRNE Agent

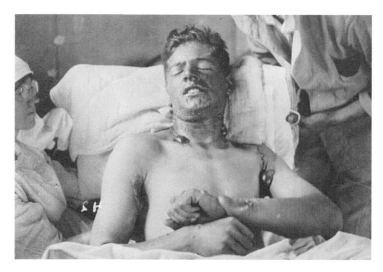

Figure 23.3 Injuries due to Mustard exposure in a soldier (Library and Archives Canada, C-080027/ Bibliothèque et Archives Canada, C-080027)

CHEMICAL AGENT – MUSTARD

"Mustard gas" (HN and HD) is a liquid chemical agent at room temperature that can be easily dispersed through vapourisation and has a characteristic odour of garlic. Direct contact with human tissue causes DNA alkylation and destruction resulting in the characteristic damage to the exposed skin and eyes, and delayed blistering of exposed skin and lung damage. Absorption into the bloodstream leads to systemic toxicity causing delayed bone marrow suppression, sepsis, and death. Inhalation can also cause rapid lung tissue destruction and impaired gas exchange that can be lethal within hours (see Figure 23.3).

Lewisite (L) is an arsenic-containing liquid vesicant which can be vapourised as a colourless and odourless gas. Inhalation can cause rapid pulmonary oedema and high mortality. Lower-dose systemic absorption occurs more rapidly than mustard causing comparatively greater pain and local tissue damage.

CYANIDES

Hydrogen Cyanide (AC) is a highly volatile gas, the archetypal "non-persistent" agent, which is readily obtainable in most industrialised communities. During WWII, hydrogen cyanide gas was used by the Japanese during invasions of Chinese territories, and hydrocyanic acid granules or "Zyklon B", from which hydrogen cyanide gas is produced as a fumigant, was used by the Nazis in concentration camps. Hydrogen cyanide gas has a subtle bitter almond odour and is colourless which makes detection difficult. Cyanogen chloride (CK) is a volatile liquid form which can be vapourised for the purpose of causing airway irritation and damage. Solid forms of cyanide include cyanogen bromide which is water soluble and could represent a potential method of poisoning water supplies. The relative ease of access to cyanide compounds in many industries makes this a prominent potential terrorist chemical weapon.

PULMONARY AGENTS AND IRRITANT GASES

Chlorine (CL) is a water-soluble chemical which is easily disseminated as a greenish-yellow gas. Chlorine gas is a potent upper airway and mucous membrane irritant and has a distinct pungent chemical odour. This easily accessible substance was utilised by terrorist insurgents in 2007 during the Iraq conflict. Five chlorine gas tankers were retrofitted with explosives and detonated over the course of two months leading to the deaths of around 350 civilians.

Phosgene gas (CG) is a highly volatile gas with an odour like that of fresh mowed hay. Phosgene gas poisoning can produce delayed respiratory effects, from hours to days, which can be easily missed by clinicians. Millions of tons of phosgene are manufactured for industrial purposes worldwide, making this substance highly accessible, however its non-persistent nature makes it difficult to handle as a chemical weapon.

Incapacitating, deliriant, and riot control agents

A variety of CBRNE agents have also been developed to specifically have non-lethal effects. Incapacitating agents, such as anaesthetics, sedatives, and narcotics, have received significant attention since their use in the 2002 Moscow Theatre Siege where individuals were deliberately rendered unconscious using a highly potent incapacitant – possibly a synthetic fentanyl derivative or anaesthetic gas. Agents such as BZ and LSD are also known to be part of military arsenals and are designed to cause mass delirium or hallucinations. The irritant riot control agents such as oleoresin capsicum (OC) and tear gas (CS) are used extensively by law-and-order organizations around the world and cause temporary incapacitation, airway, and eye irritation.

COUNTERMEASURES AGAINST CHEMICAL AGENTS

Due to the significant threat posed by chemical agents in warfare, much effort has been expended to develop medical countermeasures. Countermeasures range from simple measures such as removal from further exposure, to administration of antidotes for emergency treatment, and subsequent advanced medical treatments and therapeutics to avoid late effects (see Table 23.1).

BIOLOGICAL WEAPONS

The Center for Disease Control in the United States and the World Health Organization have identified a range of biological agents of concern for weaponisation as outlined in Table 23.2. The purpose of this section is to provide a summary of the pathogens of most significance.

Exemplar CBRNE Agent

BACTERIAL AGENT – ANTHRAX

Anthrax disease is caused by exposure to *Bacillus anthracis*, an encapsulated spore-forming bacterium. The disease naturally occurs in cattle or sheep which feed on grasses contaminated with spores. Processed anthrax spores used as a weapon can be dispersed widely, are stable in storage for long periods, cannot transmit between individuals, and only cause

Table 23.2 Major biological agent threats to human populations and society

Category A	Category B	Category C: Emerging pathogens
• Easily disseminated/ transmitted • High mortality rates	• Easily disseminated • Moderate morbidity rate • Low mortality rates	
Bacillus anthracis	Brucella suis	Nipah virus
Yersinia pestis	Salmonella	Hantavirus
Variola major	E. coli O157:H7	
Francisella tularensis	Shigella	
Hemorrhagic Fever Viruses	*Burkholderia species*	
Botulinum Toxin	Chlamydia psittaci	
	Coxiella burnetti	
	Vibrio cholerae	
	Cryptosporidia	
	Rickettsia prowazekii	
	Ricin toxin	
	Staphylococcal enterotoxin	
	Epsilon toxin – *Clostridium perfringens*	
	Viral Encephalitis viruses	

disease in those exposed. These have significant advantages as a biological weapon. Disease manifests in three alternate forms depending on the method of exposure: cutaneous, gastrointestinal, and inhalational. Inhaled or ingested anthrax rapidly grows in the body leading to septic shock and death. Untreated inhalational anthrax mortality approaches 100%, reducible to less than 50% with intensive medical care. Malicious dissemination of spores occurred in the United States in 2001 when an unknown terrorist mailed anthrax spores to political leaders and journalists. Twenty-three people exposed to the letters contracted anthrax leading to five deaths. Weaponised anthrax was accidentally disseminated in the city of Sverdlovsk in the USSR in 1979 from a biological weapons production facility leading to many deaths in the community, leading to an international outcry and investigation (Meselson et al., 1992) (see Figure 23.4).

Exemplar CBRNE Agent

TOXIN – BOTULINUM NEUROTOXIN

Botulinum toxin is the most potent toxic substance by weight known to man. The toxin is produced by the spore-forming bacterium *Clostridium botulinum* and causes flaccid paralysis by blocking neurotransmitter release of acetylcholine. Four types of botulism can occur: foodborne botulism, wound-related botulism, infant botulism, and inhalational botulism after intentional aerosolisation during a bioterrorist event. Intoxication via the bloodstream is rapid following inhalation, ingestion, or mucous membrane contamination.

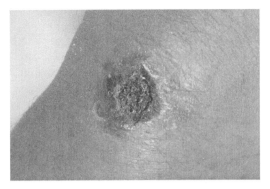

Figure 23.4 The black eschar of cutaneous anthrax (CDC/James H. Steele)

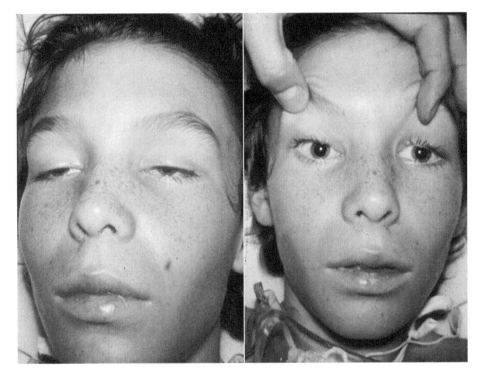

Figure 23.5 Diplopia and mydriasis due to paralysis from botulinum neurotoxin intoxication (Herbert L. Fred, MD and Hendrik A. van Dijk)

Paralysis begins with the small muscles of the face and progressively descends to involve paralysis of the entire body including the muscles of respiration resulting in what is sometimes referred to as "locked in" syndrome. Treatment consists of mechanical ventilation, intensive care, neutralisation of the toxin with intravenous antitoxin and/or human immunoglobulin, and vaccination. Survival is possible if mechanical ventilation and supportive care are maintained while affected nerve terminals recover, a process that usually takes months (see Figure 23.5).

PLAGUE

"Black plague" is a zoonotic disease caused by *Yersinia pestis*, a bacterium which commonly infects rodents. Infection can occur from flea bites, direct handling of affected animal products, and human-to-human transmission via respiratory droplets. Skin inoculation with *Y. pestis* leads to the formation of localised abscesses (buboes) within two to eight days, with subsequent infection of the blood stream (sepsis) leading to organ failure, shock, and coma within days. Untreated plague has a mortality rate of 60%. Inhalation of weaponised plague bacilli has a shorter incubation period of two to four days. Symptoms mimic many other respiratory illnesses and include high fever, headache, cough, and Smallpox transmits readily via chest pain, progressing to death in two to four days if untreated. Plague has been used as a biological weapon in WWII when Japan packaged fleas engineered to carry plague around explosive devices which were detonated in besieged cities in China. Weaponised strains of plague were also actively developed and stockpiled in the USSR.

SMALLPOX

Smallpox is a viral disease caused by the poxvirus *Variola major*. It is the only disease declared to be eradicated in humans by the World Health Assembly in 1980. Smallpox transmits readily via contact, droplet, and airborne routes with many historical examples of infection at significant distances from cases. It is highly contagious and spreads rapidly within susceptible populations. Since eradication, only intentional or accidental release of Smallpox from carefully guarded laboratory stocks at the CDC in Atlanta, USA or at the Vector facility in Koltsovo, Russia are considered to be likely smallpox threats.

RADIOLOGICAL AND NUCLEAR WEAPONS

Radiological dispersion devices (RDDs) are designed to disseminate radiological material for the purpose of contaminating an area with ionising radiation. Two types of RDDs are theorised for use during a radiologic attack: explosive and non-explosive devices. Explosive RDDs disseminate particles of radioactive material and are commonly referred to as "dirty bombs". Non-explosive RDDs disperse radioactive materials usually via an airborne mechanism. Mechanisms of injury include impalement of radioactive material from shrapnel, exposure from contaminated clothing and skin, or inhalation or ingestion of radioactive particles. Radiological exposure devices are static concealed sources of ionising radiation (usually gamma or neutron emitters) placed in high-traffic areas for the purpose of irradiation of individuals or groups.

Large-scale nuclear weapon detonations of enriched uranium or plutonium are characterised by a high-speed chain reaction resulting in massive energy production and release of radiation. Explosions from nuclear detonations produce four types of released energy: nuclear radiation, thermal, blast and shock wave, and radioactive fallout. Widespread and devastating effects within the vicinity of the blast as well as long-term radiation contamination from fallout leave affected areas devastated and uninhabitable for long periods. Attack of a stationary nuclear power plant theoretically could result in a runaway or "meltdown" nuclear reaction, or compromise of nuclear containment, causing dispersion of radioactive material and local environment contamination. The widespread effects of such an incident are exemplified by the events which took place at Chernobyl in 1986.

TERRORISM AND THE PSYCHOLOGY OF TERRORISM

"Terrorism" has become a prominent potential trigger for complex disasters and the acquisition and potential use of CBRNE weapons and "know how". As the methods, motives, and materials utilised by terrorists evolve so does the definition of terrorism. Currently, a generalisable definition is as follows: The utilisation of violent tactics via non-conventional methods by non-state actors to influence target entities to achieve a social, political, or religious goal. Over the past half-century, terrorist-related activities have proliferated and greatly impacted global foreign relations and national security measures. Much effort has been dedicated to the study of psychological impacts of terrorism from the perspective of the perpetrators and the victims.

Developing methods to understand, define, and predict the factors influencing individuals to participate in terrorist activities have proved challenging. Terrorism transcends age, gender, intelligence level, and social status. There are no consistent personality traits across societies that reliably indicate a predisposition to radicalisation. To understand the psychology of the terrorist, efforts are directed towards studying the social and political environment, early psychological development and community constructs that allow for acceptance of violent extremism. Our progress towards understanding the psychology of the terrorist is an area of active research and focus worldwide. Some researchers suggest the key to identifying individuals at risk of radicalisation and commission of terrorist acts is to focus on recruitment ideology and tactics utilised by recruiters and senior leadership of terrorist organisations.

Psychological impacts of victims of terrorism are more easily studied as the populations affected are more readily available for evaluation. Following the events of the September 2001 terror attacks in the US very early psychological support and intervention were provided across large populations. This data showed that early post-disaster stress responses were common and are considered to be normal and adaptive responses to a major event. However, some then progress into dysfunctional psychological states, one of which is post-traumatic stress disorder. For some, these events amplify pre-existent vulnerabilities to disease. Larger groups who did not directly witness the event but were exposed through the media have also been considered vulnerable to similar stress responses. Research has highlighted that certain prevailing social norms and customs in communities may influence the type and extent of psychological reactions, however generalisation to all populations is not possible.

ACTIVITIES

1. Why is prevention of proliferation a key focus of international efforts to mitigate the risks of CBRNE events?
2. How can public health systems and the broader community prepare for CBRNE and terrorist incidents?
3. How would the response to a CBRNE or terrorist event occur in your community?

KEY READINGS

Arnon, S. S., R. Schechter, T. V. Inglesby, D. A. Henderson, J. G. Bartlett, M. S. Ascher, E. Eitzen, A. D. Fine, J. Hauer, M. Layton, S. Lillibridge, M. T. Osterholm, T. O'Toole, G. Parker, T. M. Perl, P. K. Russell, D. L. Swerdlow and K. Tonat, Botulinum toxin as a biological weapon: Medical and public health management. *JAMA*, 2001. **285**(8): p. 1059–1070.

Bland, S., Chemical, biological, radiation and nuclear (CBRN) incidents. *BMJ Military Health*, 2006. **152**(4): p. 244–249.

Bland, S.A. Chemical, biological and radiation casualties: Critical care considerations. *Journal of the Royal Army Medical Corps*, 2009. **155**(2): p. 160.

Bland, S.A. Chemical, Biological, Radiological and Nuclear (CBRN) casualty management principles, in *Conflict and catastrophe medicine: A practical guide*, J.M. Ryan, A.P.C.C. Hopperus Buma, C.W. Beadling et al. Editors. 2014, London: Springer London. p. 747–770.

Bozue, J., C. Cote and P. Glass, *Medical aspects of biological warfare*. 2018. Fort Sam Houston, TX: US Army Medical Department.

Calder, A. and S. Bland, CBRN considerations in a major incident. *Surgery (Oxford)*. 2018. **36**(8): 417–423.

Cieslak, T. J. and F. M. Henretig, Medical consequences of biological warfare: The Ten Commandments of management. *Military Medicine*, 2001. **166**(12 Suppl): p. 11–12.

Dennis, D.T., T.V. Inglesby, D.A. Henderson, J.G. Bartlett, M.S. Ascher, E. Eitzen, A.D. Fine, A.M. Friedlander, J. Hauer, M. Layton, S.R. Lillibridge, J.E. McDade, M.T. Osterholm, T. O'Toole, G. Parker, T. M. Perl, P.K. Russell, and K. Tonat, Tularemia as a biological weapon: Medical and public health management. *JAMA*, 2001. **285**(21): p. 2763–2773.

Henderson, D.A., T.V. Inglesby, J.G. Bartlett, M.S. Ascher, E. Eitzen, P.B. Jahrling, J. Hauer, M. Layton, J. McDade, M. T. Osterholm, T. O'Toole, G. Parker, T. Perl, P.K. Russell, and K. Tonat, Smallpox as a biological weapon: Medical and public health management. *JAMA*, 1999. **281**(22): p. 2127–2137.

Hudson, R., The sociology and psychology of terrorism: Who becomes a terrorist and why? 1999. Washington DC, USA, Library of Congress.

Inglesby, T.V., D.T. Dennis, D.A. Henderson, J.G. Bartlett, M.S. Ascher, E. Eitzen, A.D. Fine, A.M. Friedlander, J. Hauer, J.F. Koerner, M. Layton, J. McDade, M.T. Osterholm, T. O'Toole, G. Parker, T.M. Perl, P.K. Russell, M. Schoch-Spana, and K. Tonat. Plague as a biological weapon: Medical and public health management. *JAMA*, 2000. **283**(17): p. 2281–2290.

Inglesby, T.V., D.A. Henderson, J.G. Bartlett, M.S. Ascher, E. Eitzen, A.M. Friedlander, J. Hauer, J. McDade, M.T. Osterholm, T. O'Toole, G. Parker, T.M. Perl, P.K. Russell and K. Tonat, Anthrax as a biological weapon: Medical and public health management. *JAMA*, 1999. **281**(18): p. 1735–1745.

Jones, R., B. Wills and C. Kang, Chlorine gas: An evolving hazardous material threat and unconventional weapon. *The Western Journal of Emergency Medicine*, 2010, **11**(2): p. 151–156.

Keyes, D., J. Burstein, R. Schwartz and R. Swienton, *Medical response to terrorism: Preparedness and clinical practice*. 2005, Sydney, Australia: Lippincott Williams & Wilkins.

Melnick, A.L. Biological, chemical, and radiological terrorism: Emergency preparedness and response for the primary care physician. 2008, New York: Springer New York.

Meselson, M., J. Guillemin, M. Hugh-Jones, A. Langmuir, I. Popova, A. Shelokov, and O. Yampolskaya, The Sverdlovsk anthrax outbreak of 1979. *Science*, 1994. **266**(5188): p. 1202–1208. doi: 10.1126/science.7973702. PMID: 7973702.

Mickelson, A. *Medical consequences of radiological and nuclear weapons.* 2012, Falls Church, VA: Borden Institute.

NATO. NATO AMedP 7.1- Medical Management of CBRN Casualties, 2018.

Open Society Justice Initiative. *Eastern and Western Ghouta Sarin attack.* 2021, New York:, Justice Initiative.

Organisation for the Prohibition of Chemical Weapons. Convention on the prohibition of the development, production, stockpiling and use of chemical weapons and on their destruction. 2020, United Nations.

Pastel, R. and E. Ritchie, Terrorism and chemical, biological, radiological, nuclear, and explosive weapons. In *Combat and Operational Behavioral Health*, Borden Institute Walter Reed Army Medical Center, Editor, 2011. Government Printing Office. p. 593–608. From the Textbooks of Military Medicine series; Falls Church, VA: Office of The Surgeon General, United States Army; Fort Detrick, MD: Borden Institute, 2011. https://www.academia.edu/77088060/36_Terrorism_and_Chemical_Biological_ Radiological_Nuclear_and_Explosive_Weapons

Pomper, M. and G. Tarini. *Nuclear terrorism – Threat or not?.* AIP Conference Proceedings, Conference: Nuclear Weapons and Related Security Issues. 2017. **1898**(1):p. 050001. doi:10.1063/1.5009230

Public Health England. Chemical, biological, radiological and nuclear incidents: Clinical management and health protection. 2018. London (UK): Public Health England.

Richardt, A. and T. Dawert. *CBRN protection: Managing the threat of chemical, biological, radioactive and nuclear weapons.* 2013. Weinheim: Wiley-VCH Verlag GmbH: p. 273–294. doi:10.1002/9783527650163.ch10

Secretariat of the Convention on Biological Diversity. *Cartegena protocol on biosafety to the convention on biological diversity.* 2000. Montreal, Canada: United Nations.

Sen, J. P. B., R. Sandhu and S. Bland. Chemical incidents. *BJA Education,* 2021. **21**(4): p. 126–132.

The Australia Group. The Australia Group. 2022. 2007; Available from: https://www.dfat. gov.au/publications/minisite/theaustraliagroupnet/site/en/index.html.

Tuorinsky, S. *Medical aspects of chemical warfare.* 2008. Falls Church, VA: Borden Institute.

United Nations Office for Disarmament Affairs. *Treaty of Tlatelolco.* 1967. Mexico City, Mexico: United Nations.

United Nations Office for Disarmament Affairs. *Treaty on the non-proliferation of nuclear weapons.* 1970. New York: United Nations.

United Nations Office for Disarmament Affairs. Convention on the prohibition of the development, production, and stockpiling of bacteriological (biological) and toxin weapons and on their destruction. 1972. Geneva, Switzerland.

United Nations Office for Disarmament Affairs. *Treaty of Rarotonga.* 1986. Geneva, Switzerland: United Nations.

United Nations Office for Disarmament Affairs. *Treaty of Bangkok.* 1997. Geneva, Switzerland: United Nations.

United Nations Office for Disarmament Affairs. *Central Asian nuclear-weapon-free zone treaty.* 2006. Semipalatinsk, Kazakhstan: United Nations.

United Nations Office for Disarmament Affairs. *Treaty of Pelindaba.* 2009. Geneva, Switzerland: United Nations.

Zala, B., "How the next nuclear arms race will be different from the last one." *Bulletin of the Atomic Scientists,* 2019. **75**(1): p. 36–43.

24
Pandemics

Penelope Burns, Graham Dodd, Angela Hamilton,
and Michael Kidd

The aim of this chapter is to provide a broad overview of pandemics: the evolution of pandemics, the characteristics that influence their impact, and the principles of pandemic management. This chapter is of particular relevance due to the worldwide SARS-CoV-2 (Sudden Acute Respiratory Syndrome Corona Virus 2) pandemic, also referred to as the COVID-19 pandemic, that occurred from March 2020 to May 2023, only just declared over at the time of writing this chapter. The knowledge and experience gained from this pandemic to date are summarised.

> … ingenuity, knowledge, and organization alter but cannot cancel humanity's vulnerability to invasion by parasitic forms of life. Infectious disease which antedated the emergence of humankind will last as long as humanity itself, and will surely remain, as it has been hitherto, one of the fundamental parameters and determinants of human history.
>
> (William H. McNeill, 1976: p. 291) [1]

On completion of this chapter, you should be able to:

- Describe the characteristics of pandemics.
- Demonstrate an understanding of pandemic management strategies through the Prevention, Preparedness, Response, Recovery (PPRR) disaster management cycle.
- Identify the contribution of healthcare innovation and adaptation to pandemic management.

INTRODUCTION

Micro-organisms, including worms and insects, protozoa, viruses, bacteria, fungi, and prions, cause infectious diseases. Transmission can occur from animals to humans (zoonosis), and from human to human. *Endemic disease* describes an infectious disease occurring at constant or relatively stable levels within any community. In contrast,

DOI: 10.4324/9781032626604-31

an *epidemic* is a widespread outbreak of an infectious disease in the community defined by an excess of cases in the community above that normally expected. Sometimes it will be due to the emergence of a new infectious disease.

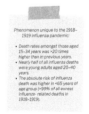

The SARS-CoV 2 infectious outbreak was declared a pandemic by WHO on 11th March 2020.

The Director-General stated: This is not just a public health crisis, it is a crisis that will touch every sector – so every sector and every individual must be involved in the fight. I have said from the beginning that countries must take a whole-of-government, whole-of-society approach, built around a comprehensive strategy to prevent infections, save lives and minimize impact.

When a novel infectious disease spreads globally across multiple international boundaries, it becomes a *pandemic*. Defining a pandemic is difficult. The International Epidemiology Association's Dictionary of Epidemiology defines a pandemic as "*an epidemic occurring worldwide, or over a very wide area, crossing international boundaries and usually affecting a large number of people*" [2]. The World Health Organisation (WHO) is responsible for monitoring and declaring when an infectious disease has become a pandemic. The term *pandemic* comes from the Greek; pan meaning *all* and dermos meaning *people*.

Lessons from history suggest that the appearance of novel and diverse infective organisms will continue as the world's human population continues to increase, with greater density and connectedness across the globe. The challenge for humans is to learn to adapt and thrive in such an evolving interconnected and interdependent health ecology.

Prior to the 2019–2023 SARS-CoV-2 pandemic[1], perhaps the most-cited pandemic, the Spanish Flu, occurred in 1918, at the end of World War I. A highly virulent and highly transmissible form of influenza emerged first in the USA and then arrived in military camps in Europe. The virus subsequently spread to every continent and many countries through the movement of people. Global population density, intercontinental travel, health standards, and the capacity to treat people have changed considerably since 1918. These factors will affect the ability of infectious diseases to spread, and the capabilities of healthcare services in response.

CHARACTERISTICS OF PANDEMIC VIRUSES

The WHO technical set of requirements in a virus for pandemic potential includes the ability to:

- Infect humans.
- Cause disease in humans.
- Spread readily between humans.

The word virus derives from Latin meaning 'poison'. Human influenza causes annual winter epidemics and is considered one of the most significant global pandemic threats. The variability of the influenza virus results in ineffective natural or acquired immunity. It continues to mutate, meaning immunity to previous strains does not prevent infection from new variations of the virus.

Phenomenon unique to the 1918–1919 influenza pandemic:

- Death rates amongst those aged 15–34 years was >20 times higher than in previous years.
- Nearly half of all influenza deaths were young adults aged 20–40 years.
- The absolute risk of influenza death was higher in <65 years of age group (>99% of all excess influenza- related deaths in 1918-1919).

Influenza is a highly infectious disease with the potential to cause significant morbidity and mortality usually amongst the very young, elderly, or immunosuppressed people. However, the characteristics of those most vulnerable can vary between strains, and as we now know, there is a high risk of threat from other viruses, including coronaviruses.

> **Situation report: SARS-CoV-2 pandemic 2019–2023 ongoing**
>
> In the years preceding publication of this textbook, March 2020 to May 2023, the world has been in an acute emergency response to the SARS-CoV-2 pandemic, also referred to as the COVID-19 pandemic. In March 2023, over 6.8 million people were reported to have died from *COVID-19*, the disease caused by the SARS-CoV-2 virus. The virus was first identified in 2019 in Wuhan, China, in cases of pneumonia due to a then-unknown organism. It was thought to have been transmitted from bats, through an intermediate animal host to humans at wet markets. In a global population of 8 billion, greater than three-quarters of a billion (759 million) documented cases of COVID-19 have been reported. True numbers are likely to be much higher. The inequitable effect of the pandemic on morbidity and mortality across countries has been compounded by many factors, including how early in the pandemic countries were first affected; pre-existing healthcare service capability; access to testing, vaccinations, and treatment; and the effects of public health measures on social and economic resilience.

UNDERSTANDING PANDEMICS AND THEIR IMPACT

Phases of a pandemic

The WHO describes pandemics in six phases with Phases 1–3 correlating with preparedness and Phases 4–6 signalling the need for response and mitigation [3]:

Phase 1: disease present in animals but no evidence of spread to humans.
Phase 2: evidence of a circulating animal disease known to have caused disease in humans, but no current evidence of human disease.
Phase 3: small number of human cases but no person-to-person spread except in rare circumstances of very close contact. There is no sustained community outbreak.
Phase 4: evidence of person-to-person spread in very small clusters involving common exposure or intimate contact. There are sustained community outbreaks.
Phase 5: large clusters of cases arising from person-to-person contact, with sustained community outbreaks in two or more countries in one WHO region.
Phase 6: increased and sustained person-to-person spread with widespread distribution of the disease across at least two WHO regions.

WHO reviewed its approach to pandemics following the experience learned from the 2009 H1N1 (Swine flu) pandemic. As seen in Figure 24.1, it now links the phases to the all-hazards principles of emergency risk management across the PPRR disaster framework.

Variability of response stages between nations

This continuum of pandemic is based on virological, epidemiological, and clinical information, and emphasises risk assessment. Response to a pandemic is global, however at any one time, different countries, and different regions within countries, are likely to be in different phases.

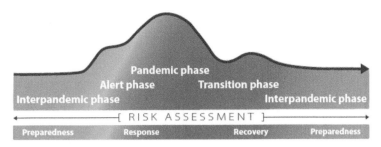

Figure 24.1 World Health Organisation pandemic phases – adapted from materials developed by CDC [4]. This continuum is according to a 'global average' of cases, over time, based on continued risk assessment and consistent with the broader emergency risk management continuum

THE IMPACT OF PANDEMICS AND EPIDEMICS

The human impact of a pandemic will depend on the characteristics of the agent, the characteristics of the community, and the effectiveness of control strategies. The interplay of these factors will directly affect the speed of the onset of the epidemic, the number of people infected, and the number who suffer significant health adverse outcomes, including death.

1. **The characteristics of the organism** determine the nature of the disease, its pathological impact (severity), and its capacity to efficiently spread (transmission).
2. **The characteristics of the population**, such as level of immunity, population density, existing health, social determinants, and equity of access to resources and healthcare services all affect susceptibility.
3. **The effectiveness of public health and community intervention strategies**. Early recognition of the disease, dependent on effective surveillance, will enable a rapid response thereby reducing the disease's impact. The extent and effectiveness of routine infection control procedures and public health preparedness within the community affect transmission.

CLINICAL SEVERITY AND TRANSMISSIBILITY

The impact of a pandemic is strongly affected by the rate of spread of the disease which is described as the *transmissibility of the organism* (how quickly it spreads); and on the *severity of the disease,* also described as the case fatality rate (CFR). Figure 24.2 estimates the difference in severity and transmissibility of previous pandemics and outbreaks, clearly demonstrating the deadly combination of high levels of both characteristics present in the Spanish Flu strain of H1N1 and the range of transmissibility and clinical severity seen in the different variants of SARS-CoV-2.

The average number of people an infected person may infect is defined as the 'R factor' of the epidemic. If the R factor exceeds one, then the epidemic will continue to expand. If the R factor is less than one, then the epidemic will decline. The pathogenicity of the agent may paradoxically limit its ability to spread rapidly. A disease which kills rapidly may be more likely to limit the mobility of infected people, and their ability to contact vulnerable individuals or populations. Equally however, using the example of Ebola, fear of the disease and the limited treatment options in hospitals, led to many more exposed individuals as patients avoided or fled hospitals, seeking care from traditional or religious healers [6].

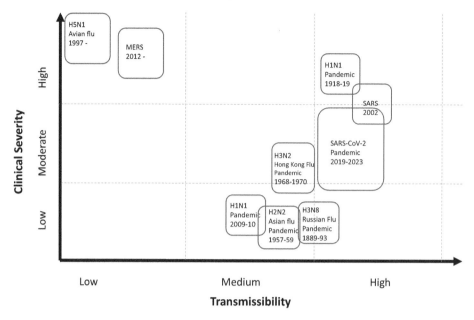

Figure 24.2 Clinical severity and transmissibility of infectious outbreaks and pandemics [5]

CASE STUDY 24.1 – THE 2019–2023 SARS-CoV-2 PANDEMIC

The 2019–2023 coronavirus pandemic involved numerous waves, and numerous variants of the virus, broadly classified and chronologically named according to the Greek alphabet in order of evolution, including most notably Alpha, Beta, Delta, and Omicron, all with their own descendent lineages. The continuous evolution of circulating variants of the SARS-CoV-2 virus required monitoring for their changing characteristics, particularly transmission rate and the severity of associated disease, for the effectiveness of public health and social measures (PHSMs), and as developed, of vaccines and therapeutic medications.

Ongoing rapid changes in the variants of SARS-CoV-2 viral lineages emphasised the need for continual surveillance and rapid distribution of data and understanding of the virus. Variants of Concern (VOCs) are those with genetic changes known to affect virus characteristics and identified as those associated with a comparative change that is of significance to global public health characterised by increased transmissibility, increased virulence, change in clinical presentation, or decreased effectiveness of public health or vaccine or therapeutic measures [7].

SARS-CoV-2 Omicron's characteristics of immune escape, where the immune system is unable to respond to the virus, for example, due to changes in the virus that make it no longer recognisable by the immune system as the same foreign substance, have resulted in the most rapid, simultaneous increase in COVID-19 incidence of the pandemic. Although acknowledging limitations in interpreting data collection during COVID-19, Figure 24.3 shows that worldwide there was a peak of over 143 million new cases of COVID-19 in the first two 28-day periods of 2022, equivalent to one-third of

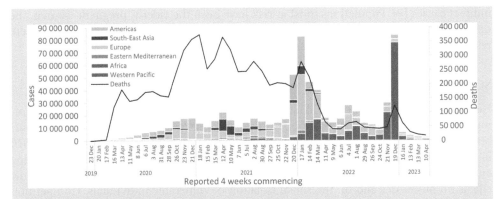

Figure 24.3 COVID-19 cases reported by WHO Region, and global deaths by 28-day intervals, 16 December 2019 to 7 May 2023 [8]

the total 433 million cases and the highest peak of the pandemic at that time. However, then in the last month of 2022 an even higher 28-day peak occurred with almost 100 million cases in one month alone. The highly transmissible Omicron VOC was the dominant strain in May 2023 at the official end of the pandemic and replaced other circulating variants. Vaccination reduced morbidity and mortality, however the unvaccinated remained at high risk of severe disease and hospitalisation. Fortunately the CFR for the Omicron VOC was lower than some of the previous SARS-CoV-2 VOCs.

CLINICAL DISEASE

COVID-19 is a multisystem disease. The health effects of COVID-19 are predominantly respiratory with cough and fatigue. The severity of health effects is influenced by the variant of SARS-CoV-2, vaccination status, age, and particular comorbidities including obesity and severe immunocompromise [9]. Infection with SARS-CoV-2 can be asymptomatic, mild, moderate or severe. Over 80% of people experience mild symptoms and recover promptly and fully. Severe disease with shortness of breath (SOB), hypoxia, and >50% lung involvement occurs in <14%; and critical disease with respiratory failure, shock, or multiorgan dysfunction in <5%. Overall case fatality varies but was around 2.3% during the first years of the pandemic.

Limited understanding exists of the longer-term effects of COVID-19 disease. Roughly 10% of people experience prolonged illness following COVID. It has been defined as post-acute COVID-19 (PAC) if it persists for over three weeks, and chronic, or *long COVID*, if it persists for over three months. As a multisystem disease, symptoms vary broadly. Remitting and relapsing cough, fever and fatigue are most common. SOB, chest pain, headache, myalgias, cognitive difficulties, gastrointestinal upset, rashes, thromboembolism, and mental health issues are also seen [10, 11].

ROUTINE HEALTHCARE ACCESS

The impact of SARS-CoV-2 on health was also indirect with reduced access to healthcare for non-COVID healthcare in many countries, as well as financial and economic effects on livelihood and access to food. It is impossible to estimate the excess mortality from indirect causes [9]. Populations most at risk have been the elderly, pregnant women, the unvaccinated, and the severely immunocompromised. In this pandemic children were relatively spared.

SOCIETAL IMPACT

New and emerging pandemics will have not only a significant effect on the health of communities, but also significant economic, social and environmental effects. The 2003 outbreak of SARS was estimated by the Asian Development Bank to have cost between US$10 billion and US$30 billion [12]. Restrictions in travel, or in movement from homes, during enforced 'lockdowns', or through self-restriction due to fear, may have profound economic effects on businesses and on the social isolation of vulnerable individuals. Competition for scarce resources may result. Loss of family and friends may have a long-term personal impact on communities and on future productive capacity.

When the Sudden Acute Respiratory Syndrome (SARS) outbreak spread to Hong Kong a cluster of cases occurred in some residential housing blocks in Amoy Gardens. Residents in those buildings reported distress from the stigma and marginalisation during the outbreak [13]. Psychosocial impacts are of particular significance to health professionals. The infectious agent may pose a risk to health professionals who may be reluctant to expose themselves and their families to the risks associated with caring for infected patients. During the SARS outbreak in Hong Kong, nearly a quarter of cases were healthcare workers, and in Canada, 65% of the 141 probable cases were healthcare workers [14].

PANDEMICS COMPOUNDING NATURAL DISASTER AND CONFLICT

In early 2023, the number of people requiring humanitarian assistance continues to increase and is now reaching 347 million [15]. More than 1% of the world's population is now displaced, and almost half of these (42%) are children [16]. Many of those displaced suffered inequity during the SARS-CoV-2 pandemic in access to vaccinations, therapeutics, infection prevention and control measures, and Water Sanitation and Hygiene resources [17, 18].

A significant adverse effect on health systems is being felt globally. Diagnosis and treatment activities for human immunodeficiency virus, tuberculosis and malaria, antenatal care, and routine childhood vaccinations have all decreased. Economies and livelihoods have also been destroyed, and education affected [17].

STAGES OF PANDEMIC MANAGEMENT

Pandemic planning across PPRR varies from country to country. A summary of Australia's Pandemic Response stages based on the Australian Health Management Plan for Influenza Pandemic is provided as an example in Table 24.1 below [19].

PRINCIPLES OF PANDEMIC MANAGEMENT

The key aims in managing a pandemic or epidemic are to:

- **Minimise transmission, morbidity, and mortality.**
- **Minimise the impact on the healthcare system.**

Table 24.1 National pandemic response planning in Australia

Stage	Activities
Preparedness	Plan, practice, and ensure resources are available. Ongoing surveillance
Response: Standby	Monitor the emergence of the disease locally with readiness to respond immediately
Response: Action Initial	Response stage when little is known about the disease and information is still being gathered
Response: Action Target	Response stage when enough is known about the disease to direct a more targeted response to specific needs
Response: Standdown	Move to post-pandemic business and revise plans for future pandemics

Epidemics and pandemics do not respect international borders. Past infectious threats posed by SARS, Ebola, MERS-CoV are global concerns. International cooperation is essential in limiting the impact. Poorer countries are most susceptible to disease outbreaks and resource shortages. They have fewer resources and less capacity to manage the economic and social impact.

WHO's international standards complement the International Health Regulations (IHR) [20]. These legally binding agreements by member states establish an agreement to work cooperatively on the management of new outbreaks at the source, not just at national borders. Most countries have pandemic preparedness plans, which are variously updated and practiced.

A major pandemic will be a disaster and managed in accordance with both national and international disaster response arrangements. Health services will play a lead role particularly in the provision of advice on system strategy and in the management of the patients. One of the lessons identified from the 2009 H1N1 influenza pandemic, which had a lower fatality rate than usual seasonal influenza, was that not all pandemics are the same. Pandemic response strategies need to be tailored to the characteristics of the particular causative organism. **Pandemics require a *proportional response* with different levels of responses for mild, moderate, and severe pandemics.**

Protection of the community against potential epidemics relies on a whole of health response. One of the key frontline professions in surveillance for emerging diseases, management of outpatient cases of infectious disease, and delivery of community vaccination programs is General Practice/Family Practice. In Australia, another lesson learned from the H1N1 pandemic was the paucity of involvement of General Practitioners (GPs), also known as Family Physicians, in the planning and preparedness, and the lack of provision of personal protective equipment (PPE) and other protection to healthcare workers based in the community, compared to their peers working in hospitals [19, 21]. During the SARS-CoV-2 pandemic the increased involvement of GPs and primary care was clearly visible [22, 23].

Protection of the community against an evolving pandemic relies on both individual and population strategies.

Hierarchy of Controls

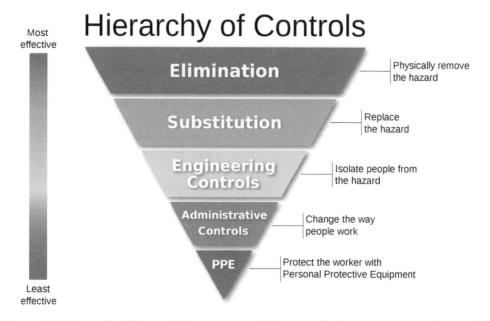

Most effective

Least effective

Elimination — Physically remove the hazard

Substitution — Replace the hazard

Engineering Controls — Isolate people from the hazard

Administrative Controls — Change the way people work

PPE — Protect the worker with Personal Protective Equipment

Figure 24.4 Hierarchy of Controls illustrates potentially more effective measures in reducing risk at the top. [By Original version: NIOSH; Vector version: Michael Pittman)] [24, 25]

INDIVIDUAL STRATEGIES

At the individual level, strategies aim to prevent infection to break the chain of transmission, and to prevent severe disease. This is achieved by ensuring maximum personal protection through immunisation; isolation and social distancing; changes to workplace environment; personal infection control and hygiene measures including use of PPE such as face masks, gowns, gloves and eye-protection; the use of prophylactic or therapeutic drugs such as anti-viral medication; and early identification and management of individual infection. Vaccination and early therapeutic medication, when available, assist in the prevention and management of severe disease, respectively.

The hierarchy of controls (HoCs) shown in Figure 24.4 was developed initially as a system for managing exposure risk of workers to occupational hazards, and first applied to the management of tuberculosis and ebola, but has been rapidly adapted and utilised by clinicians across all levels of community and hospital healthcare [26]. The HoC emphasises those controls at the top of the pyramid such as elimination and substitution of the hazard, as the most effective. Although also useful and often a key public focus, it illustrates PPE as a less effective strategy.

POPULATION STRATEGIES

At the population level, national strategies aim at reducing transmission of disease, severe disease and mortality, and the impact on the healthcare system. These strategies include surveillance, early recognition, early intervention, and rapid development of therapies and vaccines. As already mentioned, a pandemic is a global response. All countries have a responsibility under the IHR to maintain a system of disease surveillance, monitoring, and reporting to international authorities regarding the outbreak of infectious diseases [20].

For each nation a pandemic involves a whole of health response involving all levels of healthcare in a unified response. Public health systems of surveillance are active during interpandemic phases as part of normal operations in many countries. Frontline community health providers including GPs and emergency departments (EDs) contribute to surveillance. Maintenance of laboratory capacity ensures timeliness of accurate diagnosis to aid both recognition and management. Rapid case investigation and response by public health teams minimise the potential spread of individual cases.

Public health mitigation and strategies were shown to be effective in the reduction of COVID-19 cases, hospitalisations, and deaths [7]. Quarantine was used to isolate early positive cases through restriction of movement in monitored residences in hotels or on cruise boats. Decisions to limit viral transmission in 'hotspots', discrete populations, or areas of high circulating virus, resulted in various levels of 'lockdowns' with restricted movement of people outside their homes for weeks at a time. The effectiveness of these measures in reducing transmission needs to be balanced by their adverse economic and social impacts. As illustrated in Figure 24.5 efforts to slow the spread of the virus attempt to 'flatten the curve' by slowing the rise in infection rate in the population and thereby delay the peak in cases during waves of the epidemic with a key aim of decreasing the risk of overwhelming healthcare services. This was successfully used in some countries during the SARS-Co-V2 pandemic, but unachievable in others.

As pandemics evolve, containing transmission may no longer be possible, and aims may change to focus on the reduction of severe disease and mortality. Identification of those most at risk will allow the initiation of increased protective measures for those groups, including prioritised vaccination and therapy, and further PHSMs.

Convening and adapting expert scientific advisory groups linked systematically to government decision-makers provides evidence-based decision-making which may be swiftly updated as greater understanding of the virus and its characteristics emerge and

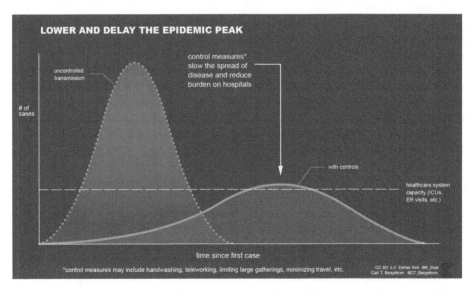

Figure 24.5 Flattening the curve and slowing the spread (CC BY 4.0 Esther Kim & Carl T. Bergstrom) [27]

change. Where the evidence doesn't exist then expert consensus input may be required to support decision-making. Global knowledge and expertise sharing supports this evidence-informed approach.

ADAPTION AND INNOVATION IN HEALTHCARE SYSTEM RESPONSES

Consideration of creative management options is part of pandemic preparedness planning in most countries. During the SARS-Co-V2 pandemic considerable innovation and adaptation were seen in the healthcare system responses in many countries to increase existing healthcare system capacity. Augmentation of healthcare service capacity was rapid, creative and arisen at both frontline clinician levels as well as national, state and local jurisdictional levels.

Strategies for managing the surge in numbers during the usual winter flu season can be increased for pandemics. GPs, EDs, and hospitals manage much of the usual seasonal influenza, or other smaller infectious outbreaks as normal operations. Functional surge management often involves the reduction in non-critical healthcare, such as postponement of non-urgent surgery or patient consultations, and in some countries the difficult necessity to triage those who are provided hospital beds and ICU admission.

General practitioner-led respiratory clinics (GPRCs)

GPs can help minimise the impact of a pandemic on an already burdened emergency and acute care system. In Australia, GPRCs were developed rapidly in response to SARS-CoV-2 as a model of healthcare provision to fill an identified gap. They are a network of GP-led COVID medical clinics staffed by GPs and nurses. Although these have been used on a much smaller scale previously, such as during the 2009 H1N1 pandemic in Australia and New Zealand, this was the first time such a substantial new healthcare service was activated to provide surveillance for, examination and assessment, management, and treatment, of those with potential COVID-19 cases who might otherwise overwhelm EDs and hospitals [28]. GPRCs also protect surge overwhelming General Practice and ED resources, supporting these health facilities to continue to see non-infected patients for more routine care.

Over 150 GPRCs were employed nationally across Australia during the SARS-CoV-2 pandemic, their function evolving with the phases of the pandemic. Such cohorting of patients provided several benefits: streamlined rapid early identification, triage, and initial management of potential cases; preservation of access to usual healthcare services for uninfected patients; reduced quantity of PPE required; and provision of a dedicated workforce for use in other roles as the pandemic evolved including vaccination.

Stockpiles

Some countries have the capacity to stockpile stores including antiviral agents, PPE, vaccines, and equipment required during an epidemic. They include physical stockpiles, such as those stored in warehouses, or imbedded stockpiles that at any time are in the manufacture, distribution, supply, and storage pathways. In the event of an outbreak, it may be important to identify the latter and secure this stockpile for priority usage.

A crucial aspect of stockpile management is a system of rapid sustained distribution to frontline healthcare workers. In British Colombia, Canada, during the SARS-CoV-2 pandemic, delays in distribution, with the exhaustion of private supply lines, left some General Practices exposed, resulting in the closure of health services due to staff safety concerns. The issue was resolved through partnerships between local family doctor organisations and local health authorities with the development of a provincial system to distribute PPE at no cost. However, costs of other office modifications such as extra cleaning, plexiglass barriers, and reduced office in-person visits were borne by community physicians and other private community healthcare businesses.

Virtual home care

Pandemic-associated public health mandates during the SARS-CoV-2 pandemic resulted in changes to the way health services were delivered. The impetus to reduce transmission of the disease and protect vulnerable populations meant that face-to-face medicine was often no longer possible. This brought about a rapid and dramatic increase in virtual healthcare consultations via telephone, video and mobile applications. The sudden increase in COVID-19 cases during outbreaks required rapid escalation of resources, development of models of care, integration of new health pathways and the use of novel technologies for managing COVID-19 cases in the community. In Australia, one of the models developed was heavily reliant on telehealth [29] and the distribution of clinical tools including pulse oximeters for remote monitoring of patients. The data gathered from these sources was then used to risk stratify and guide management with the goal of providing the best patient care and preventing hospitalisation. While a full clinical picture is often difficult to ascertain via telephone or video, telehealth models of care were critical in reducing stress on healthcare systems.

Service delivery rework

Rapid change in the healthcare delivery environment during the SARS-CoV-2 pandemic saw the use of carparks, community halls, churches, and drive-throughs for healthcare delivery; the use of garbage bags for gowns and cabbage leaves for masks for PPE; and streamlining of reduced contact patient flow through services.

Mass vaccination

With the rapid development of effective vaccines against SARS-Cov-2, rollout strategies prioritising high-risk individuals and essential workers were implemented as variable, fluctuating access to vaccines occurred. These rollouts were on the background of continuing management of recurrent hotspots or outbreaks of the disease and balancing the complex competing needs of preventing the spread of COVID-19, managing the socio-economic repercussions of lockdowns and ensuring the community's other acute and chronic healthcare needs were met.

COVID-19 vaccinations were deployed to Australia in early 2021 and various key stakeholders were required to rapidly develop and implement policies and procedures to ensure they were delivered efficiently and effectively.

At a national level this involved federal and state government organisations, the Australian Technical Advisory Group on Immunisation and the Therapeutic Goods Administration to provide approvals, guidance on risks and benefits, advice around vaccination for various groups and education about novel vaccine types.

On a local level vaccination clinics proceeded through GPs, GPRCs, and pharmacists, as well as mass vaccination clinics in major hospitals. The rationale for this model was multi-fold. Firstly, these vaccines were delivered in multidose vials (a formulation that has often been used as more doses can be delivered rapidly). Secondly the mRNA vaccine required extremely different cold chain management due to the low temperatures required to maintain viability. Thirdly, the required speed of vaccination in an attempt to achieve herd immunity required thousands of people to be vaccinated at each site daily. Finally, delivery through local general practices and pharmacies, in urban and rural areas across the nation, was to ensure that vaccines were available close to where people live. In major metropolitan areas this included centrally located mass vaccination centres.

Multi-disciplinary teams of nurses, GPs, paramedics, pharmacists, students, administration staff, dentists, staff specialists, and a wide array of allied health professionals were assembled to create these hospital mass vaccination programs. The challenges faced by the teams included rapidly changing guidelines, enforcement of public health mandates, dealing with a supply and demand mismatch, public healthcare mistrust, and administration of novel therapies, while simultaneously gathering data on efficacy and safety to modify guidelines.

Key challenges for healthcare services during pandemics are to ensure an organised and comprehensive approach to prevention and management with clear consistent communication of information and coordination of services and resources. A crucial issue in any disaster, including pandemics, is **communication**; clear, consistent, accurate up-to-date information that is reliable and regularly distributed across all responders and affected communities. This is true for those in authority who are making decisions on population management; for health professionals who need to be clear about their local role, and how those infected with the disease are to be managed; and for concerned members of the community who wish to remain safe and healthy.

The media also has a clear role in this area. Regular, clear, and consistent communication is likely to decrease the potential psychosocial impact. In pandemics with higher fatality rates, dealing with grief and bereavement for families and communities can contribute to mental health effects. Healthcare workers in particular may be dealing with stigma and fear in working closely with those infected. The impact of social media as an information source needs to be considered early in the pandemic.

One of the key challenges, particularly in larger countries where healthcare is under multiple provincial jurisdictions, and where the epidemiology of the pandemic may differ across local regions, is apparent, or real, inconsistency across national and local jurisdictional messages in regards to public health restrictions and strategies. So national advice on the national news may need to be varied for the local context in the local jurisdiction. Clear, consistent messaging is required with clarification on how and why the information might vary locally.

LESSONS LEARNED

Health systems must recover from disasters and pandemics. Learning from such events is an important part of system development. Evaluating outcomes and identifying issues allows the incorporation of knowledge learned into future planning and preparedness, with a key emphasis on pandemic system recovery. Facilities, personnel, resources, and health achievements lost must be restored. In particular, those involved in the care of others, healthcare workers, should be cared for in turn, and assisted as appropriate in recovery from the challenges and losses they have faced. A key lesson learned from the

COVID-19 pandemic was the importance of equity and the role of community engagement. The healthcare response was regularly termed a whole of health response with all levels of healthcare working together particularly highlighting the importance of engaging primary care in the national response.

In reviewing losses, it is important to focus equally on strengths and successes. Excess global mortality from 2020 to 2021 during the SARS-CoV-2 pandemic was estimated at 120.3 deaths per 100,000 population, with up to 300 in many countries. However, strategies to manage the pandemic have also been reported to have saved millions of lives. It is equally important to identify and incorporate these into planning and to prevent the overwhelming of healthcare systems and facilitate rapid restoration with resilience to future disasters and pandemics.

Pandemics are variable and throughout their evolution are unpredictable. The SARS-CoV-2 pandemic was a global crisis that lasted over 3 years. In May 2023, the Director General of the WHO declared the end of the COVID-19 pandemic as a global health emergency and as a public health emergency of international concern. SARS-CoV-2 variants continue to circulate.

The legacy of thousands affected by PAC is yet to be realised as we continue to research and gather scientific evidence on the effects. Each country faces different circumstances based on the epidemiological situation and the context [30]. The SARS-CoV-2 pandemic has been prolonged by discrepancy in vaccination access globally with some countries with ample supply to countries providing 4th and 5th doses of vaccines to citizens while others struggle to provide primary courses. A united global response is necessary for successful pandemic management. The impacts of this and other pandemics can be much broader than 'just health'; effects on social determinants of health through effects on education, socialisation, employment, and careers all place a large burden on future health following the pandemic.

Finally and critically we need to remember that SARS-CoV-2 is unlikely to be the last pandemic seen in most people's lifetimes and so we need to be prepared for a global united response to our next global infectious outbreak to protect our families, our 'communities, our societies, our economies' and our world, through 'safe scalable clinical care in resilient health systems' [31].

ACTIVITIES – SELF-ASSESSMENT AGAINST LEARNING OUTCOMES

1. What makes a pandemic more severe and how is that relevant to the management of the pandemic?
2. If you are in the position of Chief Medical Officer when the next pandemic is emerging what are the key elements of your pandemic management plan?
3. Consider the coronavirus pandemic or other pandemics you may have experienced. What are the most substantive healthcare management changes that occurred within your health profession during the pandemic?

KEY READINGS

Organisation for Economic Co-operation and Development. Ready for the Next Crisis? Investing in Health System Resilience. Paris: Organisation for Economic Co-operation and Development; 2023. Available at: https://www.oecd.org/health/ready-for-the-next-crisis-investing-in-health-system-resilience-1e53cf80-en.htm

Note

1. A pragmatic decision was made to designate 2019–2023 as the time period of the SARS-CoV-2 pandemic despite the pandemic being declared by WHO between 2020 and 2023. This was in the light of the widespread use of 'Covid-19' as the name of the disease caused by the SARS-CoV-2 virus, which derived from the timing of diagnosis of the first global cases in 2019.

References

1. McNeill, W., *Plagues and peoples*. 1st ed. 1976, Garden City, NY: Anchor. 368 p.
2. Porta, M., *A Dictionary of epidemiology*. 2008, USA: Oxford University Press.
3. World Health Organisation. *Pandemic influenza preparedness and response a WHO guidance document*. 2009 [cited 2023 25 March 2023]; Available from: https://www.ncbi.nlm.nih.gov/books/NBK143061/.
4. World Health Organisation. *The continuum of pandemic phases*. 2016 [25 March 2023]; Available from: https://www.cdc.gov/flu/pandemic-resources/planning-preparedness/global-planning-508.html.
5. Department of Health. *Australian health sector emergency response plan for novel coronavirus (COVID-19)*, Department of Health, Editor. 2020, Canberra: Department of Health.
6. Schultz, J., et al., Disaster ecology, in *Textbook of disaster psychiatry*, R. Ursano, et al., Editors. 2017, Cambridge (UK), New York (US), Victoria (AU); Delhi (IN), Singapore (SG): Cambridge University Press. p. 44–59.
7. World Health Organisation. *Tracking SARS-CoV-2 variants*. 2022 [cited 2022 14 April 2022]; Available from: https://www.who.int/en/activities/tracking-SARS-CoV-2-variants/.
8. World Health Organisation, Weekly epidemiological update on COVID-19 - 8 March 2023 Edition 133, in *Weekly epidemiological update on COVID-19*, World Health Organisation, Editor. 2023, Geneva, Switzerland: World Health Organisation.
9. McIntosh, K., COVID-19: Clinical features, in *UpToDate*. 2022, Wolters Kluwer: The Netherlands.
10. National COVID-19 Clinical Evidence Taskforce. Care of people with post-acute COVID-19, in *Clinical flowcharts*, N.C.-C.E. Taskforce, Editor. 2021, Melbourne, VIC: National COVID-19 Clinical Evidence Taskforce.
11. Greenhalgh, T., et al., Management of post-acute covid-19 in primary care. *BMJ*, 2020. **370**: p. m3026.
12. Robertson, J., *The economic cost of infectious diseases*, Canberra: D.o.P. Library, Editor. 2003. https://apo.org.au/node/6961
13. Lee, S., et al., The experience of SARS-related stigma at Amoy Gardens. *Social Science & Medicine*, 2005. **61**(9): p. 2038–2046.
14. Emanuel, E.J., The lessons of SARS. *Annals of Internal Medicine*, 2003. **139**(7): p. 589–591.
15. Reliefweb. *Global humanitarian overview 2023, January–February update (snapshot as of 28 February 2023)*. 2023 [25 March 2023]; Available from: https://reliefweb.int/report/world/global-humanitarian-overview-2023-january-february-update-snapshot-28-february-2023?_gl=1*1442i05*_ga*MjEyMDYyOTIyMC4xNjc5MTg1OTU5*_ga_E60ZNX2F68*MTY3OTE4NTk1OS4xLjEuMTY3OTE4NTk5C4yNS4wLjA.
16. UNICEF. *Child displacement*. 2023 [25 March 2023]; Available from: https://data.unicef.org/topic/child-migration-and-displacement/displacement/.
17. United Nations, *Global humanitarian overview 2022*, U. Nations, Editor. 2022, Geneva: United Nations.
18. World Health Organization, *COVAX calls for urgent action to close vaccine equity gap*, W.H. Organization, Editor. 2022, Geneva: World Health Organization.
19. Australian Government, *Australian health management plan for pandemic influenza*, D.o. Health, Editor. 2019, Canberra: Commonwealth of Australia. https://www.health.gov.au/sites/default/files/documents/2022/05/australian-health-management-plan-for-pandemic-influenza-ahmppi.pdf
20. World Health Organisation. *International health regulations (2005)*. 3rd ed. 2016 [25 March 2023]; [Available from: https://www.who.int/publications/i/item/9789241580496.

21. Patel, M.S., et al., General practice and pandemic influenza: a framework for planning and comparison of plans in five countries. *PLoS One*, 2008. **3**(5): p. e2269.
22. Kidd, M.R., Five principles for pandemic preparedness: lessons from the Australian COVID-19 primary care response. *British Journal of General Practice*, 2020. p. 316–317.
23. Desborough, J., et al., Australia's national COVID-19 primary care response. *Medical Journal of Australia*, 2020. **213**(3): p. 104–106.
24. Pittman, M., *Hierarchy of Controls*, H.o.C.B. NIOSH, Editor. 2015: Wikimedia Commons. p. By Original version: NIOSHVector version: Michael Pittman - Original version: JPEG file by NIOSH: CC0, https://commons.wikimedia.org/w/index.php?curid=90190143.
25. NIOSH, *Hierarchy of Controls*, H.o. Controls, Editor. 2023, Atlanta: The National Institute for Occupational Safety and Health.
26. Hor, S., et al., How Australian general practices managed infection prevention and control during the SARS-CoV-2 pandemic: An interview study. *BMJ Open*, 2022. **12**(9): p. 1–11. doi:10.1136/bmjopen-2022-061513
27. Kim, E. and C.T. Bergstrom, *Flattening the curve - coronavirus disease 2019 epidemic infographic.jpg*, SlowTheSpread.png, Editor. 2020, Wikimedia Commons.
28. Roberts, L., et al., Integrating General Practice into the Australian COVID-19 response: A description of the GP Respiratory Clinic Program in Australia. *Annals of Family Medicine*, 2021. **20**(3): p. 273–276. doi:10.1370/afm.2808
29. Dykgraaf, S.H., et al., "A decade's worth of work in a matter of days": The journey to telehealth for the whole population in Australia. *International Journal of Medical Informatics*, 2021. **151**: p. 104483.
30. World Health Organisation, COVID-19 weekly epidemiological update edition 87, in *COVID-19 Weekly Epidemiological Update*, W.h. Organisation, Editor. 2022, Geneva: World Health Organisation.
31. World Health Organisation, *Strategic preparedness, readiness and response plan to end the global COVID-10 emergency in 2022*, W.H. Organisation, Editor. 2022, Geneva: World Health Organisation.

25

Complex humanitarian emergencies

Nahuel Arenas-García

INTRODUCTION AND OBJECTIVES

While it is recognized that all humanitarian crises are complex, there are particular contexts in which an acute crisis is the result of a combination of factors including violence, hunger and displacement, and in which political considerations are fundamental for the implementation of humanitarian operations and, ultimately, the resolution of the crisis. This chapter focuses on the particularities of complex humanitarian emergencies (CHEs) in which there is a complex interplay of causative factors and impacts, including situations when hazards of natural origin or biological hazards further aggravate a context of threats and fragility. The chapter is structured as follows: Section I introduces the basic conceptual considerations to understand the particularities of these complex scenarios and, Section II, discusses some of the operational challenges and implications for the implementation of interventions in contexts of complex emergencies.

On completion of this chapter, you should be able to:

1. Describe the particular characteristics of CHEs.
2. Demonstrate an understanding of the complex interaction of risks that characterize major events.
3. Demonstrate an understanding of the particular importance of humanitarian principles in contexts of complex emergencies as well as some of the approaches required to ensure these events are effectively managed.

SECTION I: CONCEPTUAL CONSIDERATIONS

Complex Humanitarian Emergencies

The concepts of complex political emergencies, CHEs, or, in short, complex emergencies, was first used after the end of the Cold War to describe crises resulting from the interaction of a multiplicity of political, economic, and socio-cultural factors (e.g., the cases of civil conflicts in Mozambique and Sudan) [1]. One of the defining characteristics of CHEs is the total or substantial breakdown of national or regional authority due to multiple causes, with a far-reaching impact on people's lives, wellbeing, and dignity. CHEs are

DOI: 10.4324/9781032626604-32

typically the result of multi-dimensional phenomena in which large numbers of people are affected by conflict, displacement, disease, and/or hunger, resulting from widespread damage to societies and economies. There is, therefore, a requirement for massive multi-faceted humanitarian assistance to address the needs of affected populations, which may include lack of clean water, malnutrition, poor sanitation, and low health care and vaccine coverage, among other compound factors, coupled with "intensive and extensive political management and coordination." [2]

CHEs, as defined above, are characterized by the central role of conflict and the wide-ranging consequences of acute violence [3]. While the response to any emergency entails a level of complexity, we should not confuse CHEs with a disaster or epidemic response that takes place outside a context of conflict, violence, and profound institutional fragility. According to Albala-Bertrand [4] "the key feature of a long-lasting complex emergency is the societal/institutional weakness that fails to accommodate entrenched and violent competing identity groups." By definition, in a CHE, local and national capacities to respond to the relief needs of affected population are inadequate. According to Allen and Schomerus [5]

> More often than not, these emergencies are not unforeseen, but have been either politically created or, in fact, have been in an emergency-like state for a rather long time. Aid agencies today deal with cases where an emergency was declared years ago and yet the 'immediate action' either took a long time to be realised or the emergency situation has changed so little that the state of emergency has become a permanent one.

In today's highly inter-connected world, we are increasingly challenged by compounding and interrelated environmental, socioeconomic, and political crises. Risks become systemic and multi-hazard scenarios are increasingly common. The COVID-19 pandemic, for instance, has combined with a number of other threats to human life and livelihoods including conflict, displacement, climate-related disasters, all aggravating structural poverty and inequality in many parts of the world [6]. Climate disasters are now causing more displacement than conflict [7]. On the other hand, displaced populations face an increased risk of infectious disease outbreaks [8]. As pointed out in the United Nations Global Assessment Report [9],

> multiple interacting risks within a system, or complex risk, are present within all contexts, and the manifestation of this complexity is unique to each specific context. At different times within a given context, different combinations of risk may become more or less salient.

We will present below some considerations related to addressing multi-faceted or inter-dependent elements in contexts of violence and fragility, to explore their complexity in more detail.

Natural hazard-related disasters and displacement in the context of fragility

Climate-related disasters are projected to increase globally, driven by climate change. Higher temperatures, for instance, are increasing the frequency and intensity of droughts in many parts of the world. Increased land degradation and desertification, soil salinity, and reduced soil fertility generate pressures on local populations that may lead to conflict over limited water and food. Such a combination of stress and vulnerability increases complexity [10].

This has been the case in countries like Chad, Iraq, Sudan, and Somalia, for example, where conflict and climate risks are high and have resulted in mass displacement of large populations, generating additional pressure and competition over natural resources [9, 10]. Nordqvist and Krampe [11] have analyzed the relationship between climate change and security risks in Iraq, Lake Chad and Yemen, and conclude that such crises require responses that span multiple security sectors, such as economic, political, military, and environmental security, with a highly contextual approach. In Iraq, security risks are worsened by drought and food insecurity. Hassan, Born and Nordqvist [12] argue that the combination of hydrological limitations, increasing temperatures, and extreme weather events heighten communal tensions and increase local support for terrorist groups. The Darfur conflict in Sudan cannot be fully understood without considering the past of prolonged droughts and environmental degradation that led to population movement and increased tensions between farmers and pastoralists.

Climate change-induced migration can also promote conflict in areas receiving migrants. Competition over resources can ignite ethnic tensions, generating distrust between displaced and host populations, and exacerbating existing socioeconomic fault lines [13]. Somalia, a country affected by decades of conflict and political instability, is also highly disaster-prone, having endured several severe droughts in recent decades [9]. According to UNHCR, close to 650,000 new internal displacements were recorded in Somalia, from January to July 2018, which were caused by flooding (47%), drought (29%), and conflict (23%).[1] Pakistan, one of the foremost host countries for refugees in the world, and challenged by its own internal conflict in the Khyber Pakhtunkhwa (KP) province, also suffers from recurring disasters in the context of chronic poverty. This, in turn, limits the ability of vulnerable households to recover and resulting in additional displacement and humanitarian needs [14].

These examples show how natural hazard-related disasters can play a role in igniting social tensions that may result in violence. At the same time, there is a heightened complexity in addressing needs when natural hazard-related disasters impact violence-affected regions. In addition, displacement can further exacerbate the vulnerabilities of affected populations.

Communicable diseases in complex emergencies

Damaged infrastructure and limited functioning of government services in conflict situations can deeply affect the health of the population. In Syria, for example, after more than a decade of conflict, local populations have 40% less drinking water than they had before the war. According to the International Committee of the Red Cross, only 50% of water and sanitation systems function properly [15].

The movement of populations and their resettlement in places that may be overcrowded and/or lack basic hygiene and sanitation infrastructure can also contribute to communicable disease transmission. Other contributing factors are the poor nutritional status that may result from food shortages and the overall limited access to health care in the context of complex emergencies. Absent or overwhelmed public services and infrastructure hamper the overall capacity to implement prevention and control programmes, with a consequent rise in vector-borne diseases including malaria, yellow fever, and other vaccine-preventable diseases [16].

Violence, or the threat of violence, can be an impediment to vaccination. Even where access is possible, large gatherings could be targeted by violent groups, putting people (especially women and children) at risk. Health workers and those involved in the logistics of mass vaccination could also be at risk. In these cases, decisions need to consider not only epidemiological and vaccine considerations, but also ethical and political aspects that are specific to the context in which the emergency is unfolding [17]. Armed conflict in the Arab Region, for instance, has resulted in damaged healthcare facilities, and the death or fleeing of healthcare workers, greatly impeding the health response to COVID-19 [18].

All factors promoting disease transmission interact synergistically, especially exacerbating the "risk of communicable diseases including diarrhoeal diseases, acute respiratory diseases, measles, meningitis, tuberculosis, HIV, viral haemorrhagic fevers, hepatitis E, trypanosomiasis and leishmaniosis" [19]. In most complex emergencies, communicable diseases, often in combination with malnutrition, are the major cause of illness and death [16]. Diarrhoeal diseases are a major cause of morbidity and mortality in complex emergencies, particularly in camp situations or in contexts where the quality and quantity of water and of other hygiene and sanitation conditions are inadequate. According to Connolly et al. [16], "in camp situations, diarrheal diseases have accounted for more than 40% of these deaths in the acute phase of an emergency, with over 80% of these deaths occurring in children aged under 2 years."

SECTION II: ETHICAL AND OPERATIONAL CONSIDERATIONS

The multi-dimensional nature of the emergencies described in this chapter, and their long-term impact on societies, require integral and multi-faceted approaches. Operating in highly politicized and complex contexts may present ethical dilemmas and particular challenges, some of which we present below.

Humanitarian principles

Most humanitarian actors are guided by the four humanitarian principles of humanity, impartiality, neutrality, and independence, as shown in Table 25.1. These principles have

Table 25.1 Humanitarian principles

Humanity	Impartiality	Neutrality	Independence
Human suffering must be addressed wherever it is found, without discrimination. The purpose of humanitarian action is to protect life, alleviate suffering, and respect the dignity of human beings.	Humanitarian action must be carried out on the basis of need alone, giving priority to the most urgent cases of distress and making no distinctions on the basis of nationality, race, gender, religious belief, class, or political opinions.	Humanitarian actors must not take sides in hostilities or engage in controversies of a political, racial, religious, or ideological nature.	Humanitarian action must be autonomous from the political, economic, military, or other objectives that any actor may hold with regard to areas where humanitarian action is being implemented.

gained broad acceptance and consensus across humanitarian actors and, thus, provide the foundations for humanitarian action.

These principles are derived from the core principles which have long guided the work of the International Committee of the Red Cross and the national Red Cross/Red Crescent Movement. The humanitarian principles have also been formally enshrined in two General Assembly resolutions: 46/182, which was adopted in 1991, and endorses the principles of humanity, neutrality and impartiality, and General Assembly resolution 58/114, adopted in 2004, and which added independence as a fourth key principle underlying humanitarian action.

In addition to their consequential value to guide decisions and inform strategic choices within the framework of humanitarian assistance, promoting and respecting these principles is also fundamental to build trust with affected populations and parties of a conflict, understand their needs and perspectives, and gain the required access to help those in need. These and other principles are further developed in the Humanitarian Charter,[2] which also summarizes the key commitments widely agreed upon by humanitarian agencies to guide their work, including adherence to the Code of Conduct for the International Red Cross and Red Crescent Movement and non-governmental organizations (NGOs) in Disaster relief, and to minimum quality standards (to know more, see Core Humanitarian Standard on Quality and Accountability – CHS).[3]

The Sphere movement was started in 1997 by a group of humanitarian professionals from NGOs, along with the Red Cross and Red Crescent Movement, to frame a series of rights, obligations and principles that should guide humanitarian response (the Humanitarian Charter), as well as to develop a set of universal minimum standards in core areas of humanitarian assistance. Its aim is to improve the quality of assistance provided to people affected by humanitarian crises and to enhance the accountability of the humanitarian system in humanitarian response. See – https://spherestandards.org

---

Some international organizations involved in humanitarian action and advocacy, like Oxfam, do not adhere to the principle of neutrality. This is because they understand that not every party to violence is always equally to blame and because they believe they cannot call themselves neutral while at the same time taking a stand on the causes of humanitarian need and proposing policy changes to solve them [20]. The ICRC, however, does not believe that neutrality prevents it from taking steps to get perpetrators of international humanitarian law violations to stop their illegal actions [21]. The reality is that humanitarian contexts are complex, each situation is different, and applying humanitarian principles is in essence challenging and poses ethical dilemmas.

According to ICRC [21]:

If applied with consistency and intelligence, the principles provide a formidable guide for delivering humanitarian assistance and protection in the most extreme circumstances, as demonstrated [in] Afghanistan. In this context, the consistent application of the principles has allowed the ICRC to maintain its presence throughout decades of conflict and to operate across multiple frontlines. [...] This acceptance and the access it made possible – at times benefiting other actors such as WHO – was not a straightforward process [...]. The situation required perseverance, consistency and creativity in the way the ICRC applied the principles to demonstrate to all sides the benefits of having a neutral intermediary in the midst of conflict.

Humanitarian principles provide an operational framework that help navigate or overcome the challenges and dilemmas inherent to delivering aid in complex environments [22]. Notwithstanding certain differences in conceptual and operational approaches, all humanitarian interventions must be guided by strong ethical and legal principles as well as by professional and quality standards, putting affected populations' lives and dignity at the centre of humanitarian action.

Coordination and multi-faceted response

Affected populations (including refugees or internally displaced populations) in contexts of CHEs often depend on governments (or rebel factions) with very limited capacities to assist them (provided they want to in the first place). The delivery of humanitarian aid is mostly in the hands of external actors, including UN agencies such as UNHCR, WFP, WHO and UNICEF, international NGOs, and the ICRC among others. The role and capacities of local NGOs, community-based organizations, volunteer networks, the local Red Cross/Red Crescent chapter, and local faith-based organizations, among others, are critical to reach the most in need. Different organizations have different mandates and expertise, on which they base their interventions, from operational assistance at the community level to sectorial policy at the national level, to political negotiation and advocacy at the international level. At the national and local levels they would coordinate among themselves participating in sectorial clusters that seek to ensure gaps are identified, complementarities are maximized and overlaps are prevented. OCHA has the role of supporting humanitarian coordination, while different sectoral experts (UN Agencies, NGOs, etc.) lead the different clusters. Local authorities, including those from different sectors, may also participate, co-lead or even chair these coordination efforts, depending on the context. There is a global call to ensure that local actors are part and parcel of these coordination mechanisms, participating in the design and accessing funds to implement humanitarian action.

Emergency relief operations can be largely effective in saving lives and preventing hunger and excess morbidity. Humanitarian actors can help deliver quality water, food, provide adequate shelter and sanitation, and health services (among others). Their effectiveness will depend on many factors including the access to resources (funding and staff to support the humanitarian operation) and supplies, access to affected populations, caseload and extension of the affected areas (e.g., whether the humanitarian crisis is taking place in a small or large geographical area, whether it is affecting the entire country or is it a cross-border/regional situation), conditions of the terrain (e.g., for transportation, availability of sources of water, etc.), security of its staff and existence of coordination mechanisms to ensure complementarity of capacities and efficiencies across humanitarian actors. According to Connolly et al. [16] "available interventions need to be implemented more systematically in complex emergencies with higher levels of coordination between governments, UN agencies, and non-governmental organizations."

A mass population movement or a spike in hunger in the framework of a conflict, for instance, are often acute emergencies in the context of a protracted crisis. For humanitarian aid agencies, this may require shifting modes of operation. For example, while emergency food distribution might be required and pertinent during an acute emergency to save lives, it may not be an appropriate strategy in the medium and long term, since it could contribute to aid dependency, may hamper the functioning of the local economy and agricultural system (particularly if the food distributed is imported), among other risks and unintended consequences – in cases of functioning local markets, cash-based interventions may be a better choice.

In any case, understanding the local context with its political complexities is of critical importance to deliver aid in the context of CHEs. This requires constant monitoring and (re) assessing the situation to ensure the interventions match the priorities of the affected populations, do no harm and minimize risks.

Accessing affected populations and providing humanitarian assistance in an environment of genuine danger is, of course, a key challenge. In these complex contexts aid could be seriously impeded, delayed, or prevented by politically or conflict-motivated constraints [2], posing significant risks for humanitarian relief workers [23]. Even if security risks are managed, there might be important operational challenges. For example, in contexts of internal conflicts it might be difficult to have a centralized strategy in the face of an epidemic outbreak [24].

Since CHEs are essentially political and politicized, an effective response would normally require active political support for humanitarian interventions, usually from the Security Council or the UN in general, and a coordinated response among humanitarian and political organizations.

Long-term considerations

An acute crisis may be a short-term manifestation of deep-seated political, social, ethnic, cultural, and economic fractures. If the underlying factors resulting in a crisis are not understood and addressed, the symptoms will continue to manifest time and again. While saving lives and alleviating suffering is the humanitarian imperative, humanitarian relief must be provided in a way that is conducive and supportive of recovery and long-term development. General Assembly resolution 46/182, which created a framework for humanitarian assistance and coordination, indicates that "the rehabilitation phase should be used as an opportunity to restructure and improve facilities and services destroyed by emergencies in order to enable them to withstand the impact of future emergencies." [25]

While the term *rehabilitation* refers more narrowly to the measures aimed at restoring normal living conditions, basic services and facilities interrupted or degraded as a consequence of the emergency, the term *recovery* focuses on restoring the

> capacities of the government and communities to rebuild and recover from crisis as well as to prevent relapses into conflict. In so doing, recovery seeks not only to catalyze sustainable development activities, but also to build upon earlier humanitarian programmes to ensure that their inputs become assets for development.
>
> [26]

As mentioned earlier in Chapter 3, the goal is not only to restore, but also to *improve* livelihoods and health, as well as economic, physical, social, cultural and environmental assets, systems and activities; in other words, "build back better" to avoid recreating the conditions that led to the conflict or disaster in the first place [27].

Early recovery is an approach that addresses recovery needs that arise during the humanitarian phase of an emergency; using humanitarian mechanisms that align with development principles. It enables people to use the benefits of humanitarian action to seize development opportunities, build resilience, re-build capacities, and contribute to solving, not exacerbating long-standing problems that may have contributed to the crisis [28].

Given the profound level at which conflicts and disasters affect societies, their consequences can last for generations. Clearly, the rehabilitation phase cannot be approached with short-term isolated measures but with an integral approach that contributes to peace, security, and development. In the aftermath of a conflict, this may involve measures geared towards reconciliation and the rebuilding of the legitimacy of the state and its institutions. In the words of Green [29] "Rehabilitation after war — or rehabilitation during a lull in recurrent conflict to avert its reappearance — is a process interacting with reconciliation and is rarely stable, continuous or predictable." If the conflict creates mass displacement, the priority of most of the displaced populations will be to return home and regain their livelihoods in a context of security. This means supporting institutions to restore law and order, as well as supporting and resourcing national priorities to ensure access to basic services and infrastructure. This also applies to contexts of disasters. The Sendai Framework for Disaster Risk Reduction 2015–2030, in its priority 4b, encourages to "utilize the recovery to invest in capacity for greater resilience and preparedness for future crises." There is a direct connection between the targets of the Sendai Framework and the Sustainable Development Goals (particularly SDG1, 11 and 13). Without addressing risk and vulnerability, development efforts can never be sustainable.

Unfortunately, many countries are caught up in a continuous recovery mode, being struck by crisis after crisis that deepens their vulnerability with limited time and capacity to fully recover and build resilience (e.g., Haiti). The COVID-19 pandemic can also be an opportunity to build back better if stimulus packages are geared to reducing risks and enhancing preparedness. Every opportunity must be taken to fully consider risks into recovery planning and implementation, with a holistic and systemic approach, so that these efforts contribute to building societal resilience.

FINAL NOTES

Today, human, social, political, economic and environmental systems are in complex interaction. Our global interconnectedness creates an interdependence of challenges like climate change, biodiversity loss, conflict, pandemics, urbanization, and population growth among others. Crises and humanitarian emergencies are seldom the result of an isolated event but the manifestations of structural deficiencies and governance failures that interact with multiple stressors. Natural and social hazards, the COVID-19 pandemic, economic shocks, political fragility and conflict can all become concurrent drivers of complex emergencies that challenge local capacities and peoples' resilience [6]. The current context reflects a landscape of hybrid risk, in which many man-made threats interact in an environment of extreme weather and climate events, as well as with underlying societal risk drivers, including poverty, inequality, lack of access to basic services, etc. [30]. Our effectiveness in responding to this challenge will ultimately lie in our capacities to overcome siloed thinking and embrace holistic and systemic approaches, which require enhanced collaboration across multiple sectors and actors, and strengthened partnerships. Addressing complexity requires developing flexible and adaptive preparedness and response mechanisms that are built on local knowledge and capacities and are conducive to building resilience in the long term.

ACTIVITIES

1. Identify a current CHE and consider all the possible underlying factors that contribute to the crisis.
2. Consider all the actions needed to save the lives, alleviate the suffering and respect the dignity of displaced populations in the context of a complex emergency.

KEY READINGS

Inter-Agency Standing Committee (IASC). Definition of Complex Emergencies. Working Group XVIth Meeting. 30 November 1994.

The Humanitarian Charter – https://spherestandards.org/humanitarian-standards/humanitarian-charter/

Notes

1. Cited in UNDRR, 2019: 409.
2. https://spherestandards.org/humanitarian-standards/humanitarian-charter/
3. https://spherestandards.org/humanitarian-standards/core-humanitarian-standard/

References

1. Perez de Armiño, K. and M. Areizaga, Emergencias complejas, in *Diccionario de Acción Humanitaria y Cooperación al Desarrollo*, K. Perez de Armiño, Editor. 2008, Spain: Icaria/Hegoa. https://dialnet.unirioja.es/servlet/libro?codigo=653996
2. Inter-Agency Standing Committee, Definition of complex emergencies, in *Working group XVIth meeting*. 1994.
3. Macias, L., *Complex emergencies*. 2013, Austin: Center for Climate Change and African Political Stability.
4. Albala-Bertrand, J.-M., Complex emergencies versus natural disasters: an analytical comparison of causes and effects. *Oxford Development Studies*, 2000. **28**(2): p. 187–204.
5. Allen, T. and M. Schomerus, *Complex emergencies and humanitarian responses.* London: University of London, 2008. **2790162**.
6. Kruczkiewicz, A., et al., Compound risks and complex emergencies require new approaches to preparedness. *Proceedings of the National Academy of Sciences*, 2021. **118**(19): p. e2106795118.
7. IDMC, *Global report on internal displacement 2021*. 2021, Geneva: International Displacement Monitoring Centre. https://www.internal-displacement.org/sites/default/files/publications/documents/IDMC_Internal_Displacement_Index_Report_2021.pdf
8. Spiegel, P.B., et al., Occurrence and overlap of natural disasters, complex emergencies and epidemics during the past decade (1995–2004). *Conflict and Health*, 2007. **1**(1): p. 1–9.
9. UN Office for Disaster Risk Reducation. *Global risk assessment report (GAR)*. 2019, Geneva: UNDRR.
10. UN Office for Disaster Risk Reducation. *GAR special report on drought 2021*. 2021, Geneva: UNDRR.
11. Nordqvist, P. and F. Krampe, *Climate change and violent conflict: Sparse evidence from South Asia and South East Asia*. 2018, Solna: SIPRI (Stockholm International Peace Research Institute). https://www.jstor.org/stable/resrep39819
12. Hassan, K., C. Born, and P. Nordqvist, Iraq: Climate-related security risk assessment, in *Expert working group on climate-related security risks*. 2018, Stockholm International Peace Research Institute. https://www.preventionweb.net/publication/iraq-climate-related-security-risk-assessment
13. Reuveny, R., Climate change-induced migration and violent conflict. *Political Geography*, 2007. **26**(6): p. 656–673.

14. USAID. *Pakistan: Complex emergency and drought. factsheet N°2.* 2019, Washington DC: USAID. https://www.usaid.gov/sites/default/files/2022-05/09.30.19_-_USAID-DCHA_Pakistan_ Complex_Emergency_and_Drought_Fact_Sheet_2.pdf

15. International Committee of the Red Cross. *Syria water crisis: Up to 40% less drinking water after 10 years of war.* 2021; Available from: https://www.icrc.org/en/document/syria-water-crisis-after-10-years-war.

16. Connolly, M.A., et al., Communicable diseases in complex emergencies: impact and challenges. *The Lancet*, 2004. **364**(9449): p. 1974–1983.

17. World Health Organisation. *Vaccination in acute humanitarian emergencies. A framework for decision making.* 2017, Geneva, Switzerland: World Health Organisation.

18. UN Office for Disaster Risk Reduction. *Increasing global resilience to systemic risk: Emerging lessons from the COVID-19 pandemic.* 2021, Geneva: UNDRR.

19. Hammer, C.C., J. Brainard, and P.R. Hunter, Risk factors and risk factor cascades for communicable disease outbreaks in complex humanitarian emergencies: A qualitative systematic review. *BMJ Global Health*, 2018. **3**(4): p. e000647.

20. Oxfam. *Oxfam's role in humanitarian action.* Oxfam Policy Compendium Note, 2013.

21. International Committee of the Red Cross, Principles guiding humanitarian action. *International Review of the Red Cross*, 2016. **97**(897–898): p. 183–210.

22. Sphere Association. *What applying humanitarian principles and standards looks like in real life.* 2016; Available from: https://reliefweb.int/report/world/what-applying-humanitarian-principles-and-standards-looks-real-life

23. Inter-Agency Standing Committee, *Introduction to humanitarian action: A brief guide for resident coordinators.* 2015, New York & Geneva: OCHA.

24. Maher, O.A., et al., COVID-19 response and complex emergencies: The case of Yemen. *Disaster Medicine and Public Health Preparedness*, 2020. **14**(4): p. e27–e28.

25. United Nations, General Assembly Resolution 46/182. Strengthening of the coordination of emergency humanitarian assistance of the United Nations, in *78th plenary meeting.* 1991, New York (NY): United Nations.

26. UNHCR. *Refugees: Master glossary of terms. Status determination and protection information section.* 2006, Geneva: United Nations High Commissioner for Refugees.

27. United Nations Office for Disaster Risk Reduction. *UNISDR terminology on disaster risk reduction.* 2009, Geneva: United Nations.

28. GCER. *Guidance on early recovery coordination.* 2016, Geneva: Global Cluster for Early Recovery.

29. Herbold Green, R., Rehabilitation: Strategic, proactive, flexible, risky? *Disasters*, 2000. **24**(4): p. 343–362.

30. UN Office for Disaster Risk Reduction., *A Green and Resilient Recovery for Europe. A working paper.* 2021, Geneva: UNDRR.

Part 8

Strategic considerations

26

Leadership

Colin Myers and Elizabeth Rushbrook[1]

INTRODUCTION & OBJECTIVES

Disaster health leadership is far more than a response during an event. Although this is the part that is most remembered – it gets the media attention, attracts interest and funding; and is subject to the closest scrutiny during the immediate aftermath of any major incident.

Disaster health leadership spans the full spectrum of the *prevention, preparedness, response and recovery* (PPRR) cycle and is equally important across all phases.

Additionally, leadership is not only the purview of the 'person at the top'. Leadership is important at all levels of disaster health management – whether it be leadership of the team that keeps 'the business as usual' functional whilst others respond, a small local response team, regional responses or those undertaken at the state, national and/or international levels.

The breadth of skills required during different phases of a disaster can be demonstrated by the Cynafin Leadership Framework first described by David J Snowden in 2000 [1] and adapted for healthcare in 2017 by Kempermann [2] (Figure 26.1).

In essence leadership practiced in the Preparation, Preparedness and Recovery phases will operate within the complex or complicated domains while crisis response will operate almost exclusively within the Chaotic domain – a domain which requires actions to be taken while there is still great uncertainty about the true nature and magnitude of the disaster.

Since the skills required in the four phases described above are different it follows that leadership will also require differing skills and qualities based on the phase of the disaster – largely depending on the degree of urgency and/or strategic vision required in each phase. For example, a leader in the response phase will need to be able to manage a high degree of urgency and uncertainty in a defined portfolio. A leader in other phases usually has less urgency, but needs to take a strategic view, knowing that their actions (or inactions) could significantly impact the cost, and the success or failure of this or a later disaster response.

Appointed persons (particularly those in Government, key Non-Government Organisations or relevant philanthropic organisations, will, as a consequence of their appointment, have a leadership role across several or all the PPRR phases even when they may not necessarily be the best person for the job at all phases of the event. Considerations should

DOI: 10.4324/9781032626604-34

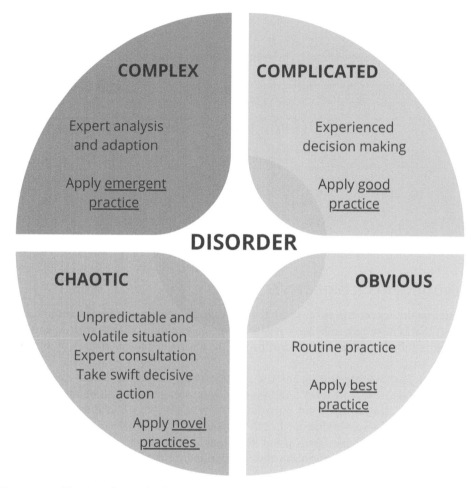

Figure 26.1 The Cynafin Leadership Framework consists of 4 domains which together categorise any event, and its leadership response, into Simple, Complicated, Complex and Chaotic (adapted from Kempermann, 2017)

always be given to ensuring that the best person for the job is leading or has a key role within any particular phase, particularly when the phases are overlapping (as is often the case in response and recovery).

In an emergency management context, leadership operates at all levels from each individual response team to the local, regional and state incident controller, and ultimately through to the department head and the Minister (or responsible elected official). Each level of this continuum has a distinct role and responsibility, but the fundamental elements are the same. In general, team leaders must have a tactical[2] focus, operational[3] context as well as a strategic[4] awareness of such factors as training, resources, mitigation measures, planning and alliance building. In contrast, incident controllers must have a tactical awareness, operational focus and strategic engagement. Ultimately, Department heads and Ministers need to have a strategic focus, good operational awareness and no tactical role (but they still need to understand the tactical level). The key to success is obviously a strong network of transparent and connected relationships between leaders at all levels, underpinned by trust and common goals.

This chapter aims to contextualise leadership in disaster management rather than discuss in detail the characteristics of leadership on which countless words and volumes have been written. At the end of this chapter, you should:

1. Have a comprehensive understanding of the qualities of effective leadership styles during all phases of disaster management.
2. Understand that leadership occurs at all levels and is not limited to 'those in charge'.
3. Understand the difference between crisis (*response*) leadership and consequence (*prevention, preparedness and recovery*) leadership.
4. Be inspired to be more aware of your own and others' leadership style and future development opportunities.
5. Understand the steps organisations need to take to identify and develop future leaders.

THE LEADER – QUALITIES

Are leaders *born or made*? In our view it is a combination. All great leaders need and have excellent interpersonal skills. This is related to innate personal qualities such as values, personality and presentation – the result of the nature of the person along with growth and experience. However, good leaders need to hone their skills; increase their understanding of the subject area in which they are working; increase their knowledge of the contemporary environmental conditions in which they work; and know and understand their stakeholders, especially their needs and priorities.

There are a multitude of books and articles written about leadership and many hundreds of leadership development programs. Prospective leaders can find many sources for learning the basics of leadership, studying such concepts as the various *leadership styles* (directive, visionary, affiliative, participative, pacesetting, coaching). Some sources for those who wish to pursue these concepts are listed in the further reading section.

Leadership qualities that are especially applicable during emergency management or emergency events include:

1. **Taking responsibility in both good and bad times** for those people and programs they are leading.
2. **Make the hard decisions** whether determining who gets what training/resources or deciding a behavioural matter within the team.
3. **Demonstrate self-reflection and self-awareness** to understand the strengths and weaknesses of the team, the activity or the operation.
4. **Measure and build emotional intelligence competencies** including self-awareness, social awareness, self-management and relationship management.
5. Ensure **connectedness with the teams** and fully understand their skills and needs.
6. Be able to **work with the political and social system**.

WHY IS LEADERSHIP IN DISASTER MANAGEMENT DIFFERENT?

Disasters are not a theoretical construct. They are real events typified by uncertainty, commonly involve short periods of extreme intensity, long periods of recovery, are not able to be prevented and they are highly public. They are often separated by long periods with no disaster. It follows therefore that leaders in this environment require honed skills.

There are a few simple rules to consider:

- Publicly recognise and, if necessary, take responsibility and accountability for the problem early.
- Act in a timely manner. There is ample time for analysis. A great response two weeks too late is ineffective.
- Show empathy with those impacted by the disaster and don't be afraid to express genuine emotion.
- Know the facts and voice them clearly.
- Communicate regularly and often. Then communicate again.

Over recent decades disaster management has become increasingly a mainstream consideration of most departments and organisations. They are supported by emergency service agencies – government/state, corporate and non-government. This became increasingly so following the 9/11 attacks on the World Trade Centre and the Bali bombings in 2002, followed by the 2003 Canberra fires, the 2004 Indian Ocean Tsunami, the Japanese earthquake and Tsunami, the 2005 Hurricane Katrina and the 2006 Cyclone Larry. Awareness of these natural disasters coinciding with increased terrorism risk has meant that emergency management is now everybody's business.

In recent years many organisations (both business and government) have developed the concept of risk 'management' to incorporate Disaster Management and Recovery into the broader concept of Business Continuity. In health this continuum is also described as

CASE STUDY 26.1 – TWO DIFFERENT LEADERSHIP STYLES

Captain Bligh steers the ship in face of adversity [Davis, 2011]	*How not to do it [Owen, 2011]*
Premier Anna Bligh, Queensland	Tony Hayward, CEO of BP
<ul><li>Was in control</li><li>Took ownership</li><li>Knew the name of each town already impacted by the flood and which towns were under threat</li><li>Could talk accurately about river heights, and the response and recovery arrangements.</li></ul> A key factor was that she did not try to hide the fact that people were likely to die and the community should prepare for that possibility. *'It might be breaking our hearts … but it will not break our will',* she said.	<ul><li>Was not in control</li><li>Did not take ownership</li><li>Was not sympathetic to those impacted by the disaster</li></ul> *'What the hell did we do to deserve this?'* (April 29) *'I want my life back'* (May 31) *'I think the environmental impact of this disaster is likely to be very, very modest,'* *'I don't feel my job is on the line'* (May 31).

Business Continuity, Disaster and Emergency Management arrangements or plans. Business Continuity can be defined as the capability of an organisation to continue to deliver products or services at acceptable levels during a major disruptive incident and is discussed in more detail in Chapter 6. There is a continuum between Business Continuity and Disaster recovery (BCDR) hence a leader in Emergency Management will also be deeply involved within the process of Business Continuity. As BCDR has developed the leadership roles within Disaster Planning and Emergency Management have become ever more public.

Leaders in emergency management are now under more intense public scrutiny; particularly with social media leaving the impression that our unforeseen crises are no longer disasters but instead political and media 'events'.

From the community perspective greater connectivity, increased inter-dependencies, just-in-time supply chains and increased urbanisation have led to greater community vulnerability so that previously *normal* disasters have much greater impact. Climate change and geopolitical events have created disasters not previously encountered (e.g., in the last 15 years Nations have variously received disaster-affected evacuees; evacuated citizens from various countries; responded to terrorism events and threats; responded to huge fires and floods; and provided major assistance in other countries' disasters.

Against this backdrop, more than ever before today's environment has created more complexity and placed greater responsibility on the shoulders of emergency management leaders. Disaster managers no longer have to solely focus on the incident, they need to deal with an equally large, demanding and complex situation created from the constant need for senior briefings, media briefings, community expectations and reassurance. Some of the compounding factors that require clear, strong leadership include:

- Changing **demographics** including cultural and linguistic diversity, urbanisation and the ageing population.
- **Climate change** and environmental protection focus.
- International and domestic **political interest** – a very high degree of political interest; politicians want to be more involved and therefore place more demands on managers and leaders for accurate information and well-developed plans.
- **Instant media and social commentary** – particularly as a consequence of immediate access to information, not necessarily facts.
- **Community and political expectations** – both expect more data, more quickly, and have greater performance expectations of managers.
- **Enhanced emergency management** – many more agencies/stakeholders have a role in emergency management than ever before.
- **Standards** – There has been slow development of International and National standards over the past few decades.
- **Non-routine events** – campaign events such as fires burning for months; slow-onset events (nine-year drought); ripple tsunami events; terrorist attacks, industrial mishaps and prologued pandemics all require much more sophisticated responses than the standard floods and fires.
- High likelihood **of post-incident commissions or inquiries** and a search for scapegoats and culprits – post-event inquiries/reviews, while important to enable lessons to be identified, they frequently result in finger-pointing and blame-allocation (often stimulated by the media).

CRISIS (RESPONSE) VS CONSEQUENCE (RECOVERY) LEADERSHIP

The single most important consideration of any leader with responsibilities in a disaster situation is the recognition that they have two responsibilities. Firstly, they must address the disaster event itself – plan for it, prevent it, mitigate it and bring it to an end. Secondly, they must address the consequences of any event – recover from it, be better in the future.

In any emergency, the government's priority is to save lives and restore public faith in the government and the future. The community and their political masters expect leaders to be able to clearly articulate what is going on (and why), explain what this means, describe what is being done about it and be clear about what is expected of others.

To do this the leader needs to create confidence and purpose by moving from the known to the unknown, making sense of the event, establishing a coalition of agencies/services, knowing and understanding the community's priorities, risks, information needs and manage the now while anticipating the future.

In other words, they need to deliberately and calmly RESPOND to the immediate critical events, whilst also predicting and addressing the CONSEQUENCES of the event and providing a clear vision of the way forward.

Finally, they also need to define the strategy to resolve the issues and then COMMUNICATE with their team, the media, the community, their political masters and other agencies to ensure a shared vision and an agreed pathway to recovery.

CRISIS LEADERSHIP (RESPONSE PHASE)

The critical phase of a major incident can be very short. Within four days of the 2002 Bali bombings, all Australians were repatriated and admitted to hospitals across Australia, however elements of the recovery phase continued for some ten years. In contrast, some disasters can continue for a lengthy time (sometimes being referred to as a *campaign event*). Severe bushfire seasons are one example, and the COVID-19 pandemic response is another. When a disaster starts it may not always be obvious whether it will be short-lived or will continue.

Whatever the disaster, speed matters. Time is a leader's nemesis in a crisis. When a crisis looms, the usual system responses and decision-making processes need to be suspended and decisions made in ways that reassure key stakeholders that its leaders understand that there is a problem, take it seriously and are immediately taking steps to address the issues. This does not mean that consultation is not required but that consultation must be carried out rapidly and often informally before 'best guess' decisions are made on limited information and then updated in real time as an understanding of the depth and complexity of the disaster becomes more apparent.

There are a number of principles that must guide a crisis leader to inform his/her actions and priorities:

1. **Primacy of life**. The first priority in crisis decision-making is to protect the life of employees, emergency workers and community members.
2. **Community protection**. The protection of communities and their assets and infrastructure is an important part of crisis management. Failure to do this adequately significantly contributes to the cost of recovery and the impact on those people affected.

3. **Multi-agency/all hazards**. Dealing with emergencies requires engagement with and input from all agencies, government departments, the community and the private sector.
4. **Community engagement**. The community is best informed and positioned to identify how and what is required to restore them to the new normal before, during and after an emergency. The preparedness and resilience of a particular community will inform this.
5. **Accountability and constant improvement**. All actions and decisions will be reviewed after the crisis, so it is critical to record them to understand both how that crisis was managed and to inform better management of future crises.

Leaders must ensure they are effectively communicating with all the key stakeholders involved in a crisis. They should have a crisis communication plan in place that is not only mainstream media-centric, but uses all available channels to reach key stakeholders, particularly the affected community. Communication should be two-way. Special attention should be paid to communication with the families and loved ones of any victims involved in an event.

Crisis leaders should be aware that following any incident, questions will be asked about what could or should have been done to prevent or at least mitigate the consequences and speed of recovery from the incident in question. These are reasonable questions and leaders should be prepared to address them early.

CONSEQUENCE LEADERSHIP (PREVENTION, PREPAREDNESS AND RECOVERY PHASES)

Consequence management is a broad term encompassing measures to protect the community's health and safety, restore essential services, and provide relief to governments, businesses, and community members affected by an event. By definition, it requires a multi-function, all-agency response coordinated by a nominated leader. Consequence management occurs *before* a crisis through prevention and preparedness and *after* the crisis during the recovery phase. These roles are perhaps the most difficult and the most time-consuming for emergency management leaders.

Prevention and Preparedness. During the *prevention and preparedness* phases, leaders need to be able to establish and maintain the involvement of key stakeholders. This is because effective crisis response requires trust and prior trust enables leaders to make the time-limited decisions that must be made.

This is true within an organisation and even more critical in a multi-agency environment such as government where different priorities exist and where familiarity is more difficult. Relationships can't be developed in the heat of an incident. Building these relationships and maintaining them (particularly within their communities) is therefore one of the highest priorities for emergency management leaders in the *prevention and preparedness* phases.

This can be particularly difficult during periods of less frequent incidents when budget, political and social priorities move community and government focus away from disaster preparedness and response.

The current level of government and community focus on disaster management will be directly proportional to the magnitude of the last disaster and inversely proportional to the time since that last disaster occurred.

Recovery. The recovery phase often very quickly disappears from the public eye. This can lead to a diminution of resources available for the recovery of communities affected by a disaster. This is often driven by the 24-hour media cycle but may also occur because another crisis has occurred, or sometimes disaster fatigue means that people move on. This has proven to be particularly difficult for communities affected by major infrastructure losses who feel abandoned as the focus shifts rapidly away from their plight.

A key element for a *recovery* leader is to ensure that recovery aspects are included while the *response* is still unfolding. This situates the recovery plan within and integral to the original crisis and ensures that critical decisions enable, rather than burden recovery efforts and outcomes.

As recovery proceeds, the clarity of the intended outcome diminishes as complications begin to occur. For example, if a building collapses from an earthquake, the immediate focus is clear – rescue survivors with little regard to cost. As time progresses, those affected (physically, psychologically and financially) need to be cared for – and at this time, complexity and cost begin to be considered. Communities sometimes compare the treatment of those affected to those from other disasters where different priorities and strategies were applied. Perceived differences will always be critically and publicly discussed.

WHO recognises that the actual time taken for a community to recover from a major disaster can be in the order of 20 years. In contrast, the news cycle will have moved on within 20 days, and most centralised resources designed to assist recovery with be withdrawn within 20 months

Recovery leaders need to be able to establish and maintain engagement over an extended timeframe, sometimes for many years, even decades. This, by necessity, includes establishing effective and efficient systems that are independent of any particular individual. Finally, recovery leaders must ensure that what they learn is used to inform not only future recovery operations, but also the prevention, preparedness and response aspects of future events. Comprehensive record-keeping and post-event debriefs are therefore essential.

Personal Disaster Leadership – developing 'your own style'
The influence of a great leader goes beyond words or actions. They not only know what to say and do, but they influence how team members operate, how teams of teams work together by multiplying their influence and others repeat their words and live out their values.

Petrie [3] suggests as leaders progress through their leadership development they should:

---

1. Focus more on their leadership development process and less on actual *leadership content*.
2. Make their leadership development and their work inseparable.
3. Create strong development networks.
4. Make their leadership development a process not an event.

In addition, leaders should ensure that they are well prepared for their role. Leaders need to continuously cultivate their personal readiness by:

1. Analysing learnings from previous events.
2. Broad research and reading (*Leaders are Readers*).

3. Identifying their own vulnerabilities as well as their team's.
4. Identifying their own skillsets.
5. Rehearsing – practice, practice, practice.

Put simply, disaster leadership can be described as everyone's responsibility. Whether it be in your own household, at work or in your community. Those who wish to hone their leadership skills should make leadership development part of their everyday plans, goals, and actions.

Organisational disaster leadership – what does it look like?

Hudson [4] is a global recruitment and talent management leader. Surveys of more than 100 human resource business leaders in Australia and New Zealand conducted by Hudson in 2015 and 2016 show that leadership development was their highest priority in both years. These surveys also showed that only 54% of organisations actually had their own clearly articulated leadership strategy.

Leadership is not an exact science but any organisation can improve the quality of their leadership. Hudson [4] describes four key factors in building leadership in an organisation:

1. Define what good leadership looks like in your organisation (capability) that can be used to guide recruitment and development.
2. Plan for the future, update annually.
3. Identify the people you need then develop assessment methodologies to understand their development needs and evaluate potential leaders.
4. Develop the capability of your leaders.

WHOLE OF COMMUNITY APPROACH

It is fitting that the final part of this chapter views emergency management leadership from the end-user perspective: the community.

Leaders must see the community as partners in dealing with disasters, although the direct role of the community (largely untrained and under-equipped) is more in *preparedness* and *recovery* rather than in planning and response.

Communities need to be engaged so that they understand their risk exposure; understand what measures they can take to better prepare; and understand the recovery process. For example, communities in Japan know the risk of earthquake while communities in California and Australia understand their fire risk. As a generalisation, those communities in natural disaster-prone areas, (e.g., the rural/urban interface) understand their risk although this changes when urban dwellers shift to the *country* and vice versa. In this situation, leaders need to target messages for specific communities, rather than simply relying on a general broadcast approach.

The principles that underpin the whole of community leadership in disasters and which should be applied include:

1. People understand the risks that may affect them and others in their community.
2. People have taken steps to anticipate disasters and protect themselves, their assets and their livelihoods.

3. People work together with local leaders using their knowledge and resources to prepare for and deal with disasters.

4. People work in partnership with emergency services, their local authorities and other relevant organisations before, during and after emergencies.

5. Businesses and other service providers undertake wide-reaching business continuity planning that links with their security and emergency management arrangements.

6. Public-private partnerships are important to better serve the community and are particularly valuable with vulnerable community members.

The most underdeveloped aspect of crisis management is the final task – political and organisational lesson-drawing

CONCLUSION

Business Continuity and Disaster Recovery (BCDR) has become mainstream in large organisations in recent years. As expectations of organisations to continue to function under extreme pressure have intensified so have the expectations placed on leaders in this field. Nowhere is this more critical than in the health services.

Disaster management leaders have a very complex role which may come under microscopic, universal scrutiny at any time. They must be able to analyse, plan and lead in the complex and at times chaotic environment created by a disaster. The rewards for a job well done, if recognised, are great but they can be sure that perceived mistakes or missteps will attract opprobrium.

Only by preparing themselves, their teams and their communities; by learning the lessons from previous events; and by adopting a sound, logical approach, underpinned by well-established networks and evidence-based decisions can they be sure that they have provided the best service to the communities who rely on their expertise.

ACTIVITIES

1. Consider the various phases of disaster management across the continuum of the PPRR cycle and produce a table which captures the different leadership traits you think may be appropriate to each stage.

2. How would you evaluate the effectiveness of a leader or a leadership team in crisis management?

3. Develop your own study plan with appropriate readings, exercises and courses to further develop appropriate leadership skills for your area of interest and occupation.

ADDITIONAL READINGS

Anthonissen, P., *Crisis communication: Practical PR strategies for reputation management and company survival*. 2008, London: Kogan Page.

Bernstein J., *Manager's guide to crisis management*. Briefcase Books Series. 2011, New York: Mc Graw-Hill Education.

Birkland, T.A. *Lessons of disaster: Policy change after catastrophic events*. American Governance and Public Policy Series. 2006, Georgetown: Georgetown University Press.

Boin, A. The new world of crises and crisis management: Implications for policymaking and research. *The Review of Policy Research,* 2009. **26**(4): p. 367–377.

Cantwell, J. *Leadership in action.* 2015, Melbourne: Melbourne University Press.

Channel Ten. We will rebuild [Internet]. 2011 [updated 2011 Jan 13; cited 2015 Dec 10]. Available from: https://www.youtube.com/watch?v=nfPXmEtyKrA

Cohn, R., *The PR crisis Bible: How to take charge of the media when all hell breaks loose.* 2008, North Charleston: Book Surge Publishing.

Correia, Dean, *Business continuity playbook,* 2nd ed., 2013. Amsterdam: Elsevier.

Dezenhall, E., *Damage control: The essential lessons of crisis management.* 2011, Westport: Prospecta Press.

Fink, S., *Crisis communications - The definitive guide to managing the message.* 2013, New York.

Fink, S., *Crisis management: Planning for the inevitable.* 2000, New York: American Management Association.

Garcia, H.F. Effective leadership response to crisis. *Strategy & Leadership.* 2006. **34**(1): p. 4–10.

Harari, O. *The Powell principles: 24 Lessons from Colin Powell, A legendary leader.* 2013, New York: Mc Graw-Hill.

Hardie, G., and M. Lazenby, *The emotionally healthy leader.* 2013, Carlton North: Monterey Press.

Lane, P., R. Clay-Williams, A. Johnson, V. Garde, and L. Barrett-Beck, Creating a healthcare variant CYNEFIN framework to improve leadership and urgent decision-making in times of crisis. *Leadership in Health Services,* Aug 2021.

Lehane, C., M. Fabiani, and B. Guttentag, *Masters of disaster: The Ten commandments of damage control.* 2014, New York: Palgrave Macmillan.

Moore, J., and P. Crocetti, What is BCDR? Business continuity and disaster recovery guide. techtarget.com.

Owen, J. BP oil spill crisis management: How not to do it. *CBS News* [Internet]. 2011 Jun 11 [cited 2015 Dec 10]. Available from: http://www.cbsnews.com/news/bp-oil-spill-crisis-management-how-not-to-do-it/

Phillips, B. *The media training Bible: 101 Things you absolutely, positively need to know before your next interview.* 2012, Washington (DC): SpeakGood Press.

Raphael, B. *When disaster strikes: How individuals and communities cope with catastrophe.* 1986, New York: Basic Books.

Snowden, D., and M. Boone, A leader's framework for decision making. *Harvard Business Review,* November 2007

Susskind, L, and P. Field, *Dealing with an angry public: The mutual gains approach to resolving disputes.* 1996, New York: Free Press.

Notes

1. With acknowledgement to previous authors Dudley McArdle, Peter Channells & Bob Jensen.
2. Disaster management tactics: carefully planned actions to be undertaken by an individual or team contributing to strategic outcome through coordinated operation(s).
3. Disaster management operations: coordinated (sequential or simultaneous) actions aimed to achieve strategic outcomes.
4. Disaster management strategy: the ultimate high-level plan of actions across the PPRR to achieve the outcome of minimising impact of disaster.

References

1. Snowden, D. Cynefin, a sense of time and place: an ecological approach to sense making and learning in formal and informal communities, in *KMAC* 2000. The University of Aston.
2. Kempermann, G., Cynefin as reference framework to facilitate insight and decision-making in complex contexts of biomedical research. *Frontiers in Neuroscience*, 2017 Nov 14. **11**: p. 634. doi: 10.3389/fnins.2017.00634.
3. Petrie, N., *Vertical leadership development - Part 1: Developing leaders for a complex world*. 2014, Center for Creative Leadership. p. 1–13.
4. Hudson, *Hudson 2015 Leadership survey results: HR leaders reveal top people priorities for 2016*. Available from: http://au.hudson.com/talent-management/hudson-2015-leadership-survey-results.

27

Evaluation and lessons management

Colin Myers and Diane Bretherton[1]

INTRODUCTION AND OBJECTIVES

Evaluation is a critical part of all that we do. Evaluation means assigning value, and this follows a process of critical and comparative analysis in which the effectiveness of what we do is compared with *best practice* or *prior knowledge and experience*.

Therefore before, during and after a disaster there is a need to evaluate what happened, why things happened as they did and to identify what could be done in the future to minimise adverse impacts, promote good practice and leverage opportunities for improvement.

The impacts of a disaster at their broadest levels are evaluated within the framework of their effects on the community – health services, infrastructure, environment and the economy. The key challenge of evaluation is to identify useful frameworks that will clearly indicate what should be evaluated, how it should be evaluated and what benchmarks or best practices will be used as a comparison. This is then compared against the performance of the system, i.e., what actually happened. This ongoing cycle of post-event analysis, evaluation and subsequent continuous improvement and review is contemporaneously known as **Lessons Management.**

Lessons management in its components and forms has been a part of post-disaster psyche for centuries, however, only relatively recently, have organisations and agencies combined knowledge management and lessons management disciplines. Leadership now faces major adverse events with a greatly expanded knowledge and capacity. Well-developed plans and recurrent coordinated disaster exercises have now replaced personal knowledge as the basis of a system-wide response. The increasing prevalence and experience of disasters have also generated higher community expectations of governments in all phases of disaster; particularly where events occur in the same location in close successions and comparisons can readily be made. This in turn generates higher levels of accountability for agencies to 'learn the lessons' from previous events in order to focus their actions and spending on resilience activities that will reduce the impact of future events.

Key to lessons management is the evaluation of system performance as a whole, through the applications of plans, processes and procedures. There has been much work within the high-risk safety, aviation and healthcare systems to implement a shared culture of

DOI: 10.4324/9781032626604-35

accountability to ensure honesty and responsiveness of all staff involved in their evaluation of errors or poor outcomes. This 'No Blame Culture' acknowledges the Swiss Cheese Model of Error first described by James Reason in 1990 [1] and seeks system-wide solutions. Enlightened organisations take up the mantra of, 'all are accountable, no one is to blame' [2].

As with many evaluations of performance, the processes of post-disaster evaluation and reporting can, if mismanaged, become adversarial, especially where serious shortfalls are perceived or readily apparent. Individuals or agencies may seek to absolve themselves of responsibility for failure to prepare and plan. Focussing on individual blame rather than failures of policy, planning and responsiveness within the system will cause strategic lessons to be overlooked, not understood and certainly not applied as the passage of time dims memories.

Note: Lessons management and continuous improvement is a foundational component of organisational resilience. Refer to Chapter 5 for an understanding of Organisational Resilience.

The aim of this chapter is to:

1. Outline the lessons management approach used in disaster health and review its implications on the future development of health policy and organisational structure, as well as disaster arrangements and performance.
2. Demonstrate the interrelationships between Health Disaster Planning, Disaster Response and Business Continuity and knowledge management within a Continuous Improvement Cycle.

On completion of this chapter, you should be able to:

1. Describe the Continuous Improvement Cycle and Lessons Management approach used in disaster healthcare.
2. Outline the processes and mechanisms of lessons management including debriefing, data collection analysis, evaluation and reporting.
3. Identify how the lessons identified from disasters may be used to assist the future development of health policy, organisational structure, arrangements and performance.

THE CONTINUOUS IMPROVEMENT CYCLE

General

Continuous improvement, sometimes called continual improvement, is the ongoing improvement of products, services or processes through incremental and breakthrough improvements. These efforts can seek 'incremental' improvement over time or 'breakthrough' improvement all at once.

Among the most widely used tools for the continuous improvement model is a four-step quality assurance method – the plan-do-check-act (PDCA) cycle[2]:

- **Plan:** Identify an opportunity and plan for change.
- **Do:** Implement the change on a small scale.
- **Check:** Use data to analyse the results of the change and determine whether it made a difference.
- **Act:** If the change was successful, implement it on a wider scale and continuously assess your results. If the change did not work, begin the cycle again.

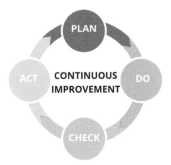

Figure 27.1 The PDCA cycle

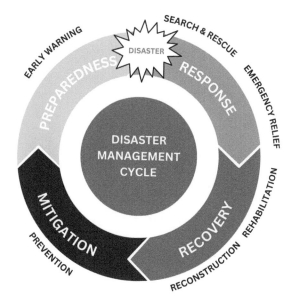

Figure 27.2 The PPRR model

Other widely used methods of continuous improvement, such as Six Sigma[3], Lean[4] and Total Quality Management[5], emphasise employee involvement and teamwork, to measure and systematise processes, and reduce variation, defects and cycle times.

The PDCA Cycle (Figure 27.1) closely approximates the PPRR model (Figure 27.2) which describes a continuous improvement model within Disaster Management. In this model the PPRR stands for Prevention (Mitigation), Preparedness (Planning), Response and Recovery.

LESSONS MANAGEMENT CONCEPTS, PRINCIPLES AND STANDARDS

Lessons management is useful to assess health system performance in response to a disaster event. It acts as a learning tool, gives credibility to and validates previous work. The evaluation should address contextual issues, desired outcomes, strategies, performance indicators, data sources, findings, outcomes, evaluation and recommendations (Figure 27.3).

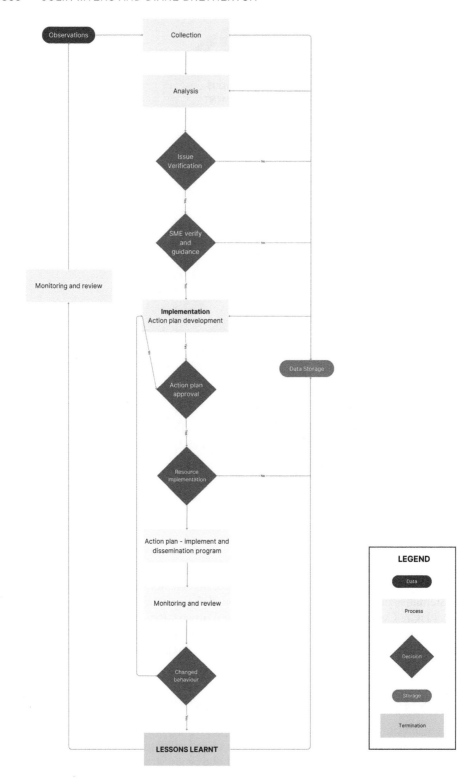

Figure 27.3 Elements of a lessons management system (adapted from Australian Emergency Management Handbook 8: Lessons management)

Leaders in disaster management at *strategic levels* including political officeholders, agency leaders and other senior executives need to ensure that the lessons that should be learnt from each event are identified and used to transform future preparedness and responses. At the *tactical/operational* level of incident commanders and operations managers, there is a need to identify and imbue meaning into the events and impacts of what has happened and to advocate for the appropriate development of systems and plans.

A recent review of major disasters in Australia conducted by the Monash Injury Research Institute identified six major strategic issues impacting the continued development of research and evaluation in disaster management [3].

1. State emergency management arrangements.
2. Understanding, awareness and assessment of risk.
3. Critical infrastructure.
4. Community communications and empowerment.
5. Research.
6. Defining disaster resilience for the community.

Health Services are involved in every one of these areas so as health practitioners we must all contribute to the work required to develop solutions which are appropriate to the areas and countries within which we live.

BUSINESS CONTINUITY PLANNING (BCP)

BCP is another lens by which to understand disaster planning and is discussed in more detail in Chapter 6. It is particularly helpful because it emphasises the requirement for a business or service to continue to function and provide critical services even under the significant stress of an unsuspected major incident or disaster. It involves developing practical plans to ensure that a business or service (including health) is prepared for and can continue to operate during and immediately after an incident or disruption and subsequently return to normal functioning. It allows a business or service to:

- Identify and prevent or reduce risks where possible (prevention or mitigation).
- Prepare for risks that can't be controlled (preparedness).
- Respond and recover when an incident or crisis occurs. (response and recovery).

Preparing a business continuity plan will help a health service to maintain critical services during an incident and recover more effectively once it has occurred.

As with any disaster planning a business continuity plan should be regularly exercised and updated to ensure continued relevance.

CONCEPT OF EVALUATION AND EVALUATION FRAMEWORKS

The process of evaluation (which sits within a continuous improvement cycle), seeks to make sense of what has occurred and to ascribe meaning that can inform future directions in regard to prevention, preparedness, response and recovery from disasters. Evaluation should occur throughout the entire cycle of disaster management focussed around a structure of assessing inputs, processes, outputs and subsequent outcomes.

In 2003, the World Association for Disaster and Emergency Medicine published *Guidelines for Evaluation and research in the Utstein style* [4]. This was the first attempt to standardise the conceptual framework, terminology and approaches to investigations into the medical and public health aspects of disasters. This framework was updated in a series of articles published in the journal Prehospital and Disaster Medicine. In introducing those articles, Birnbaum et al. [5] identified a framework based on two broad research approaches, **epidemiological** and **interventional,** which are transcended by five frameworks for medical and public health aspects of disasters:

- **Conceptual framework** recognises the causal linkage between hazards, events, impacts and consequences.
- **Longitudinal framework** describes the chronological continuum throughout the pre-event, event and post-event.
- **Transactional societal framework** recognises the complexity of interactions between 13 societal systems that underpin the risk and consequences of disasters, and which interact with each other through a fourteenth system of coordination and control.
- **Relief/recovery framework** provides the basis for understanding the effectiveness of interventions during the response phase.
- **Risk-reduction framework** detailing the effectiveness of risk-reduction strategies.

PRINCIPLES OF LESSONS MANAGEMENT

There are generally accepted principles underpinning the use of lessons management which provide a framework for its application. These include:

- **Useful:** That the evaluation is useful to the stakeholders.
- **Practical:** That the evaluation is able to be done effectively without disrupting the normal functions of the community and its recovery and is cost-effective. Evaluation may need to include both qualitative and quantitative approaches.
- **Ethical:** That the evaluation respects people's rights but also maintains perspective.
- **Accurate:** That the evaluation is conducted objectively and is reliable.
- **Engaged:** That the evaluation involves the perspectives of those affected and in turn reports outcomes to them.

The application of lessons management and thematic analysis provides a way to understand issues arising out of a disaster response, particularly when recurrent, and to develop the means to identify and highlight them. In a submission to the Victorian Bushfire Community Recovery Committee in 2010 following the 2009 Black Saturday Bushfire Disaster in the state of Victoria, Australia, t'Hart [6] identified six common themes through post-event evaluations which were found to have severely impacted the performance of the state's response and recovery systems. These were:

1. **The planning syndrome**. The tendency to focus on the plan as the outcome and to be restrained by its limitations when the unstructured and unpredictable nature of disasters may result in *pervasive surprise, uncertainty and overwhelming scale.*
2. **The obsession with full information**. Full information will never be available initially, if at all. The search for full information can paralyse decision-making and assessment.

3. **Communication breakdowns.** Evaluations always focus on communication breakdowns. The nature of crises is such that communication is difficult and restrained not only by incomplete information, but also by the intensive and complex nature of the disaster environment.

4. **Total reliance on command and control.** Modern complex societies, particularly in western democracies have challenged traditional views of command and control. Emergent behaviours and emergent leadership facilitated by access to social media may undermine traditional approaches leading to breakdowns in organisation which may appear chaotic while paradoxically improving local outcomes.

5. **Underestimating the key concept that the medium is the message.** The relationship between disaster managers and the media is often fraught if not adversarial during a disaster. In reality working with the media and enlisting their support as an ally to communicate with the population is a far more productive collaboration. The internet and social media have fundamentally altered the media's role, and the ability of anyone to control information.

6. **Underestimating the crisis after the emergency.** The post-response phase is the most complex and challenging period as the public's attention wanes, but the managerial challenges expand. Other players including lawyers, insurers, politicians and academic commentators will buy into the critical analysis, often with incomplete information or in the words of John F Kennedy 'we enjoy *the comfort of opinions without the discomfort of thought*' (J F Kennedy, Yale University, June 11 1962).

Since 2010, these themes have continued to be relevant. Serious Bushfires have been experienced in Australia, the USA, Canada, Russia and Europe while floods have occurred in South America, Europe, India, Africa, Asia and Oceania.

Disasters that could have been prevented, or at least mitigated are inevitably followed by recriminations and cries of '*how could this have happened*', and '*it must never happen again*'. Comprehensive evaluation following a disaster is a powerful tool to identify gaps in systems and structures and plan future training and operational needs. However, recurring themes following disasters continue to be identified leaving the question, ***do we ever learn?***

Table 27.1 Recurring themes of Australian bushfires

Major Australian bushfires 1939–2009
Emphasis on prevention activities and risk reduction, resources and activity, education and awareness, clearing of fuel around buildings, track access and fuel reduction   • Failure to recognise the value of volunteers and their contribution to the community   • Complacency before every fire   • Inadequate resources   • Communication and telecommunication infrastructure failures   • Failure to utilise local knowledge   • Lack of understanding of the roles and responsibilities of local government   • Role and responsibilities of the insurance industry

Table 27.2 Recurring themes of NASA space shuttle accidents

Challenger and Columbia space shuttle accidents

- NASA's safety system had failed
- Organisational problems
- Fundamental problem within the culture of NASA
- A deeply flawed risk philosophy preventing investigation of anomalies during previous shuttle flights
- Adopting the position that because nothing happened during previous missions and the same risk existed prevented NASA from sufficiently rectify risks or delay missions.

PROCEDURE FOR THE EVALUATION OF DISASTER OPERATIONS

The literature provides countless case studies and analyses of disasters and best practices for responding to and recovering from their impact [2, 7–18]. Drawing upon this literature, the authors offer a procedure for evaluating the response and recovery operations following a disaster. These steps allow all actors involved to identify gaps in the PPRR cycle and provide opportunities to improve structures and systems and community resilience.

1. **Sense-making:** How well did communication flow within and between systems and organisations involved? Did this hinder warning messages and the ability to provide an appropriately resourced response? Did organisations work in collaboration with each other? Were there conflicts? How were conflicts resolved?
2. **Meaning-making:** Were reports and public accounts of what was happening, why it was happening and what was being done to rectify or mitigate the situation appropriate? How were the media (including social media) used and did this hinder or assist the response?
3. **Decision-making:** Were strategic policy judgements appropriate? Were there any gaps in policy that impeded decision making? Did the response and recovery have an agreed authoritative decision-making and conflict-resolution structure?
   a) **Diagnosing and deciding:** At the strategic, tactical and operational levels, was there an understanding of the nature and extent of the situation? Were responses sensible, feasible and continually updated as the situation evolved, and new information became available?
   b) **Informing and empowering:** Was the dissemination and flow of information – up, down and out of the crisis response structure and into the community accurate, timely, and actionable? Did the information allow *informed crisis response decisions* to be made?
4. **Coordinating:** Was communication and collaboration at a strategic level appropriate? Did each agency work effectively together at all levels? Was this sustained throughout the response and recovery? Was this reflected within and across public, private and community sectors?
   a. **Mobilising and organising:** Were the necessary resources to meet demand available? Were resources deployed appropriately and in a timely manner?
   b. **Containing and mitigating:** Were available resources used in the most effective and efficient way to minimise loss of life and damage to property?

5. **Consolidating:** Was there any loss of attention and/or momentum during the transition from response to recovery and normal operations? Were immediate, short-term, mid-term and long-term services delivered appropriately and equitably?
6. **Account-giving:** Was the media managed appropriately? Were legislative processes adhered to? Were responsibilities clarified and accepted?
7. **Learning:** Were there opportunities for the operational agencies and the community to participate in critical, non-defensive briefings during and debriefings following the response and recovery phases? Were responders provided a safe forum to reflect on the response/recovery without recrimination? What were the lessons to be learnt from this disaster? What needs to be done to prevent the same errors and omissions from being repeated in the future?
8. **Remembering:** Were lessons identified from previous disasters learned or were the same errors and omissions repeated?

REAL-TIME DATA COLLECTION, RECORDING AND REPORTING

The process of evaluation necessarily involves the collection of data that may inform not only reporting of what has occurred but also enable a far more effective evaluation of the preparation and management of the event. The challenge is to obtain this data while not permitting the process of data collection to become an impediment to providing critical relief. The scope of required data must necessarily focus on the key components for any evaluation including:

- The nature and extent of the impact.
- The activities that occurred in responding.
- The opinions of those involved and of experts.
- Key decision-making by who and when.
- Objective measures of outcomes and comparison with benchmarks if available.
- Recording of any adverse incidents and experiences during the event.
- Resources, equipment and facilities used, their quantum and suitability.
- The people involved in the management of the event.

In developed countries operational-level data is now collected automatically as part of normal operations of the combat agencies (Ambulance, Police and Fire and Rescue Services). In addition, most health services now use an electronic medical record. This is operational data which can be consolidated to provide tactical decision-making.

In a major disaster additional information can be captured using GPS, aerial surveillance pictures (including drones) and texts, Email, photos and even videos from suitably equipped and trained people on the ground.

From the perspective of an Emergency Operations Centre (EOC) there is increasing use of computers and software to document and coordinate all incoming and outgoing information as well as discussions and decision-making within the EOC. Examples of this software include platforms such as Noggin and Web EOC. This is tactical data that can be consolidated to provide strategic information.

This computerised data collection assists response management and immediate reporting to other agencies and levels of government, but also forms a clear record for later evaluation, audit and report composition. It also provides community assurance that the response is being well coordinated and managed.

While the above is ideal in developed countries and urban environments the challenge of collecting real-time accurate data becomes more difficult as resources decrease, distances increase, and communications become more difficult. For example, the reporting and data collection on the initial phases of a tsunami in a remote location will be extremely difficult and inaccurate. The number of people affected is unknown and widespread damage makes physical access and immediate on-scene assessment impossible, yet the level of response required, and the resources needed to provide medical care are dependent on the numbers affected and the injuries sustained. Patient and situation assessment in this environment is much more complex and time-consuming. Data collection will likewise be hampered by a lack of automated record keeping, resource scarcity, poor communications and a justifiable clinician focus on patients rather than data.

The response to this situation will be described in more detail in Chapter 22 on Complex Humanitarian Emergencies.

Debriefing

Identifying and recording lessons requires organised and structured approaches of which debriefing is an important aspect. An opportunity to identify issues and lessons to be learnt and to allow some degree of mutual support, debriefing has traditionally been of two broad types:

1. **Hot or operational debriefing** focuses on the clinical or management team's immediate response to the situation and is designed to be protective and reassuring to frontline staff while gleaning any appropriate immediate observations for later review.
2. **Post-event or cold debriefing** is more frequently undertaken by staff working at the strategic level and focuses more on the performance of systems and structures and the strategic lessons to be learnt.

Formal debriefing should be professionally facilitated and conducted in an objective manner. Participation must be voluntary and offered to multiple agencies. There can be no judgement or assignment of blame. Both can be used to quietly identify staff likely to be at psychological risk and to confidentially offer these individuals additional support [19].

Performing objective response evaluations also has the benefit of reducing the inappropriate propagation of disaster myths particularly around public health issues. These myths have led to numerous inappropriate plans and responses which have endangered life and property in past events [20].

SCOPING AND MANAGING AN EVALUATION

Any event may result in a formal review. Most organisations will seek to identify the impact the event has had on them, and the effectiveness of the actions taken so that the lessons identified may inform future planning and preparedness. It is important for organisations to do these reviews but in doing so to ensure that they are effectively managed. Poorly managed reviews may fail to identify objectively the key findings or become distracted by internal political matters. Equally a poorly managed review may be destructive to individuals within the organisation or to the organisation as a whole resulting in secondary damage.

REPORTING

It is inevitable that as a society we will reflect on major events seeking to understand what happened, how it happened, how prepared we were, how we managed the incident and how well society has subsequently recovered. Thus, consideration must be given to how those experiences can be captured and communicated. The process of incident evaluation and reporting of those findings enables others to use those lessons to inform their preparedness.

Those tasked with responsibilities for managing disasters throughout the PPRR continuum, also have both personal and professional responsibilities to report on what has occurred. That responsibility also derives from any official position within an organisation and is required to assist in informing any subsequent enquiry, to meet professional accountabilities, to help with incident management and to inform future planning and preparedness. Reports will rely on the availability of reliable information as described above.

Any report should meet relatively simple criteria:

- **Objectivity** of analysis and comment.
- **Analytical** to examine reasons why things occurred as they did and to identify remedial action if necessary.
- **Respectful** of the privacy of individuals and of the performance of other responders.
- **Relevant** to the context and purpose.

The format for a report is often determined within a particular jurisdiction, however in broad principle they should follow a simple structure which will include what happened, what impact it had, how it was managed, what was learnt and what remedial recommendations should be taken.

MANAGING AND CONTRIBUTING TO EXTERNAL REVIEWS

Incident evaluation is also of particular importance because of the level of scrutiny applied either through media attention or more formally through subsequent official enquiries. Additionally, communities of any size may seek to conduct a society-wide review. The terms of reference of that review may be narrow (focussed on particular elements) or broadly based. In theory such reviews should be focussed on identifying the lessons to be learned but unfortunately, they are often captured by sectional interests pushing political agendas. These may include identification of fault to use for political purposes or as grounds for compensation.

There is now considerable experience with formal community-wide reviews and enquiries some of which are legally constituted and will have widespread compulsive powers to attend and give evidence with penalties imposed for failure to cooperate or the provision of false information. Such reviews or commissions are of considerable public interest and draw daily media attention and may necessitate defensive action by those whose actions are likely to be the focus of the review. Thus, they become a highly formalised legal process. A formal review conducted at government level is further complicated by the requirement to integrate the reports and submissions from multiple departments and organisations into a single final set of recommendations and actions.

SUMMARY AND RECOMMENDATIONS

1. Data collection and management are vital to learning lessons from each disaster response.
2. Automation of data collection will reduce the impact on clinical response and increase the validity of records for later review.
3. Using a continuous improvement model known as lessons management and based on the PPRR (Prevention, Preparedness, Response and Recovery) disaster planning model will best support ongoing learning and development of disaster plans.
4. Disaster response should no longer be based on previous individual experience but on well-developed plans based on the prior learnings created and refined within the disaster management system.
5. Modern disaster planning should be located within the context of the BCP Framework of any organisation including health.

ACTIVITIES

Imagine you have been asked to prepare terms of reference for an enquiry into a major flood, fire or other incident in which your service was involved.

1. Draft brief terms of reference.
2. Identify the data required for the enquiry and where you are likely to be able to access it.
3. Write the framework for a report based on the principles of BCP.

KEY READINGS

Department of Homeland Security. Chapter 5, *The Federal Response to Hurricane Katrina Lesson Learned*. 2006, US Government.

Voss, M. and K. Wagner, Learning from (small) disasters. *Natural Hazards*, 2010. **55**: p. 657–669. https://doi.org/10.1007/s11069-010-9498-5

Lange, A., J. Hernantes, and J. Mari Sarriegi, Analysis of disasters impacts and the relevant role of critical infrastructures for crisis management improvement. *International Journal of Disaster Resilience in the Built Environment*, 2015. **6**(4): p. 424–437. https://doi.org/10.1108/IJDRBE-07-2014-0047

Qian, H., C. Connolly Knox, and N. Kapucu, What have we learned since September 11, 2001? A network study of the Boston marathon bombings response. *Public Administration Review*, **74**(6): p. 698–712. https://doi.org/10.1111/puar.12284.

Department of Homeland Security. Chapter 5: Lessons learned. in *The Federal response to hurricane Katrina: Lessons learned*, Department of Homeland Security, Editors. 2006. Washington, DC: United States Government.

Hu, Q., C. Connolly Knox, and N. Kapucu, What have we learned since September 11, 2001? A network study of the Boston marathon bombings response. *Public Administration Review*, 2014. **74**(6): p. 698–712.

Lange, A., J. Hernates, and J. Mari Sarriegi, Analysis of disaster impacts and the relevant role of critical infrastructures for crisis management improvement. *International Journal of Disaster Resilience in the Built Environment*. 2015. **6**(4): p. 424–437.

Raphael, B., and J. Wilson, Psychological debriefing: Theory, practice and evidence. 2012, United Kingdom: Cambridge University Press. ISBN13 9780521647007

Voss, M., and K. Wagner, Learning from (small) disasters. *Natural Hazards*. 2010. **55**: 657–669.

Notes

1. With acknowledgement to previous authors Gerard FitzGerald & Marie Fredriksen.
2. https://asq.org/quality-resources/pdca-cycle
3. https://asq.org/quality-resources/six-sigma
4. https://asq.org/quality-resources/lean
5. https://asq.org/quality-resources/total-quality-management

References

1. Reason, J., *Human error*. 1990, Cambridge: Cambridge University Press.
2. Stern, E., Crisis and learning: A conceptual balance sheet. *Journal of Contingencies and Crisis Management*, 1997. **5**(2): p. 69–86.
3. Goode, N., Spencer, C., Archer, F.L., Salmon, P.M., Mcardle, D., & McClure, R.J. (2011). Review of *Recent Australian Disaster Inquiries*. Melbourne: Monash University Accident Research Centre, Department of Paramedicine.
4. Sundnes, K.O. and M.L. Birnbaum, Health disaster management: Guidelines for evaluation and research in the Utstein style. *Prehospital and disaster medicine*, 2003. **17**(Supplement 3): p. 31–55.
5. Birnbaum, M.L., et al., Disaster Research/Evaluation Frameworks, Part 1: An Overview-RETRACTED. *Prehospital and Disaster Medicine*, 2022. **37**(3): p. E3–E14.
6. t'Hart, P. *Organising for Effective Emergency management; Submission to the Royal Commission on the Victorian Bushfires*. 2010; Available from: https://www.amsa.gov.au/.../Paul%20t'Hart%20Organisaing%20for%20E.
7. Boin, A. and P. 't Hart, Organising for effective emergency management: Lessons from research 1. *Australian Journal of Public Administration*, 2010. **69**(4): p. 357–371.
8. Boin A, M.A., and P. 't Hart, Crisis leadership, in *Political and civic leadership: A Sage reference handbook*, Couto RA, Editor. 2010 p. 229–239, London: Sage.
9. Deverell, E., *Crisis-induced learning in public sector organizations*. 2010, Stockholm: Elanders Sverige.
10. Flin, R., P. O'Connor, and M. Crichton, *Safety at the sharp end: A guide to non-technical skills*. 2008, Aldershot: Ashgate.
11. Boin, A., A., McConnell, and P. 't Hart, eds. *Governing after crisis: The politics of investigation, accountability and learning*. 2008, Cambridge: Cambridge University Press.
12. Rodriguez, H., E.L. Quarantelli, and R.R. Dynes, eds. *Handbook of disaster research*. 2006, New York: Springer.
13. Boin, A., P. 't Hart, E. Stern, and B. Sundelius, eds. *The politics of crisis management: Public leadership under pressure*. 2005, Cambridge: Cambridge University Press.
14. Bos, C.K., S. Ullberg, and P. 't Hart, The long shadow of disaster: memory and politics in Holland and Sweden. *International Journal of Mass Emergencies & Disasters*, 2005. **23**(1): p. 5–26.
15. Flin, R., and K. Arbuthnot, eds. *Incident command: Tales from the hot seat*. 2002, Ashgate: Aldershot.
16. Hilliard, M., *Public crisis management: How and why organizations work together to solve society's most threatening problems*. 2000, Lincoln: Writer's Club Press.
17. Birkland, T., *After disaster: Agenda-setting, public policy, and focusing events*. 1997, Washington: Georgetown University Press.
18. Flin, R., *Sitting in the hot seat: Leaders and teams for critical incident management*. 1996, New York: Wiley.
19. Raphael, B. and J. Wilson, *Psychological debriefing: Theory, practice and evidence*. 2012, Cambridge: Cambridge University Press.
20. de Ville de Goyet, C., Stop propagating disaster myths. *Disaster Prevention and Management: An International Journal*, 2000 Aug 26. **356**(9231):p. 762–764. doi: 10.1016/s0140-6736(00)02642-8. PMID: 11085709

28

Education, training, and research

Gerry FitzGerald, Vivienne Tippett, and Stacey Pizzino[1]

INTRODUCTION AND OBJECTIVES

To avoid the esoteric debate around the differences between education and training, this text will refer to the terms as one. Nevertheless, it must be recognised that education is traditionally considered as developing knowledge and understanding while training develops skills.

Previous chapters have emphasised the critical importance of the development of capability and the contribution to this made by education and training. They have also identified the need for policy and practice to be based on the best available evidence. However, the system-wide challenge lies in how to take an organised and disciplined approach to capturing the evidence and translating it into practice through policy, standards, education, and training.

It is vital to establish resilient, integrated, and standardised approaches to education, training, and research as a foundation for effective disaster management practice. Traditionally there has been little consistency in education and training for disaster management. Additionally, disaggregation of policy responsibility and leadership at government levels in many countries makes it increasingly difficult to identify and adopt a standardised approach. On the other hand, there is considerable value in standardising core aspects of training and education to support interaction, while ensuring flexibility in delivery to enable adaptation to different contexts. This balance between standardisation and flexibility is the key to a resilient training and education framework.

This chapter examines the principles and concepts that underpin effective education, training, and research. It is not intended to explore individual programs or define content but rather focusses on the educational and research strategy. On completion of this chapter, you should

1. Have a broader understanding of the principles and concepts that underpin effective disaster management training, education, and professional development programs.
2. Be able to conceptualise, design, and organise the delivery of training and educational programs including desktop and field exercises.

DOI: 10.4324/9781032626604-36

3. Understand the use of evidence-based research to improve health disaster health management policy and strategies and to strengthen actions at all levels.
4. Direct and design an appropriate and progressive research agenda in disaster health management.

EDUCATION AND TRAINING FRAMEWORKS

There are innumerable training and educational programs in disaster health management provided by a broad range of organisations including government bodies, service providers, universities and other educational institutions, NGOs, commercial entities, and individuals. There are also a number of approaches to the delivery of training and education including e-learning (online), simulation and table-top exercises, workshops, and didactic lectures. This diversity provides variety for those seeking training and educational opportunities, but conversely, such diversity weakens the strength of capability development, inevitably leading to duplication and wasted effort, and reduces the prospects for interoperability and standardised approaches.

Current education and training provisions can be classified into the following categories:

- **Credentialed courses** that result in the attainment of a qualification through the achievement of learning objectives or the demonstration of competence. Such programs may be found across the full spectrum of educational offerings from Certificates to University Doctorates. These programs may be either inherently theoretical or a mixture of theory and its practical application.
- **Non-credentialed short programs** that focus on the development of specific skills or competencies and also assist with broadening understanding.
- **Continuing professional development** programs which aim to update and extend an individual's capability.

Following the 2010 Haiti earthquake, there was a clear recognition by many of those involved in the response, of the need for a global consensus on international standards for educational and training of personnel, particularly international healthcare workers. The challenge to date has been to achieve consistency in educational outcomes and to provide mechanisms so participants can follow a structured hierarchical approach to training and education.

In 2010, an Australian national network of disaster health educators recommended a structured approach to disaster health education and training [1]. This framework proposes seven levels of education and awareness. These are outlined in Table 28.1.

However, it may be considered that this approach of standardising programs is input (course) focussed while a more appropriate approach would be competency focussed. Two reviews of expected competencies [2, 3] have sought to create competency outcomes as the foundation for the standardisation of education and training frameworks. Limitations include imprecise and inconsistent terminology and structure, a lack of universal acceptance, and a relative absence of lack of validation (Daily 2010). These impede their translation and applicability into practice, and cohesion in one standardised framework.

On the other hand, the scope and content of educational and training programs must necessarily take into consideration the local context and the level and roles of individuals. Thus there is a need for considerable flexibility. However, this flexibility is difficult to deliver in pragmatic terms.

Table 28.1 Framework for education and awareness

Strategy
General public awareness of threat, impact and broad principles of disaster management and community resilience.
Introduction to principles of disaster management arrangements and practice designed to provide health workers with a common understanding
Intended to create awareness amongst health workers likely to be involved in major incident responses. Includes the principles and practice of disaster response and the roles and responsibilities of key individuals and organisations.
Targets leadership with key roles in preparedness or response. Addresses detailed PPRR arrangements and the skills required to manage those arrangements.
Targets individuals responsible for leading the development of preparedness and response arrangements. Level provides an in-depth understanding of the principles and practice of disaster health management.
Aimed at the future educators and system designers. Intended to provide candidates with an extensive understanding of both the principles and practice of disaster health management and in-depth awareness of specific components.
Individuals who are leading the innovation and creative edge.

FitzGerald et al. [4] developed Generic Emergency and Disaster Management Standards for education and identified eight broad themes organised into three domains of knowledge, skills, and application. Domains organised in that may guide the development of content. The level in each domain is to be determined by the level of the program (Figure 28.1).

The first two domains focus on the 'what' and 'how' that providers require in this field of study. Graduates need to apply these skills to the solving of complex problems through the use of domains of professional practice and critical thinking. However, it must be emphasised that any attempt to describe the complex inter-relationships that characterise emergency and disaster management is by its nature a simplification intended to aid understanding.

From a more operational perspective, the current emphasis is on ensuring programs are both generic and context-specific, both academically and operationally focussed, multi-disciplinary, and adapted to both domestic and international responses.

For example, consider the training needs of responding medical teams. Members of such teams have two broad needs.

1. **Broadening of knowledge** for all team members on general disaster and humanitarian principles and practice: security, logistics, water/sanitation, relevant general health epidemiology, culture, and communities.
2. **Development of technical skills specific to the deploying context** for the individual roles within the team (doctor, nurse, team leader, data manager, logistician).

CONSIDERATIONS IN TRAINING

Response teams and coordination

Develop knowledge of all team members on general disaster and humanitarian principles and practice.

Develop technical skills specific to deployment context for individual roles.

Within these broad conceptual frameworks, the task for disaster health leaders is to develop an integrated program of education and training. Such an integrated program

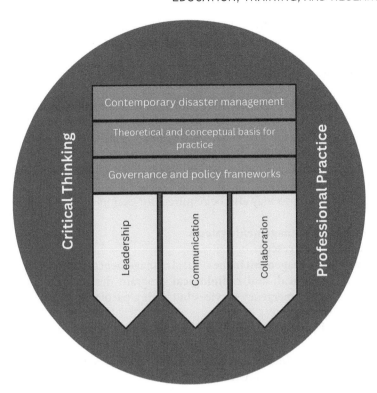

Figure 28.1 Themes and domains of education and training (Adapted from FitzGerald, G., J. Rego, V. Ingham, A. Cottrell, I. Manock, A. Surjan, L. Mayner, C. Webb, B. Maguire, H. Crawley, J. Mooney, S. Toloo, F. Archer, Teaching emergency and disaster management in Australia: Standards for higher education providers. *AJEM*. 2017. **32**(3), p. 22–23

should ensure a consistent understanding of core principles that permeate all elements of the program. It should also recognise the needs for variability determined by context and by the specific needs of various roles in an integrated response. The principal elements of any integrated program should include:

- **Core principles of disaster health management** and the organisational and governance arrangements required for planning, preparedness, and response.
- **Clinical care in disasters** in both the immediate and long term and addressing both physical and mental health needs including primary care.
- **The management of mass casualties** within the local context. For example, a mass casualty incident in a country with a developed healthcare system and extensive pre-hospital medical services will be approached very differently to a similar incident in a country with a less developed healthcare system and resource infrastructure.
- **Public health protections** following disasters including sanitation, food and water safety, and environmental health.
- **The roles and responsibilities of various players** in the disaster response throughout the continuum of preparedness, response, and recovery.

- **Mutual-aid**, including the role of national and international organisations/teams and their integration with local culture and health guidelines and resources, population health strategies, and clinical practice.
- **Health logistics** and the supply of consumables and services.

In addition to any tiered approach to the underpinning principles and practice, there is also a need for task-specific training relating to a particular role. For example, international response teams will need to be trained in the principles and practice of disaster management to an appropriate level for their role. This may then need to be complemented by specific training in the role and its responsibilities and by context-specific briefing relating to the particular deployment.

Finally, special programs may also be required, for example:

- **Major incident management systems.**
- **Urban search and rescue.**
- **Mass casualty management** in the clinical management of victims of major incidents.
- **Chemical, biological, and radiological** program designed to complement programs offered by emergency services but with a particular emphasis on the health impact of CBR.
- **International assistance program** targeting health teams that offer international assistance.
- **Pandemic preparedness program** for public health workers.
- **Mental healthcare and disasters.**

The scope and level of training and education programs needs to focus on the role of the individual and their functions within the health system. Consideration may be required for specific roles including Team leaders, evaluators, planners, and policy makers.

The approach to all education and training within disaster and emergency management should have a three-tiered approach, each tier is of equal importance:

1. Training relevant to **the individual** (e.g., specific healthcare training).
2. Training relevant to **the team** and adapted to the context (e.g., team-focussed operational simulation training).
3. Training relevant to **the organisation** (e.g., training on specific security procedures or integration in the humanitarian system).

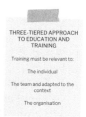

THREE-TIERED APPROACH TO EDUCATION AND TRAINING

Training must be relevant to:

The individual

The team and adapted to the context

The organisation

Finally, it is worth reviewing the myths outlined by Burstein regarding disaster education [5].

1. People need to know special things in disasters. Disaster responses should be based on normal, but context and resource-appropriate practice.
2. We are smart; hearing it once is enough. One off courses provide only a temporary boost to knowledge and performance, this type of work needs to be continually professionalised.
3. A drill now and then is enough. Drills need to be applied to various contexts and continually repeated to refresh and maintain awareness.

4. The government will take care of it. The government is a key player and must be supported by the international community, but mostly, it is the local community that will respond.
5. It is impossible to be prepared. Putting aside the digital nature of this myth (it is never all or nothing), people, organisations, and communities can be prepared.

EXERCISES AND SIMULATIONS

One of the most effective means of testing an organisation's preparedness and response capability is through context-specific exercises. Most organisations are familiar with fire drills and evacuations, but few conduct regular disaster management exercises. In particular, health organisations find it difficult to suspend routine activities to test their capabilities for non-routine events.

In emergency management, exercises are important to ensure personnel are aware of possible situations and to develop their experience and expertise. Simulation exercises are also important to ensure policies, plans, and procedures are tested and evaluated in as near to real environment as possible. Creative and innovative ways may be necessary to find opportunities to test preparedness and response capabilities. Some may use large-scale activities designed for another purpose as an opportunity to test their capability. For example, moving into a new facility may be used to test evacuation capabilities and a mass crowd event may be an opportunity to test preparedness and planning.

Exercises may be desktop or live and those involved may be players, controllers, and observers. Exercises need to be well-designed and as near to real time as possible.

- **Desktop or table-top exercises** are indoor facilitated discussions with no operational response. They may take the form of discussion exercises designed to tease out the elements of a problem or functional exercises replicating the real-world environment without its physical or visual clues. Table-top exercises typically involve a small number of people and concentrate on a specific aspect of the plan. They can easily accommodate complete teams or a single representative from each of several teams. Typically, participants work through a simple scenario and then discuss specific aspects of the plan.
- **Live exercises** are usually simulations to test parts of the plan against a scenario. They are often conducted outdoors and require an operational response. Live exercises are difficult to organise, and they consume resources. They may be difficult to justify on economic or clinical grounds as they do distract resources for normal operations. The value of live exercises is that they are high-profile events that genuinely test responses in a real-time environment but at the same time may raise awareness.
- **Virtual exercises** using facilitative technology. These may range from relatively low technology systems such as the Emergo Train System[2] or potentially complex system that use gaming technology to simulate real-world scenarios.

Such exercises may be simple and focussed on a particular element of the disaster response or they may be complex (real world) exercises that test all elements of response including coordination and control elements. A complex exercise aims to have as few boundaries as possible. It incorporates all the aspects of a medium exercise. The exercise may be presented within a virtual world, but maximum realism is essential. This might include no-notice activation, actual evacuation, and actual invocation of a disaster recovery site.

CASE STUDY 28.1 – EXERCISE NUGENTS

Exercise NUGENTS was developed following the 2010/2011 flood events in QLD, Australia. A large-scale live exercise, NUGENTS was conducted over three days from 30 November 2012. NUGENTS was designed to enhance the readiness of disaster management groups by practising disaster management arrangements in the context of an extreme weather event. Developed to incorporate the key elements of disaster preparedness and response, NUGENTS enabled participants to build and validate disaster management capability by providing participants with the opportunity to:

- Trigger the activation of disaster management arrangements.

Practice
- Procedures to initiate different warning mechanisms including those that do not rely on electricity and the SMS alert approval process.
- Safety messaging and media interviews.
- Handover briefs, shift change and 2nd roster.

Exercise
- Disaster management group relationships and engagement at the local and district level.
- Support between councils.
- Disaster coordination centre capacity to deal with high-volume calls.
- Evacuation plans and sub-plans, including those involving facilities in which residents require assistance to evacuate, and plans for evacuation centres.
- Re-supply arrangements and other specific arrangements for communities isolated by disaster.
- Exercise and evaluate the effectiveness of software in facilitating the communication flow between disaster management groups.

Prior to the live exercise, a planning meeting where participants were encouraged to identify areas within their jurisdiction to be exercised was held. Flexibility was built into NUGENTS design to allow participants to exercise as fully as resources permitted while continuing business as usual. An overview of the exercise was presented at a pre-exercise briefing and discussion exercise. Attendees were presented with two severe weather events similar to the scenarios used in the NUGENTS exercise. Participants worked through the scenarios in their respective disaster management groups to formulate strategies to manage the situation. Feedback from participants was that this was a worthwhile desktop exercise identifying a number of issues. Answers provided were used as a basis for NUGENTS serials, 670 serials were written for the exercise.

Serials were aligned with participants' identified objectives and the call centre component of the exercise. These included vulnerable clients, assisted evacuation, call centre capacity, isolated communities, resupply, council-2-council, and community inventory.

The lessons identified provided invaluable information for future education and training and provided participants with the opportunity to revise/refine their disaster management arrangements and plans. Particularly in relation to improving coordination, clarifying roles and responsibilities and fostering cooperation among agencies.

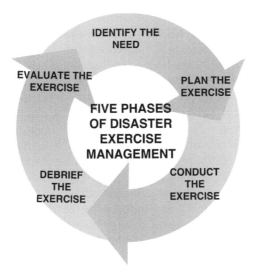

Figure 28.2 Exercise Management Cycle

Thunderbolts are no-notice, internally run exercises that focus on specific portions of an organisation or a specific process. They are usually of short duration and are a key tool for a leader to test his/her team.

The disaster exercise management cycle includes five phases:

1. **Identify the need**: All exercises begin with a specific need to test, evaluate, and validate plans, assess performance, practice or train, and identify issues. It is important that the any exercise has a clearly defined purpose. The identified need should be analysed to determine the aim and objectives for the proposed exercise.
2. **Plan the exercise**: All exercises need to be planned in detail and in as close to a realistic context as possible. The plan needs to be documented so that each of the key controllers is aware of their role. The information available to participants needs to be provided in as close to real time as feasible.
3. **Conduct the exercise**: Conducting the exercise involves the pre-exercise activities including briefing, starting, managing, and finishing the exercise and debriefings.
4. **Debrief the exercise**: Debrief is the process of critically analysing the conduct of the exercise.
5. **Evaluate the exercise**: Evaluation should include the design and conduct stages of the exercise as well as the participants' response to the developing scenario. Evaluation may take the form of an after-action review and should include an evaluation of any recommendations for subsequent action.

Finally, all exercises need to incorporate an evaluation program that identifies the elements to be evaluated, the criteria to be used in the evaluation and the standards expected.

RESEARCH PROGRAMS IN DISASTER HEALTH

The ultimate purpose of research in any field of endeavour is to improve outcomes for people through better policy and practice. The conversion of research outputs (publications and reports) into action is dependent on many factors including the quality of the research, its relevance to the real-world problems confronting the industry and the presence of mechanisms whereby the research can be evaluated and translated into action.

Effective research is dependent on a comprehensive understanding of the available literature and the use of appropriate methods to address the research questions. New research efforts should be focussed on addressing current gaps in the field and should build on previous research. Disaster literature has developed considerably over the past several decades. This body of work has discredited disaster myths; described the actual responses of people and various groups; discussed the challenges of multi-agency coordination; and examined issues in disaster preparedness, response, and management. There is now an understanding that during disasters, individuals, and communities often respond in different ways to what is anticipated [6].

Contemporary advances in technology and communications open extensive opportunities for new inter-disciplinary and industry partnerships to address the challenges associated with community and organisational preparation, response, and recovery.

The WHO [7] has developed guidance for research methods in health emergency and disaster risk management with the aim of improving the quality of research, increasing research capacity, and strengthening collaboration. This was complemented by the creation in 2018 of the WHO Thematic Platform for Health EDRM Research Network to promote collaboration amongst researchers. Key themes emerging from this group included taking a holistic approach, identifying populations at risk, standardisation of assessment means, multidisciplinary and multisectoral approaches; and connecting research to policy and decision making.

Conceptualising a research program?

While there is undoubtedly a place for spontaneous and opportunistic research-driven enquiry, there is also a place for a sustained and targeted effort that may be driven by priority-driven funding schemes and structures (research centres) that build a critical mass of capable people from multiple disciplines. However, any cohesive program must be based on a sound theoretical basis.

One such basis is the conceptualisation of disasters as social phenomenon. Disasters are complex social events that require an in-depth understanding of the social structures and how they change during disasters.

It is generally well-recognised that there are a number of structural social changes unique to disasters [8]. New behaviours, social relationships and community organisations will often appear after a disaster. These new relationships are also sometimes characterised by an extension of the roles and responsibilities of professionals. A better understanding of these emergent changes is essential for effective disasters management.

Some physical and psychological phenomena associated with disasters don't appear until sometime after the event [9]. Thus progressing a body of work that better understands these impacts will necessarily require longitudinal mixed methods approaches.

Organisation and role are important parts of sociological theory but to date, research has not successfully related these components of structure. Social action and social order describe the process by which an individual commits to a course of action and how social units influence the involved thoughts and behaviours.

In order to relate these concepts to disaster management, there needs to be a conceptualisation of social structure and the factors that influence these. This structure is based on the following elements, each of which gives rise to important areas of research endeavour:

1. Domains: boundaries distinguishing a group from others.
2. Tasks: including division of labour giving focus and direction.
3. Resources: capacities and technologies of individuals and collectives.
4. Activities: combines actions of individuals and social units.

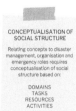

THEORETICAL FRAMEWORK
TO RESEARCH

Identify and define the problem.

Build a set of coherent and
evidence-based assumptions to
test/explore.

Select a methodology
appropriate to the nature of the
question.

An alternative way to structure a comprehensive research agenda is to consider the widely accepted phases of a disaster; before, during and after often described as Prevention, Preparedness, Response and Recovery. Though this model has been criticised by some for its assumption of a linear relationship between the stages of an incident, it nevertheless provides a reasonable theoretical platform on which to structure a disaster research program.

Regardless of the theoretical framework applied to the research, it is critical in any research endeavour to:

1. Identify and define the problem.
2. Build a set of coherent and evidence-based set of assumptions to test/explore.
3. Select a methodology appropriate to the nature of the question.

CONCEPTUALISATION OF
SOCIAL STRUCTURE

Relating concepts to disaster
management, organisation and
emergency roles requires
conceptualisation of social
structure based on:

DOMAINS
TASKS
RESOURCES
ACTIVITIES

Birnbaum et al. [10] proposed five frameworks that help structure the information and research agenda. These include conceptual, temporal, societal, relief/recovery, and risk reduction frameworks.

POTENTIAL RESEARCH TARGETS

With the increase in major disaster incidents globally, both natural and man-made, there is increasing research attention on the challenges associated with large-scale collaborative international responses. The research into COVID-19 has been massive and across a broad spectrum of biomedical, sociological, clinical and public health research. Montesanti et al. [11] explored the implications of rapid research conducted in response to COVID-19. While recognising the benefit of rapid research to help guide ongoing policy and practice, they also noted the risks of what they refer to as the 'research gold rush' in encompassing researchers with limited knowledge in the disaster field, the potential for over-research of limited value, and the potential for research to interfere with people's healing and recovery. They emphasised the need for such research to engage the affected community and to establish strong research partnership.

The scope of the research opportunity in examining the effectiveness and efficiency of response to these events is broad. Logistics and supply chains; inter-agency operations; communications; community re-location and re-establishment; policy and procedures are all areas which warrant exploration [12]. However, researchers face a number of challenges which can impede systematic analyses of this body of work.

In a rigorous analysis of disaster management research, Galindo and Batta [3] drew attention to the current lack of research in several areas. These topics include definitions of organisational networks which facilitate coordination and communication; exploration of opportunities for the development of new technologies to assist disaster preparedness and response; business continuity; infrastructure design; modelling of service allocation to disaster victims; post-disaster housing; re-establishment of community post-event; and the specific challenges facing communities in the developing world. These authors also very valuably identify flaws in many of the assumptions that researchers have brought to attempts to contribute to the development of operational management and community response to disasters.

Finally, research needs to be evaluated for its quality and effectiveness. Strahan et al. [13] explored models and frameworks for assessing the value of disaster research. Although noting the need for further refinement, they proposed the research impacts may be considered within the economic, academic, social, cultural, and environmental domains. Also, within these broad parameters impacts need to be assessed in the short, medium and long term and that any impacts need to be demonstrable, attributable, and quantifiable.

ACTIVITIES

1. Imagine you have been asked to advise your organisation on how it could improve the education and training of staff for disaster management. Prepare a brief for the governing body outlining the key element of such a program.
2. Should a research agenda be developed for disaster health or should it be left to individual researchers to set their own agenda?
3. Prepare a brief recommending the establishment of a research centre in disaster health management.

KEY READINGS

1. Burstein, J. The myths of disaster education. *Annals of Emergency Medicine*, 2006. 47(1). 50–52.
2. FitzGerald, G.J., P. Aitken, P. Arbon, F. Archer, D. Cooper, P. Leggat, C. Myers, A. Robertson, M. Tarrant, and E.R. Davis, A national framework for disaster health education in Australia. *Prehospital and Disaster Medicine*, 2010. 25(1): p. 4–11.
3. Daily, E., Padjen, P., and M.L. Birnbaum, A review of competencies developed for disaster healthcare providers: Limitations of current processes and applicability. *Prehospital and Disaster Medicine*, 2010. 25(5): p. 387–395.
4. Guidelines for evaluation and research in the Utstein Style. WADEM; Available from: http://www.wadem.org/guidelines/intro.pdf
5. Ripoll Gallardo, A., A. Djalali, M. Foletti, L. Ragazzoni, F. Della Corte, O. Lupescu, et al. Core competencies in disaster management and humanitarian assistance: A systematic review. *Disaster Medicine and Public Health Preparedness* [Internet]. 2015. p. 1–10. Available from: http://www.journals.cambridge.org/abstract_S1935789315000024
6. *WHO guidance on research methods for health emergency and disaster risk management.* 2021. Geneva: World Health Organization. Licence: CC BY-NC-SA 3.0 IGO.

Notes

1. With acknowledgement to previous authors, Amy Hughes, Nieves Amat Camacho & Peter Horrocks.
2. https://www.emergotrain.com/home/about-us

References

1. FitzGerald, G.J., et al., A national framework for disaster health education in Australia. *Prehospital and Disaster Medicine*, 2010. **25**(1): p. 4–11.
2. Daily, E., P. Padjen, and M. Birnbaum, A review of competencies developed for disaster healthcare providers: Limitations of current processes and applicability. *Prehospital and Disaster Medicine*, 2010. **25**(5): p. 387–395.
3. Galindo, G. and R. Batta, Review of recent developments in OR/MS research in disaster operations management. *European Journal of Operational Research*, 2013. **230**(2): p. 201–211.
4. Fitzgerald, G., et al., Teaching emergency and disaster management in Australia: Standards for higher education providers. *Australian Journal of Emergency Management, The*, 2017. **32**(3): p. 22–23.
5. Burstein, J.L., The myths of disaster education. *Annals of Emergency Medicine*, 2006. **47**(1): p. 50–52.
6. Misanya, D. and A.O. Øyhus, How communities' perceptions of disasters influence disaster response: Managing landslides on Mount Elgon, Uganda. *Disasters*, 2015. **39**(2): p. 389–405.
7. World Health Organisation, *WHO guidance on research methods for health emergency and disaster risk management.* 2021, Geneva: World Health Organisation.
8. Kreps, G.A. and T.E. Drabek, Disasters are nonroutine social problems. *International Journal of Mass Emergencies & Disasters*, 1996. **14**(2): p. 129–153.
9. North, C.S. and B. Pfefferbaum, Mental health response to community disasters: A systematic review. *JAMA*, 2013. **310**(5): p. 507–518.
10. Birnbaum, M.L., et al., Research and evaluations of the health aspects of disasters, part I: An overview. *Prehospital and Disaster Medicine*, 2015. **30**(5): p. 512–522.
11. Montesanti, S., I. Walker, and A.W. Chan, Improving disaster health outcomes and resilience through rapid research: Implications for public health policy and practice. *Frontiers in Public Health*, 2022 Aug 2. **10**: p. 989573. doi: 10.3389/fpubh.2022.989573. PMID: 35983355; PMCID: PMC9379345.
12. de la Torre, L.E., I.S. Dolinskaya, and K.R. Smilowitz, Disaster relief routing: Integrating research and practice. *Socio-economic Planning Sciences*, 2012. **46**(1): p. 88–97.
13. Strahan, K., A. Keating, and J. Handmer, Models and frameworks for assessing the value of disaster research. *Progress in Disaster Science*, 2020. **6**: p. 100094.

29

Future challenges

*Gerry FitzGerald, Mike Tarrant, Peter Aitken,
Marie Fredriksen, Penelope Burns, Stacey Pizzino,
and Benjamin Ryan*[1]

INTRODUCTION AND OBJECTIVES

While it is difficult to predict the future of disaster health management, we can at least reflect on what we currently know of the challenges and opportunities facing disaster managers and the communities they serve. Challenges starkly highlighted by the recent experiences with SARS-CoV-2 and how mitigation measures used or not used impacted society in different ways.

Modern societies and organisations are incredibly complex and dependent on interconnected socio-technological systems which create tremendous opportunities for improved services and products. However, at the same time societies are vulnerable because of this complexity and the reliance on others in order to function. Leaders and managers face diverse challenges characterised by an increasingly complex environment, making performance and accountability more difficult in a climate of *minimal tolerance for failure*.

Any attempt to simplify this complexity is challenging. A paper prepared for the Bushfire Cooperative Research Centre in Australia [1] identified seven key challenges facing disaster managers. Although generic in their application, these challenges are equally applicable to disaster health managers today.

1. Increased uncertainty, complexity, and convergence.
2. The disconnect between disaster risk reduction and public policy.
3. The expectations and resilience of the community.
4. Social media, networking and emergent behaviours.
5. The political-operational nexus.
6. Evaluating emergency management responses.
7. Development and capability.

This chapter explores the challenges to governance and coordination of disaster management activities throughout all aspects of disaster management, the association between disasters and development, the impact of social and technological change, the effect of macro societal issues such as climate change and emerging operational issues requiring resolution. This exploration is not intended to provide solutions or to be exhaustive, but

DOI: 10.4324/9781032626604-37

rather to use the concepts, principles and practice outlined throughout this text to help practitioners reflect on their practice and explore the complexity that characterises effective disaster health management.

On completion of this chapter, you should be able to

1. Identify and critically discuss key strategic issues confronting disaster health management and the way in which those issues may impact on the health and wellbeing of the community.
2. Identify new challenges and discuss mechanisms for analysis and evaluation of those issues and to identify potential solutions.

GOVERNANCE AND COORDINATION

In recent years governance has become an important aspect of disaster and crisis management. It reflects a body of thinking that aims to see disaster management or disaster risk management as a fundamental part of how organisations and countries function rather than as a marginal specialised activity. However, at the same time governance is becoming increasingly complex as stakeholder's demands for performance and accountabilities increase, coupled with ever-increasing pressure on resources. For example, the CEO of an organisation is accountable to the owners, the staff and customers and to a range of legislative and regulatory bodies and instruments. Larger companies may be able to afford people to ensure those accountabilities are met, but in theory those same accountabilities apply to the solo operator of the coffee cart outside your building.

Managing disaster risk has become another accountability for leaders of organisations or countries. If simply added to the other tasks, this may become an additional burden that threatens to consume scarce resources rather than enhancing resilience. While it is possible to gain the attention of the decision-makers during a crisis it is much harder for them to invest scarce resources which may not produce a return for a very long period.

Overlaying this fundamental problem there are international trends towards the disengagement of governments from service delivery. This reduces the ability of government to command the changes required to build resilience, increasing the role of businesses and individuals. Thus, governments need to rely on policy settings, financial incentives and partnerships with industry to help build resilience. Private sector companies have history and experience in the affected areas, understand supply chains, can drive innovation, growth and jobs, and the type of businesses in an area often reflect communities' needs and priorities. They do not, however, have the overarching responsibility to the community that is required and expected of government.

At the same time, at the industry and at the organisational level, globalisation is driving demands for greater efficiency and cost savings. The interconnectedness of modern complex systems is such that they are susceptible to cascades of failure and often in unpredictable ways. The growing complexity of modern organisational processes and structures has the net effect of limiting not only management's ability to understand the interconnections but also to manage those interconnections in the event of any failures of component parts.

This has been highlighted in the recent experience with SARS-CoV-2 where communities faced challenges not only to their health and wellbeing from the virus, but also the disruptions caused by panic buying, loss of jobs and failure of supply and production chains. Imagine a hospital with the responsibility to manage those injured in an earthquake when

CASE STUDY 29.1 – COVID-19

Commencing in 2020, the world experienced a global pandemic. Worldwide, Coronavirus disease (COVID-19) threatened human health and wellbeing and the economy of every nation impacted by this disease. The virus forced many countries to implement extreme strategies such as travel bans, closing borders and schools and a ban on all public events and gatherings. Both the disease and the measures taken to control it have had significant health, social and economic impacts. The challenge has been to balance the risks of the disease against the risks of the measures taken to control it.

the power supplied by independent companies has failed, the drug and other consumable supply companies are unable to deliver because of unusable roads, and the company that provides meals has been damaged and unable to operate. How do leaders and managers meet their objectives by finding work-around solutions and restructuring their systems and processes to fit the situation? How do leaders and managers build resilient systems that can withstand those challenges and shocks?

New means are required to work out how those accountable to the community can exact those accountabilities in the light of these modern challenges. The key lies in normalising disaster risk reduction as an integral part of an organisation or community risk management.

DEVELOPMENT AND DISASTER MANAGEMENT

There is a direct (two-way) association between disasters and development. In Chapter 2 we outlined the impact that disasters have on the economic development of nations. Disasters tend to impact most on less developed nations contributing further to their slow development. In general, the poorest communities cannot absorb repeated disaster costs and maintain development goals.

- The United Nations Development Programme's Human development report 2019 identifies the differential impact of climate change on poorer communities.

  Poorer countries and poorer people will be hit earliest and hardest. Some countries could quite literally disappear. Of all climate change's disequalising effects, perhaps none is greater than that on future generations, which will shoulder the burden of previous generations' fossil fuel-dependent development pathways. Inequality runs the gamut of climate change, from emissions and impacts to resilience and policy. Climate change is a recipe for more inequality in a world that already has plenty. [2]

- A study using data from the International Disaster Database (EM-DAT) over the period 1980–2007 found that "low-income countries are significantly more at risk of climate-related disasters, even after controlling for exposure to climate hazards and other factors that may confound disaster reporting". This implies that continued economic development may be a powerful tool for lessening social vulnerability to climate change. Disaster risk, social vulnerability, and economic development [3].

- A study in China showed that "economic development is correlated with the significant reduction in human fatalities but increase in direct economic losses from climate-related disasters since 1949". The study further demonstrated "that economic development is correlated with human and economic vulnerability to climate-related disasters, and this vulnerability decreased with the increase of per-capita income" [4].
- A study into the economic impacts of disasters for the period 1979–2007 found countries with low levels of financial sector development, natural disasters have persistent negative effects on economic growth over the medium term [5].

Essentially, investments made by poorer countries to achieve their development goals are nullified by these losses. Communities with fast-growing populations will incur larger costs to pay for the damage and losses that will occur. Indeed, the costs of disasters are challenging the very basis of these investments in development, but the impact is not restricted to poorer nations.

Poorer nations also have less capacity to respond and render aid. These nations are subject to the benevolence of richer nations which often comes with inappropriate aid or strings attached. On the other hand, wealthy communities can build more resilient systems and infrastructure and have available resources for response and recovery. They have the capacity and funding to adapt by developing alternative industries that can replace those destroyed.

This adverse economic impact can be extensive and prolonged. Consider the flow-on effects of this damage to critical community infrastructure through lost educational opportunities, risks to public health or lost employment opportunities arising from transportation failures which may not even be in the impacted area.

A study into the economic impacts of disasters in South America in the last 100 years found children are the most vulnerable to effects which include "less human capital accumulation, worse health and fewer assets when they are adults". The results demonstrate the intergenerational impact of disasters and crisis [6].

Given these facts, it is surprising that very few countries have public investment policies that include effective risk management approaches. They are yet to fully recognise that if global, sustained and equitable development is to be achieved, then disaster reduction, climate change adaptation and poverty eradication must shape future development plans for energy, water and all other strategies for the public good.

This connection is recognised by global leadership. The 2015 Global Risk Assessment Report [7] *Revealing Risk, Redefining Development* and the Sendai Framework for Action (2015) both highlighted the absence of risk-sensitive development strategies. The United Nations developed an international agreement to guide disaster management. The Sendai Framework 2015 [8] identified four priorities:

- Priority 1: Understanding disaster risk.
- Priority 2: Strengthening disaster risk governance to manage disaster risk.
- Priority 3: Investing in disaster risk reduction for resilience.
- Priority 4: Enhancing disaster preparedness for effective response and to *Build Back Better* in recovery, rehabilitation and reconstruction.

The goal therefore is to protect development investments and to save lives by building disaster risk reduction into development goals. The strategic approach is to build risk assessment and early warning systems along with education and information that builds a culture of health, safety and resilience at all levels.

At the community level, there is an important opportunity to improve the relationship with government, businesses, and the corporate community to effectively manage disaster risk through whole of community approaches. Effective management of risk builds long-term sustainability and therefore development.

This is particularly relevant to the health sector. Strategies should aim to reduce underlying risk factors to health and health systems thus building resilience for both disasters and ongoing development. Emergency preparedness arrangements should be in place for effective health response and recovery at all levels. The challenge for health systems is to broaden the focus away from relying on response to a more encompassing and inclusive approach which focuses on building resilient systems and includes reduction of risk, protection of health facilities and collaborating across sectors to meet community needs.

This text has identified the importance of effective recovery and adaptation to the impacts of disasters particularly in the longer term. Moderating those impacts can be a major contributor to economic development. Careful management of the recovery phase can ensure the development of resilience and thus minimise the economic consequences.

Economic development is not without risk or debate. There are inevitably winners and losers and individuals, communities and organisations will fight to preserve their interest against often the greater good of a broader community. Farmers will fight to retain their lands which may be required for the construction of flood mitigation works. Developers will fight for maximum return from cheap but floodable land. Delivering rational approaches in the presence of these competing interests is challenging.

THE IMPACTS OF SOCIAL AND TECHNOLOGICAL CHANGE

Changes in social structures and values may also impact on disaster management. Demographic changes, particularly population ageing, and an increasing burden of non-communicable diseases are reducing the relative workforce that is available to respond to disasters. Equally, population ageing and increasing workforce participation have resulted in fewer people being available to support volunteer agencies.

CASE STUDY 29.2 – THE IRELAND DEPARTMENT OF HEALTH AND HEALTH SERVICE EXECUTIVE CYBER ATTACK

In May 2021, a ransomware attack on Ireland's Department of Health and Health Service Executive (HSE) severely impacted the country's health services causing a nationwide shutdown of the HSE computer system. This disrupted healthcare within Ireland with loss of patient information and diagnostics due to hospitals being unable to access electronic records. This led to manual processing (e.g., paper recordkeeping) impacting patient identification and tracking. Two days into the attack, for reasons unclear, the cyber criminals provided a decryption key allowing for the recovery of services to begin. Recovery was prolonged with the restoration of IT services taking several months to complete. This incident demonstrates the importance of cyber security in patient safety, and the importance of risk management to stop or reduce the impact of a cyberattack. Risk reduction in cybersecurity will require a strong active constantly vigilant cyberspace intelligence and collaboration across industries, small businesses, and governments.

An example of how social and demographic change is impacting on disaster health management is the challenge of volunteers in Australia. Changes in society attitudes have reduced the volunteer workforce. It has not necessarily reduced the sense of compassion and preparedness to help, but it has tended to reduce individual preparedness and ability to commit in a structured way. Many people particularly the young do not want to make long-term commitments to formally structured agencies such as firefighting or other emergency services. Consider the situation of volunteer organisations such as the state emergency services in Australia. These bodies rely on community volunteers to provide a range of community response activities. At the same time, increasing accountabilities are requiring those who do participate to undertake more training and accreditation to meet health and safety standards. With increasing commitment comes decreased availability.

Other social and cultural changes include

- **Increased safety and efficiency have had an impact of reducing people's experience and tolerance for disruption or loss**. Called the safety paradox, when effective and efficient systems fail, the shock is greater.
- **People are reliant on the complex societal systems** that characterise modern society for example a multi-story residential tower. Loss of electricity renders it uninhabitable very quickly. If the power goes down, and technology fails, individuals are less able to find innovative alternatives or workarounds.
- There is an **increasing distrust of authorities** making it more challenging to communicate clearly. The use of various forms of media and the increased use of unreliable sources for information by people is influencing this change, comprising trust in authorities.
- The complexity and fragmentation of modern communities are such that there is **a decline in the sense of community**. Communities in rural areas tend still to be defined geographically while communities in the city are defined more by commonality of interest which can shift by time of day. For example, you may belong to the workplace community during working hours, the school community at pick-up time and the soccer community on weekends however you identify mainly with your online special interest community.
- The 24-hour news cycle makes it difficult to manage disasters. Modern disasters will be played out in real time on television. Bystanders have become reporters filming and distributing live footage. On the other hand there were only one or two grainy black and white film clips of a Tsunami last century; now there is enough material for people to really understand why they are so dangerous. Thus, authorities are required to provide or comment on information which they may not have.
- Increased education standards are **improving people's disaster awareness and literacy** and thus increasing their expectations.

Within many societies there is a trend towards increasing accountability alongside reduced tolerance of adversity. This apparent lack of tolerance of adversity may also result in unreasonable expectations. In a sense this is understandable because in many developed societies service delivery became extensive and very reliable. One of the great achievements of the 20th century was to build and operate extensive and reliable systems. Disasters which used to be seen as an Act of God are now seen as someone's fault. This changing conceptualisation is placing an increased burden on those responsible for disaster management.

Similarly, technological changes are having a major impact on modern disaster management. There have been vast technological advances in the past 100 years, which directly affect the risks to organisations and society as well as the disaster management capability. The rate of technological change is likely to increase, and this provides remarkable possibilities to enhance disaster management.

The consumer world is driving innovation with many services including the internet, social media, gaming, music and work emails now available in mobile form.

- Future Private, Mobile and Radio services may access a core network through mobile devices resulting in a more distributive system.
- New apps such as GIVEIT[2] have the potential to help people and organisations access resources in disasters.
- Social media platforms allow people to identify as members of communities beyond the traditional socio-cultural and geographic boundaries.

Within the disaster management sphere 'digital humanitarians' are an example of this phenomenon [9]. The movement mobilises individuals outside disaster-affected areas to provide assistance to the affected zones through the analysis of big crisis data. Practically, this can mean thousands of people who will never meet simultaneously analysing images taken by an unmanned aerial vehicle of a disaster zone to aid impact assessment and therefore relief strategies and rebuilding efforts.

In addition, the **Service-Oriented Architecture** characterises systems development and integration of systems based on functional interoperability. Therefore, different applications will be able to exchange data with one another. With all these new developments and technologies, it becomes clear that in the future, the provision of commercial offset strategies will be a key aspect of investment decisions. Where these are targeted to result in improvements in disaster response, the impact may be far-reaching and more effective than government- or non-government organisations (NGOs)-funded developments.

Information technology and social media are becoming the new norm. While it provides individuals with immediate access to vast arrays of information, it also makes it increasingly difficult to disentangle accurate information from the enormous array of inaccurate, incomplete or incorrect information. Steps are being taken to address this challenge, for example, the Indian National Disaster Management Authority is partnering with Facebook to get real-time feedback from those affected, distribute timely and rapid information and provide disaster responders with access to maps of the affected areas [10]. However, there is more work required to ensure authorities communicate clearly and consistently.

While *big data* is valuable, the sheer volume, the people power and the computing power required to perform analysis currently limits its usefulness. As computer processors and the algorithms behind predictive analytics improve the data will become manageable, but will still require integration with existing information. Importantly, movements like this are not usually led by disaster responders but by technology innovators who see a practical application of new technology. The future challenge for disaster managers is to identify these early adopters and harmonise their efforts alongside traditional information pathways. One of the very significant challenges during crises is to find the right data.

As dependence on technology increases so does the risk of technological disasters, including cybersecurity-related disasters. Cyber threat includes accidental, such as data breaches due to human error, and more concernedly, intentional malicious cyber activities, such as hacking of confidential information in ransomware attacks, and critical infrastructure attack to disrupt essential services.

Cyber security is a national priority for many governments with the risk of critical infrastructure disruption to essential services, health, utilities, transport, communications, information technologies, food and finances for prolonged periods. Worldwide, critical infrastructure networks, including health services, are being increasingly targeted by malicious cyber actors.

MACRO POLITICAL AND SOCIAL CHALLENGES

The combination of *societal and technological changes* is changing the political process. Increasingly there is political volatility. Governments sense their vulnerability to the lethal impact of social media and are becoming increasingly risk averse. Individuals are able to better manipulate the political process through social media than they ever could through traditional political organisations or through print or even electronic media which was controlled by particular sectional interests.

While enriching the democratic process it also has a restraining effect on major disaster mitigation investments. People can organise resistance to the construction of flood retention basins or to fuel reduction strategies in bushfire-prone areas. This has the effect of weakening decision-making processes which are vital to the prevention, preparedness, and recovery elements of disaster management.

The fear of adversity has created a focus which is disproportionate to the level of risk. From an historical perspective, this is one of the most peaceful times in history. Compare this Century to date with the 20th Century in which two world wars resulted in the deaths of an estimated 70 million people. Additionally, immediately after the First World War, an estimated 50 million people died around the world from the Spanish Flu. This peaceful time in many ways has resulted in complacency across sections of society, creating a lack of awareness about inherent risks and dangers. The outbreak of COVID-19 may help refocus communities on the extensive impact of natural challenges while also allowing more realistic expectations for disaster management to develop.

Climate change threatens human health and wellbeing. Changing global temperatures will impact on sea levels and on the frequency and severity of climatic events such as droughts, storms and heatwaves. Similarly changing temperatures alter the distribution of disease vectors, introducing pandemics to areas not previously at risk. Climate change drives increases in the impact and frequency of some natural hazards while risk reduction lessens disaster impacts. The latter is a development imperative that will help to anticipate events well in advance, reduce the suffering of millions and help avert catastrophes that warrant massive humanitarian responses.

However, political and economic considerations appear to have prevailed in the minds of many whereby limiting the ability of the global community to reach collective prevention and mitigation agreements. Therefore, adaptation strategies remain the only feasible actions.

CASE STUDY 29.3 – CLIMATE CHANGE

The World Meteorological Organisation report found that in the ten years ending 2019 our planet has experienced exceptional global heat, unprecedented levels of retreating ice, a record rise in sea level and higher acidity in the world's oceans. The climate is changing at an accelerated rate and this has had a detrimental impact on human health and wellbeing and the ongoing sustainability of fragile ecosystems and marine life. Globally there has been a dramatic increase in population movement and migration, the inability to safeguard food security in some regions and an increase in unseasonal severe weather-related events never witnessed in our lifetime. These include devastating wildfires in Siberia, Alaska and the Amazon rainforest, increase in severe tropical storms, erratic rainfall patterns causing widespread flooding, record heatwaves and protracted drought in many countries.

POLICY AND OPERATIONAL CHALLENGES

There are many challenges to strategic leadership in the field of disaster management. Most of these have been explored during the detailed considerations throughout this text. However, it is worth mentioning others that remain unresolved and need further exploration.

Public expectations are imposing higher levels of accountability on officials. This increases the difficulty of decision-making and has the potential to develop risk-averse practices. The result is further impeding the time-critical decision-making often required early in a disaster response. At the same time, the intense post-hoc scrutiny of disaster leaders has the potential for adverse mental health impacts on those individuals.

Health and safety of rescue and health workers in disasters. This is an area of increasing interest as individuals seek redress for any adverse impacts. At one extreme is a view that rescue and healthcare are important and by their nature, heroic and risky. Conversely, others believe rescue and recovery should occur safely and without risk to the rescuers and health workers. The need for proportionate and considered activities balancing the potential benefit against the potential risk is the most acceptable approach.

There is little known about the risks to the health and safety of emergency workers. There is on the other hand much evidence of the consequences. There is considerable evidence of the mental health consequences but less so of physical health. Additionally, there has been considerable attention paid to the direct risks of rescue and recovery but little to the indirect long-term risks associated with the preparation and recovery phases and the impact of external scrutiny including the impact of media and major public enquiries.

The **focus and scope of disaster healthcare**. There is a need to both narrow and broaden the focus of disaster healthcare simultaneously

- Narrowing it by focusing on the person experiencing the disaster and creating a person-focused/family-focused/community-focused response.
- Broadening it by expanding the time considered to constitute recovery, and by expanding the healthcare and welfare services integrated into the response and recovery effort.

There is increasing evidence that the health effects of disasters have a very long tail, in some cases years and decades and through generations. However, most of the response and recovery focuses on the first few months after the event. The news cycle moves on and decision-makers respond to new demands and problems. Long-term issues are forgotten or ignored.

Limits to the normal tiered healthcare response. Most patient care takes place at the primary healthcare level in many countries. This foundation of the health system tends to be systemically overlooked in all aspects of disaster management. Disasters separate primary carers from patients which generates very significant (health) risk but also the primary care system has to cope with a great increase in both type and scale of demand from communities after an event.

Managing conflicting priorities. Almost all managers and leaders face the daily challenge of managing conflicting priorities including managing risk. Expending resources on something that may not happen is often a challenge when compared with the expenditure of resources on things that can generate income or reduce daily costs.

The challenge of policymaking in disaster management. Many in disaster management bemoan the transitory nature of public and political interest in funding for disaster management. There are, however, two mechanisms by which disaster policy can be more easily incorporated into our systems and organisations.

Thinking about resilience evolves to address the limitations of the traditional planning model. Instead of identifying hazards and developing plans to address their impacts, resilience thinking flipped the problem around and looked to develop approaches to building the adaptive capacity of the organisation or system to shocks. The core idea is you do not know what shock may occur but investing in resilience enhances the capacity of the organisation or system to adapt. This helped mainstream the idea because it applies to any change and so was more attractive to decision-makers. That's why the work on risk management was developed in disaster management. To make this work more understandable to decision-makers in organisations and systems and within the frame of their daily work.

The use of risk management and organisational resilience approaches can be applied to any organisation or system whether it is public, private or not-for-profit. The core idea is that these approaches can help an organisation to continue to achieve its purpose under great changes including those from a disaster.

Disaster insurance and compensation. There is also considerable interest in the issues of disaster insurance and compensation. In developed economies the main impact of disasters is their distributional effects, not total loss. This is why insurance and compensation schemes are so important to address these distributional effects. Disasters are known to have considerable economic impact that can be reduced by effective disaster management. Insurance companies will look to reward customers who reduce their risk with appropriate disaster risk reduction. Each public jurisdiction also has compensation arrangements in place, but the fairness and adequacy of those arrangements have both social and financial consequences for the public and the community.

Prioritisation between funding disaster response, recovery, and mitigation. Most countries struggle with the prioritisation between funding disaster response, recovery, and mitigation. The immediacy of response and relief is very attractive to politicians where a safer community is a very abstract and not very 'announceable' product. Even though the long-term economic return from mitigation is very high. The public will often contribute generously either directly or through supporting government activity to help those affected by disaster recovery but is less generous in terms of funding the costs of mitigation works which may prevent that impact in the first place. Additionally, in most jurisdictions complex bureaucratic, social and political impediments exist to taking the whole of government approaches to mitigation.

Forging Strategic partnerships and communication with stakeholders is challenging. Disaster management is a team effort but one inhabited often by passion and egos. One of the significant failures in disaster management is to build an approach which adds value to leaders and executives who are not part of the disaster management 'family'. The role of the leader is to help provide direction and to consolidate the teamwork necessary to ensure coordinated and integrated activity when organisations and systems are disrupted. Forging the strategic partnership requires strength of leadership and the capacity to make a positive case and overcome the vested interests involved and the passions of various organisational players.

Fragmented government responsibility impedes proactive policy initiatives. Even within jurisdictions there is fragmented responsibility between various levels of government, between government organisations and NGOs, and between public, not-for-profit and private sectors.

The dispersed technical expertise required to help with policy formulation limits cohesion and collaboration. The technical expertise required for disaster management is often dispersed through an array of government organisations and NGOs.

There is also a challenge to ensure expertise is appropriate, genuine and not opportunistic. At the time of a disaster there is a tendency for an epidemic of experts; many of whom have at best transitory interest in the complexity of disasters and are informed by the wisdom of hindsight. These have been referred to in the USA as '9/12 ers' referring to the opinionated experts who arrived the day after the event and weren't present on the day much less before the event.

CONCLUSION

What does our future hold when it comes to disasters? The predictions are grim? Globally the population is increasing, there are an increasing number of extreme weather events and more frequent natural disasters which are becoming more destructive. In the future more people are going to be exposed to the adverse consequences of disasters. Furthermore, many societies are highly mobile, globally there is an estimated 1,000,000 flying at any one time which has the potential to increase the risk of a pandemic such as SARS-CoV-2. All this adds to our future challenges, every country must ensure they remain vigilant, continually monitor the threats they face and embrace cooperation and collaboration with their global partners.

Effective disaster management in its broadest context depends on predicting risks where possible and if cost-effective, implementing disaster management strategies. However, history has shown us that some things are not always predictable and are the *'unknown unknowns'* as Donald Rumsfeld described them or *'black swan events'* in risk terminology.

In fact, if assumptions underpinning predictions are not challenged the results can be very serious. While efforts can be made to identify these through scenario or *'what if'* based approaches, the likelihood of success is low by the very nature of these events. Instead the challenge is to ensure the development of a flexible, scalable, integrated system with appropriate governance and an appropriately prepared workforce that can manage these events.

The challenges for disaster management reflect the broader societal, political and economic challenges facing modern society. It is not possible for any text to identify solutions or even to unpick a detailed understanding of complex issues that continue to evolve. This chapter aimed to highlight some of those issues and to demonstrate the complexity of conceptualisation of those issues as an aid to better understanding the process by which they may be analysed evaluated and if possible, resolved.

ACTIVITIES

1. It is said we have gone past the tipping point in terms of climate change and are destined to confront its consequences throughout the later part of this Century. Outline how you would go about developing an adaptation plan in a jurisdiction with which you are familiar.
2. Discuss the relationship between economics and disasters.
3. Consider the 2020 outbreak of SARS-CoV-2 and develop a plan for improved preparedness for a jurisdiction with which you are familiar.
4. What do you see are the major future challenges for disaster health management?
5. What do you think might be the *black swan* events that we might face in the future?

KEY READINGS

Thomas, V., *Climate change and natural disasters: Transforming economies and policies for a sustainable future*. 2017, New Brunswick (USA): Transaction Publishers.

Sodhi, M.S., Natural disasters, the economy and population vulnerability as a vicious cycle with exogenous hazards. *Journal of Operations Management*, 2016. **45**(1): p. 101–113. doi:10.1016/j.jom.2016.05.010

Caruso, G.D., The legacy of natural disasters: The intergenerational impact of 100 years of disasters in Latin America. *Journal of Development Economics*, 2017. **127**: p. 209–233. doi:10.1016/j.jdeveco.2017.03.007

Notes

1. With acknowledgement to previous author Kara Burns
2. http://www.givit.org.au/

References

1. Owen, C., Bhandari, R., Brooks, B., Bearman, C., Abbasi, A., *Organising For Effective Incident Management*. 2014, Australia: Bushfire CRC. ISBN: 978-0-9875218-7-3.
2. UNDP. *Human development report 2019 beyond income, beyond averages, beyond today: Inequalities in human development in the 21st century*. 2019; Available from: https://hdr.undp.org/content/human-development-report-2019.
3. Ward, P.S. and G.E. Shively, Disaster risk, social vulnerability, and economic development. *Disasters*, 2017. **41**(2): p. 324–351.
4. Wu, J., et al., Economic development and declining vulnerability to climate-related disasters in China. *Environmental Research Letters*, 2018. **13**(3): p. 034013.
5. McDermott, T.K., F. Barry, and R.S. Tol, Disasters and development: natural disasters, credit constraints, and economic growth. *Oxford Economic Papers*, 2014. **66**(3): p. 750–773.
6. Caruso, G.D., The legacy of natural disasters: The intergenerational impact of 100 years of disasters in Latin America. *Journal of Development Economics*, 2017. **127**: p. 209–233.

7. UN Office for Disaster Risk Reducation. *Global assessment report on disaster risk reduction.* 2015; Available from: https://www.undrr.org/publication/global-assessment-report-disaster-risk-reduction-2015.

8. United Nations. *Sendai framework for disaster risk reduction 2015–2030.* 2015, United Nations: Geneva.

9. Meier, P., *Digital humanitarians: How big data is changing the face of humanitarian response.* 2015, Florida: CRC Press.

10. NDMA, *Kiren Rijiju inaugurates NDMA's India Disaster Response Summit,* 2017, New Delhi: NDMA. Accessible at https://www.indianbureaucracy.com/kiren-rijiju-inaugurates-india-disaster-response-summit/

Index

Note: **Bold** page numbers refer to tables; *italic* page numbers refer to figures.